For Dummies™

BESTSELLING
BOOK SERIES

Superfoods For Dummies

W9-BHV-736

Sheet

Superfood Shopping Tips

Shopping for superfoods isn't as difficult as getting cheap tickets to the Super Bowl or finding rare diamonds on the black market, but some superfoods may take more effort to find than others. Chapter 13 has details on superfood shopping; here are some tips to get you started:

- **Ask your doctor and health-conscious friends about their favorite superfoods and where they shop for them.**

- **Gather some recipes and plan out your meals, and then use your meal plan to create your grocery list.** You'll have the ingredients you need and minimize waste (and spend less) at the same time. Choose recipes that use superfoods for the main ingredients. See Part IV for lots of great superfoods meal ideas.

- **Don't go to the store without a list.** You'll make fewer impulse purchases — and buy less junk food — if you make a shopping list and stick to it.

- **If you're between meals, eat a snack before you go shopping.** When you're hungry, you're more likely to buy everything in sight.

- **Check out your store's organic foods, natural foods, and exotic foods sections.** As more shoppers demand healthy food options, more stores are carrying them, and you may be pleasantly surprised at what you find.

- **Stick to** ... on, the freezer section ... r in your search for sup ... od aisles that

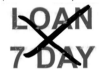

Easy Ways to Incorporate S into Your Everyday Diet

Eating superfoods becomes a habit with a little pract your day without much effort:

- Pack an apple when you brown-bag it for lunch at work or school.

- Buy baby carrots and precut broccoli florets, instead of potato chips, and serve them with veggie dip.

- Make oatmeal for breakfast.

- Toss a handful of blueberries on top of your oatmeal or breakfast cereal.

Superfoods For Dummies®

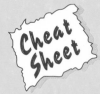

Cheat Sheet

Safely Supplementing Your Superfoods Diet

When you're unable to get enough superfoods in your diet, supplements may be the best route to take. You have tons of supplements to choose from. These are our top five:

Supplement	Superfoods
Dr. Shulze's SuperFoods Plus	Algae, soy, grains, wheat grass, spinach, and fruit extracts
FRS Healthy Energy	Green tea and quercetin (found in fruits and vegetables)
HD Food: Oranges	Multiple phytochemicals from fruit extracts, and green tea
Amazing Grass	Wheat grass
Trim Fuel Bar	Chia and soy

Focusing on Superfood Health Benefits

Superfoods have earned that distinction by having great nutritional value plus extra health benefits. If you find yourself straying from your superfoods diet, use this list of benefits to get back on track:

- **Improving your nutrition:** All the superfoods are rich in the nutrients your body needs, and they're very low in bad fats and processed sugars that can ruin a diet.

- **Strengthening your immune system:** The nutrients and phytochemicals in many superfoods keep your immune system strong so you're less likely to catch colds and the flu.

- **Fighting free radicals:** Superfoods are rich in antioxidants, which destroy the free radicals that can damage the cells in your body. This protection improves your health, reduces your risk of disease, and helps you age gracefully.

- **Reducing the risk of cancer:** The nutrients, fiber, good fats, and phytochemicals found in superfoods reduce your risk of several types of cancer.

- **Keeping your heart healthy:** Those same nutrients, fiber, good fats, and phytochemicals also protect your heart by reducing inflammation and keeping blood vessels healthy.

- **Feeling better:** Superfoods help you feel more energetic.

- **Boosting metabolism and watching your weight:** Many of the superfoods are high in fiber and low in calories, so you can load up your plate without adding many extra calories. Some of the superfoods that are a little higher in calories are rich in protein, fiber, and good fats that keep hunger at bay, and some superfoods actually increase the number of calories you burn.

- **Maintaining your youthful complexion:** The antioxidants in superfoods reduce damage to your skin, and many foods are rich in vitamin C that keeps connective tissue strong. The combination means beautiful, healthy skin.

- **Flooding you with flavor:** Who says healthy has to be dull and flavorless? Superfoods are delicious and can be used in all kinds of recipes.

For Dummies: Bestselling Book Series for Beginners

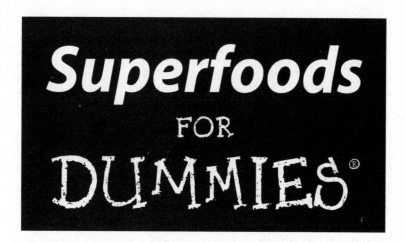

by Dr. Brent Agin and Shereen Jegtvig

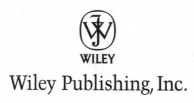

WILEY

Wiley Publishing, Inc.

Superfoods For Dummies®

Published by
Wiley Publishing, Inc.
111 River St.
Hoboken, NJ 07030-5774
www.wiley.com

WILEY

About the Authors

Brent Agin, MD: Dr. Agin was born and raised in Michigan, where he developed an appreciation for athletics and exercise at a young age. In 1989, he went off to Michigan State University, competing for four years on the MSU soccer team and earning Academic All-Big Ten honors during his junior year. He decided to pursue a career in medicine and attended Michigan State University College of Human Medicine, graduating in 1999. He headed south to finish his medical career, completing residency training in Family Medicine at the University of South Florida in 2002.

Dr. Agin's lifelong interest in sports expanded into the fields of health and nutrition. Once he entered into private practice, he implemented a practice model that allowed him to focus not only on medical care, but also on the use of diet and nutrition to improve health.

Dr. Agin co-authored the book Healthy Aging For Dummies (Wiley) while continuing to expand his diet and nutritional supplement line called Trim (www.trimlifestyle.com). He now practices wellness medicine and helps patients understand the powerful impact they have on their health and aging.

Shereen Jegtvig: Shereen Jegtvig began her first career as a chiropractor in 1990. She practiced in western Wisconsin, where she saw the effects of healthful (and not so healthful) diets on her patients every day. In order to offer the best care to her patients, she knew she needed to learn more about which foods could do the most to improve human health. Thus, her fascination with superfoods was born.

Armed with nutrition books (and eventually a new computer with dial-up Internet access), Shereen spent countless hours researching and learning about superfoods. The advent of broadband cable Internet access led her to more efficient online searches, a mild Internet addiction, and, most importantly, the opportunity to write about nutrition for the large Web site About.com in 2004.

Shereen enjoyed her newfound ability to reach a large audience that just couldn't be duplicated in a clinical setting, so she began her second career as a health and nutrition writer. She returned to college and earned a master of science degree in human nutrition with special interest in the effects of omega-3 fats on cognitive function. Today, at nutrition.about.com, she focuses on teaching readers why they need to eat superfoods as well as presenting helpful dietary tips and how-to's. Shereen knows that a pomegranate or a carton of blueberries won't help anyone's health if they never leave the refrigerator.

Dedication

Brent dedicates this book to his parents and siblings who pushed him both in athletics and academics and provided the guidance to live healthy. A special thanks to his wife Cindy and their two daughters, Emma and Grace, who have supported the long hours dedicated to his overwhelming number of projects. He can't forget his office staff — Ina, Kathy, and Zoe — for their dedication and hard work. Thanks to Shereen Jegtvig, whose extensive knowledge in nutrition and excellent writing style made writing this book a pleasure.

Shereen dedicates this book to Jim Lehman, who loves her, motivates her, and puts up with her endless hours of Internet research and writing, and to her children Kendyl and John Reis, who fill her life with happiness and wonder (and a lot of dirty dishes). And special thanks to her parents, Virgil and Becky Jegtvig.

Acknowledgments

The authors thank the following people:

To our editor, Alissa Schwipps, for her patience and expertise. Special thanks to Tracy Boggier, whose courage we appreciate and whom we hope to work with again.

To our incredible agent, Barb Doyen, for her thoughtful ideas, guidance, and special creative zest.

To Meg Schneider for her assistance and for keeping our brains and ideas on track.

Publisher's Acknowledgments

We're proud of this book; please send us your comments through our Dummies online registration form located at http://dummies.custhelp.com. For other comments, please contact our Customer Care Department within the U.S. at 877-762-2974, outside the U.S. at 317-572-3993, or fax 317-572-4002.

Some of the people who helped bring this book to market include the following:

Acquisitions, Editorial, and Media Development

Senior Project Editor: Alissa Schwipps

Acquisitions Editor: Tracy Boggier

Copy Editor: Christy Pingleton

Assistant Editor: Erin Calligan Mooney

Editorial Program Coordinator: Joe Niesen

Technical Editor: Patricia Santelli

Senior Editorial Manager: Jennifer Ehrlich

Editorial Assistants: Jennette ElNaggar, David Lutton

Cover Photos: ICHIRO

Cartoons: Rich Tennant (www.the5thwave.com)

Composition Services

Senior Project Coordinator: Kristie Rees

Layout and Graphics: Reuben W. Davis, SDJumper, Sarah Philippart, Christine Williams

Proofreaders: Laura L. Bowman, John Greenough, Joni Heredia

Indexer: Silvoskey Indexing Services

Special Help: Elizabeth Rea

Publishing and Editorial for Consumer Dummies

Diane Graves Steele, Vice President and Publisher, Consumer Dummies

Kristin Ferguson-Wagstaffe, Product Development Director, Consumer Dummies

Ensley Eikenburg, Associate Publisher, Travel

Kelly Regan, Editorial Director, Travel

Publishing for Technology Dummies

Andy Cummings, Vice President and Publisher, Dummies Technology/General User

Composition Services

Gerry Fahey, Vice President of Production Services

Debbie Stailey, Director of Composition Services

Contents at a Glance

Table of Contents

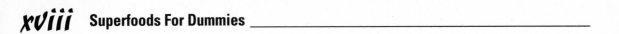

Introduction

· ·

*T*he power of the foods you eat to help you or hurt you is quite amazing. We've both seen the health of patients improve dramatically when they break their junk-food habits and turn to healthful foods instead. And we know that when patients understand the importance of nutrition, they're more likely to support a healthful diet.

We want to help you feel healthier too, so we wrote *Superfoods For Dummies* to show you which foods give you the most bang for your dietary buck — our *superfoods*. We think these foods are extra-special because they can improve your health and prevent disease, and we have the science to back these claims up. Most of our superfoods are easy to find, and you'll be quite comfortable with them. But we also introduce you to some lesser-known superfoods.

So what's in it for you? Maybe you want to be more energetic, lose weight, reduce your cholesterol, or lower your blood pressure. No matter what your reason for being interested in superfoods, we know that once you feel the benefits, you'll want to keep these superfoods in your diet for a lifetime — a very long and healthful lifetime.

About This Book

If we tried to write down everything there is to know about food, nutrition, diet, and health in this one book, you'd have to add a new room onto your home just to store it because such a book would be enormous. So, in the interest of practicality, we give you a quick overview of nutrition, then jump right into the superfoods. We do much more than just give you a list of healthful foods, though. We explain how you can benefit from adding super-foods to your diet and give you tips and how-to's for buying your superfoods. Then we tell you how to prepare them so they'll continue to be super — no unhealthy cooking methods here — and how to serve them so they'll be absolutely delicious.

Here are a few of the points that we explore:

- ✔ **Why you and your family need superfoods:** The rationale for eating them
- ✔ **What makes each superfood so super:** The science behind the food
- ✔ **Where you can find superfoods:** Grocery stores, specialty shops, and online sources
- ✔ **How to prepare and enjoy superfoods:** Cooking instructions and easy-to-prepare superfood recipes

With *Superfoods For Dummies,* you can start at the beginning of the book or pick any chapter from the table of contents and dig in. Every chapter is written to stand on its own, and we've included lots of examples and tips so you can start eating more superfoods right away.

Conventions Used in This Book

The following conventions are used throughout the text to make things consistent and easy to understand:

- ✔ We use monofont for Web sites. *Note:* When this book was printed, some Web addresses may have needed to break across two lines of text. If that happened, rest assured that we haven't put in any extra characters (such as hyphens) to indicate the break. So, when using one of these Web addresses, just type in exactly what you see in this book, as though the line break doesn't exist.
- ✔ New words or terms are in *italics,* and they're closely followed by an easy-to-understand definition.
- ✔ **Bold** is used to highlight the action parts of numbered steps and key words and phrases in bulleted lists.
- ✔ When we discuss scientific research, we give you the source of that research; titles of medical and scientific journals are in *italics.*

What You're Not to Read

We've written this book so you can find the information you need easily and quickly. All the chapters provide you with important information, but some sections offer greater detail or tidbits of information that you can skip if you like. We encourage you to read this information along with the regular text, but if you want to focus on the main points of the chapters, you can always come back to these sections another time.

You can skip the following items without feeling guilty:

- ✔ **Sidebars:** Sidebars are shaded boxes that give detailed examples or explore a tangent in more detail. Ignoring these won't compromise your understanding of the rest of the material.

- ✔ **The stuff on the copyright page:** No kidding. You'll find nothing here of interest unless you're inexplicably enamored of legal language and Library of Congress numbers.

Foolish Assumptions

This book is for anyone interested in exploring foods that not only taste great but have the potential to make you feel better and live longer — which should be you! In writing this book, we assume that you, the reader, fall into one or more of the following categories:

- ✔ You're a parent looking for some guidance on nutrition and the right foods to create a balanced diet for healthy kids.

- ✔ You're a personal trainer, health instructor, or otherwise involved in healthy living, and you want to expand your knowledge of how you can help your clients improve their diets.

- ✔ You have medical conditions that may improve by eating superfoods.

- ✔ You're over your ideal weight and want to find out how eating superfoods can help you lose weight.

- ✔ You're underweight and you're searching for healthful ways to add calories without eating junk foods.

- ✔ You already eat right, but you're looking for some new foods that can add more vitamins, minerals, and antioxidants to your diet.

- ✔ You're a chef or a restaurant owner who wants easy ways to add superfoods to your recipes to make your dishes even healthier.

- ✔ You're willing to make dietary changes and stick with them until eating healthful foods becomes a good habit.

How This Book Is Organized

Superfoods For Dummies is divided into five parts that are packed with important information to make you superfood-savvy in no time. We organized these parts so you can easily navigate through the book to find whatever topic you're looking for. Here's a quick look at what each part covers.

Part I: Getting the Skinny on Superfoods

Part I is a primer on nutrition and superfoods. We start with the basics of good nutrition and then explain why you need superfoods. Superfoods can help you feel better now and reduce your risk for diseases — like heart disease, cancer, and diabetes — later. Part I also discusses the role of dietary supplements in a superfoods diet.

Part II: From Apples to Wheat Grass: A Look at the Superfoods

Part II provides the nuts and bolts of the superfood machinery that can help you live a healthier life. The chapters in this part look closely at the foods that made it onto our superfoods list. We tell you why these foods are super and describe the research and science behind them. We also give you tips for finding, storing, and preparing them.

Part III: Launching Your Superfoods Lifestyle

This is where the saying, "Actions speak louder than words," becomes very important. In Part III, you discover how to take action and get superfoods into your lifestyle. We show you how to incorporate superfoods into your diet both at home and when you're eating out. We give you tips on getting your family to hop on the superfoods bandwagon and offer advice on shopping for superfoods. We even include a chapter on growing your own superfoods.

Part IV: Putting Superfoods on Your Table

This part is all about the eating. We show you the best ways to prepare superfoods (you'll be amazed at how quickly you can become a superfoods chef). From breakfast to dinner, we share great superfood recipes for every meal. We even include snacks, side dishes, and desserts. With these easy recipes, there's really no excuse for not adding superfoods to your culinary regimen.

Part V: The Part of Tens

The Part of Tens is designed to present lots of information in quick, easy-to-read segments. We offer four "top ten" lists in this part, starting with the best of the best, or the super-duper superfoods. We also give you our top super-food supplements and ten (or so) tips for getting those superfoods into your diet. Last but not least, we include a list of our top ten almost-superfoods — foods that don't quite make the super cut, but that are good for you and won't blow your diet.

Icons Used in This Book

This book uses *icons* — small graphics in the margins — to help you quickly recognize especially important information in the text. Here are the icons we use and what they mean:

This icon appears whenever an idea or item can save you time, money, or stress as you add superfoods to your diet. These include cooking and shopping tips, plus ideas for incorporating superfoods into some of your favorite dishes.

Any time you see this icon, you know the information that follows is so important that it's worth reading more than once.

This icon flags information that highlights dangers to your health or well-being.

 This icon points out recipes that are vegetarian.

Where to Go from Here

The *For Dummies* books are organized in such a way that you can surf through any of the chapters and find useful information without having to start at Chapter 1. We (naturally) encourage you to read the whole book, but this structure makes it very easy to start with the topics that interest you the most.

If you already know a lot about superfoods, turn to Chapters 16–19 for some great superfood recipes. If you're curious about what superfoods can do for your overall health and sense of well-being, start with Chapter 2. If you're a gardener, check out Chapter 14 for tips on starting your own superfoods garden.

Chapters 4–10 let you familiarize yourself with specific superfoods and their particular benefits. Or you can get tips and ideas for incorporating superfoods into your life by reading Chapter 11. No matter where you go in *Superfoods For Dummies,* you're sure to discover a lot and gain a healthy attitude toward eating right!

Part I

Getting the Skinny on Superfoods

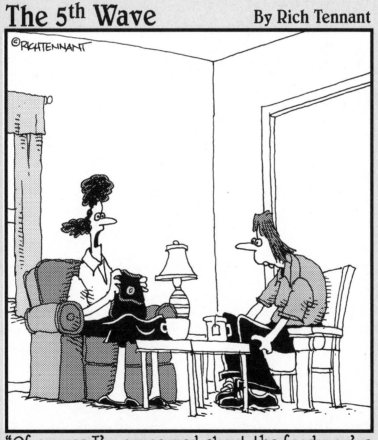

The 5th Wave   By Rich Tennant

"Of course I'm concerned about the food you're serving your family. Let's face it, you named your first three children Twinkie, Ding Dong, and Fluffernutter."

In this part . . .

Before you get started on your superfoods diet, it's helpful to understand why superfoods are so good for you. In this part, we start with a primer on nutrition and how your body uses the foods you eat, and we show you the differences between regular foods and superfoods. We also explain how superfoods can improve your own health and your family's health.

Finally, we discuss dietary supplements and what they can — and can't — do for you. Supplements are often touted as shortcuts to good nutrition, but they don't always live up to expectations. We show you what to look for and how to use supplements properly.

Chapter 1

Nourishing Your Body with Superfoods

*B*efore we get started on the superfoods, it's important to understand what a superfood is as well as the basics of good nutrition and a sound diet. The superfoods all have super health benefits; however, they'll have a bigger impact if you improve the rest of your diet as well.

In this chapter, we introduce you to superfoods and give you the basics of good nutrition. We help you figure out how many calories you need every day, and we show you examples of how superfoods fit into a well-balanced diet.

Understanding the Difference between Foods and Superfoods

What are superfoods? Your body requires food for essential nutrients and energy. But some foods are better than others. Some foods are bad for your health, and eating them can raise your risk of certain diseases. In contrast, some foods are good for you because they give you the energy you need and a few nutrients. At the top of the heap are *superfoods,* which are rich in nutrients and natural substances that have been shown by research studies to improve your health and reduce your risk for disease.

Disease is an impairment of health by a condition of the body or mind that causes dysfunction. *Health* is a condition of well-being free from disease. Eating foods that have poor nutritional value leads to *malnutrition,* which can cause dysfunction of the body and therefore is a form of disease. You need to eat foods that have the correct nutrients to help keep yourself in good health.

Superfoods have been shown to be especially good for you because they're rich in vitamins and minerals, plus they have extra compounds that have a positive impact on your health. These compounds may include good fats like omega-3 fatty acids and monounsaturated fats, a variety of phytochemicals (natural chemicals found in plants), and dietary fiber. All our recommended superfoods have been involved in scientific studies that back up the health claims.

Adding a few superfoods to your diet can improve your health by keeping your heart healthy, boosting your immune system, making it easier to lose weight, fending off diabetes, preventing some cancers, and much more. Eating a superfoods-rich diet also allows you to age gracefully and beautifully.

Boning Up on Basic Nutrition

The foods you eat supply your body with the energy you need to get through the day, along with the raw materials to keep all your organ systems running smoothly. Eating a diet with the right amounts of nutrients accomplishes just that, and superfoods do it in spades.

When you eat a diet with too many calories and unhealthful foods, you're at great risk of becoming obese. Not only do bad foods fail to give you all the nutrients you need, but they also damage your body. While the occasional candy bar or bacon cheeseburger with fries probably won't hurt you, making a daily habit of eating these kinds of foods will. Superfoods contain lots of nutrients, so eating superfoods makes it easy to get the nutrients you need without unwanted calories and unhealthy ingredients.

Picking out foods is easier when you understand what nutrients are and what they do for your body. *Nutrients* are the substances in food that your body uses for energy and to build tissues. There are big nutrients, small nutrients, and special nutrients called phytochemicals. The following sections tell you what you need to know about each type.

Introducing the big nutrients you need: Carbs, proteins, and fats

Macronutrients is the technical term for the big nutrients: carbohydrates, protein, and fats. You need to eat foods that contain all three of the macronutrients in a healthful balance every day. Eating superfoods helps you maintain this balance because superfoods contain healthy ratios of these macronutrients and high amounts of the healthiest nutrients.

Low fat versus low carb: Which is best?

Low-fat diets became popular in the 1980s. They emphasized cutting back on unhealthy, high-calorie, fatty foods, thereby helping people to lose weight. Unfortunately, food manufacturers began making low-fat and non-fat foods that were still high in calories. Of course, these products became very popular and people stopped losing weight.

In the 1990s, low-carb diets became all the rage, and, again, people lost weight when they cut high-calorie sugary foods out of their diets.

Then low-carb, sugar-free foods arrived, but they, too, were high in calories, so Americans continued to gain weight.

So which is best? We think the answer lies in the middle, with a balanced diet and the right amount of calories. That means reducing the amount of bad fats (like the low-fat diets), but keeping the good fats. It also means dumping the sugar (like the low-carb diets), but keeping whole grains and healthful fruits and vegetables.

Coping with carbohydrates

Carbohydrates include simple sugars and complex carbohydrates (starches), and we put fiber in this category, too. Dietary carbohydrates are found in foods that come from plant sources. Your body uses carbohydrates as fuel, so a large part of your diet should be made up of carbohydrates. In fact, about half of your daily calories should come from carbohydrates — but some are better than others.

All carbohydrates are made up of some combination of three simple sugars officially known as *monosaccharides* (single sugar units). These three sugars are galactose (milk sugar), fructose (fruit sugar), and glucose (the type of sugar your body uses as fuel).

Sucrose (table sugar) and lactose (milk sugar) are other types of simple sugars called *disaccharides* (two-sugar units). Lactose is made up of glucose and galactose and is formed in the mammary glands in breast tissue. Sucrose is made up of glucose and fructose. It doesn't matter whether the sugar is white, brown, or raw *(turbinado);* they're all the same. Sucrose molecules are broken down and digested very quickly. Your body either uses the resultant fructose and glucose molecules as energy or converts them to fat and stores them on your body, usually on your belly, butt, or thighs.

Starch (a complex carbohydrate) is made up of long chains of glucose molecules. Starch isn't broken down as quickly as sucrose, but it's still metabolized efficiently. And, just like simple sugars, extra starch is converted to fat.

Fiber is plant material that you can't digest, but it's very important for good health. Insoluble fiber doesn't dissolve in water; instead, it absorbs it. Insoluble fiber remains in solid form, adding bulk to your stool, which helps the muscles of the colon move stool through the digestive system. Soluble fiber dissolves in water, forming a protective gel that also adds bulk (and works as a natural stool-softener) and has other important health benefits such as lowering cholesterol.

So which carbohydrates are good and which ones are bad? The refined carbohydrates that aren't accompanied by any (or only very little) fiber are usually bad, with table sugar and high fructose corn syrup (HFCS) being the worst. They're highly refined, so they add a lot of sweetness but don't provide any nutrition other than calories. Diets high in sucrose and HFCS lead to obesity, heart disease, and diabetes.

Refined flour is just a step or two above refined sugar. Refined flour has had most of the fibrous parts (along with a good bit of the nutrition) removed. Most flour is enriched, however, which adds several vitamins back. Foods like regular pasta, white bread, and crackers are made from refined flour. Choose whole-grain (unrefined) products whenever possible to increase the amount of fiber in your diet because, unlike refined grains, whole grains retain the parts of the plant that contain the healthy fiber content.

Good carbohydrates are usually accompanied by a good dose of fiber. Besides whole grains, good carbohydrates are found in fruits, vegetables, legumes, nuts, and seeds, many of which have attained superfood status. Fiber slows down the digestion and absorption of carbohydrates, which helps to regulate your blood sugar level (which is good for energy and for preventing diabetes) and keeps you feeling full. The best part is that fiber has zero calories.

Fruit juices are high in natural sugars and low in fiber (unless you leave in the pulp), but they're also rich in vitamins and minerals, so they're good carbohydrates. One bit of caution if you're watching your weight: The natural sugars in fruit juice are absorbed quickly and can be high in calories. Eat whole fresh fruits whenever you can.

The best carbohydrates are found in most of our superfoods. They are unrefined carbohydrates accompanied by nutrients and phytochemicals (see the upcoming section "Zeroing in on superfoods nutrients: Phytochemicals"), and/or are high in fiber.

Pondering proteins

Proteins are chains of little chemical building blocks called *amino acids*. After you eat protein, the chains are broken down into individual amino acids, which are absorbed into your blood. Your body takes the amino acids, builds new proteins out of them, and uses them as the raw material to maintain and repair almost every part of your body.

All animal products contain protein, including meats, fish, poultry, eggs, and dairy products. The proteins in animal products are called complete proteins because they contain all the *essential amino acids* (amino acids that need to come from the diet because your body can't make them on its own). Plant foods contain proteins, too — especially nuts, seeds, and legumes — but most plants are missing one or more of the essential amino acids and thus are called *incomplete proteins.* This is important for vegetarians and vegans to know so they can find the right combination of foods to get all the amino acids. Fortunately, some food plants, like soy, are complete proteins, and, if you eat a variety of plant foods — grains, nuts, seeds, and veggies — every day, you can get all the amino acids you need.

Apart from being complete or incomplete, there isn't much difference in the proteins you eat. What makes proteins good or bad is the type of fat that accompanies them. For example, red meat with lots of saturated fat isn't a good source of protein and should be limited. Lean meats are better, and fish that are rich in healthy fats (see Chapter 7) are the best. Plant proteins are always a healthful choice because they're accompanied by good fats and fiber.

Cooking methods can make a difference, too. A piece of baked fish is good for you, but deep-fat fried fish is not.

You don't need large amounts of protein. In fact, only about 15 to 20 percent of your calories should come from protein. Our superfood proteins include legumes and whole grains (see Chapter 8) and nuts and seeds (see Chapter 6).

What's the fuss about fats?

The fats and oils in the foods you eat are made up of individual molecules called fatty acids. Your body needs some fats; in fact, they should comprise about 30 percent of the calories you take in daily. Fats are important for lubrication of body surfaces, formation of hormones, energy storage, and insulation from cold. Limited amounts of fat help protect internal organs, and fats also carry the fat-soluble vitamins that are necessary components of the membranes that surround all the cells in your body.

But not all fats are created equal. Some are very good for you, whereas others are bad for your health:

- **Saturated fats:** These fats are found mostly in animal products like red fatty meats, eggs, and dairy products. They're solid at room temperature. Coconut and other tropical oils also contain large amounts of saturated fat. Eating saturated fats causes your level of cholesterol (a type of blood fat) to go up and promotes inflammation. Diets rich in saturated fats are associated with both an increased risk of heart disease and an increased risk of some cancers. Our superfoods are all low in saturated fats.

  Keep your consumption of high-fat red meats to only two or three meals per week. Choose more fish, lean poultry, legumes, nuts, and seeds.

- **Trans-fats:** Most trans-fats are created by forcing hydrogen into vegetable oils to make them more solid. Some stick margarines, for example, undergo this process. (Dairy products have a natural trans-fat, but it doesn't seem to be as harmful as the artificial kind.) The process, called *partial hydrogenation,* alters the structure of the fatty acids to look more like saturated fats. Unfortunately, trans-fats are worse for your health than saturated fats, and you should avoid them whenever possible. Trans-fats are most commonly found in processed snack foods, oils that are used for deep frying, and pastries, as well as some brands of margarine. The superfoods don't have any trans-fats.

Read the labels on packaged foods to be sure they don't contain any trans-fats.

✔ **Monounsaturated fats:** These fatty acids are found in abundance in some plants. Olive oil is the best known example, but canola oil, peanuts, and avocados also contain some monounsaturated fatty acids. Monounsaturated fats are liquid at room temperature and are good for you. Eating monounsaturated fats in place of saturated fats has been shown to reduce the risk of heart disease. Monounsaturated fats lower your cholesterol, reduce inflammation, keep your blood vessels healthy, and may reduce your risk of some cancers. Many of the superfoods contain large amounts of monounsaturated fats.

✔ Choose monounsaturated fats often — every day if possible. Use olive oil for cooking and as a salad dressing.

✔ **Polyunsaturated fats:** These fats are liquid at room temperature and are abundant in plant oils and fish. There are two types of polyunsaturated fats: omega-3 fatty acids (found in fish, flax seeds, and chia seeds) and omega-6 fatty acids (found in most vegetable and seed oils). Both of these fatty acids are important for good health. They're called essential fatty acids because you have to get them from your diet — your body can't manufacture them from other fats.

There's one problem with polyunsaturated fats, though. Most people get plenty of the omega-6 fatty acids in their diet; in fact, most people get too many because vegetable oils are common in many foods. The opposite is true for the omega-3 fatty acids — most people are deficient. Eating too many of the omega-6s and too few of the omega-3s leads to an imbalance that promotes inflammation in the body. Eating the right amount, about a 4 to 1 ratio of omega-6s to omega-3s, helps to reduce inflammation and improve your health. The typical ratio in the Western diet is 15 or 16 to 1.

Many of our superfoods are rich in omega-3 fatty acids, especially our fish (see Chapter 7), flax and pumpkin seeds (see Chapter 6), and chia seeds (see Chapter 10).

Getting to know the little nutrients you need: Vitamins and minerals

Micronutrients (the little nutrients) include vitamins and minerals. You don't need large amounts of these nutrients compared to the macronutrients, but you do need small amounts on a regular basis to keep your body working at its best. Most of the superfoods are rich in some of the micronutrients, but none are rich in all of them — that's why you need a balanced diet.

When you eat a variety of fruits, vegetables, whole grains, nuts, seeds, legumes, fish, lean meats, and low-fat dairy products, you get the vitamins you need every day. When you make sure some of those foods are super-foods, you get even more nutrition plus all the powerful fats, fiber, and phytochemicals that keep you feeling young and healthy.

Becoming versed in water-soluble vitamins

Water-soluble vitamins dissolve in water and aren't as easily stored by the body as fat-soluble vitamins. The foods you eat must supply the eight B complex vitamins and vitamin C every day because your body consistently eliminates them (except for vitamin B12). Water-soluble vitamins also are more fragile and can be destroyed during cooking. By eating a healthful superfoods-rich diet, you're able to get plenty of these vitamins.

The B complex vitamins include thiamine (B1), riboflavin (B2), niacin (B3), pantothenic acid, pyridoxine (B6), folate, cobalamin (B12), and biotin. The B vitamins are found in a wide variety of foods (except for B12, which is only found in animal products). B vitamins help you convert the macronutrients from the foods you eat into energy, plus they're necessary for many other normal body functions.

Vitamin C is found in fruits and vegetables, especially citrus fruits, strawberries, and peppers. Vitamin C is needed for normal immune system function, speedy wound healing, and strong connective tissue.

Finding the fat-soluble vitamins

Fat-soluble vitamins are stored in fatty tissues and your liver, so you won't become deficient in these vitamins as quickly as with the water-soluble vitamins. Vitamin A is needed for normal vision and cell growth and is found in both plant-based foods and animal products. Vitamin E is found in nuts and seeds and works as an antioxidant to protect the cells in your body from free-radical damage. Vitamin K is found in leafy green vegetables and is essential for normal blood clotting.

A healthful, balanced diet provides just the right amounts of these vitamins, except for vitamin D, which is made by your body after your skin is exposed to sunlight. You need about 5 to 20 minutes of sun exposure to your face, arms, or legs twice each week to form a sufficient amount of vitamin D. Some foods (like milk) are fortified with extra vitamin D, or you can always get vitamin D through supplements. The American Academy of Dermatology recommends utilizing fortified foods and supplements for vitamin D rather than sun exposure because of the risk of skin cancer.

Minding the major minerals

Major minerals include calcium, magnesium, phosphorus, chlorine, potassium, sodium, and sulfur. They're called *major* because you need to replenish them with amounts greater than 0.01 percent of your body weight every day. Major minerals are found in a variety of foods. A healthful diet contains all the minerals you need, although calcium is commonly taken as a dietary supplement.

Calcium is important for many processes in your body and is especially important for strong bones, muscle function, and normal blood clotting. Magnesium and phosphorus are also important for bone health, and magnesium is present in your muscles, too. Potassium, chloride, and sodium are called *electrolytes:* They work to keep your body fluids in balance, which affects your blood pressure. Sulfur is used in making some proteins.

Many of the superfoods are rich in calcium, magnesium, and potassium, while remaining low in sodium. Although sodium is necessary for good health, most people consume way too much of it, which can lead to high blood pressure.

Tackling the trace minerals

Trace minerals include iron, iodine, cobalt, copper, fluoride, manganese, molybdenum, selenium, vanadium, and zinc. You don't need quite as much of the trace minerals as you do the major minerals; however, they're just as important for maintaining a healthy body.

Iron, copper, and cobalt are necessary for normal red blood cell production; iodine helps your thyroid; fluoride is good for your teeth; molybdenum, vanadium, and zinc are cofactors in many chemical reactions; and selenium is an antioxidant.

Our superfoods provide varying amounts of the trace minerals, especially iron, selenium, manganese, and zinc.

Zeroing in on superfoods nutrients: Phytochemicals

Phytochemicals are plant chemicals that offer a variety of health benefits, and all our plant-based superfoods are rich in phytochemicals. There are several different types of phytochemicals (we go into details for each superfood in Chapters 4–6 and 8–10). Here's a basic rundown:

- **Polyphenols** are a family of related phytochemicals that includes bioflavonoids, tannins, and lignans.

  - **Bioflavonoids** are produced in plants and include some of the pigments found in red, blue, purple, and black fruits, vegetables, and legumes. Bioflavonoids like quercetin, anthrocyanadins, and cate-chins help to reduce inflammation, protect your heart, and reduce your risk of some cancers.

- **Tannins** are found in tea and red wine. Tannins may help to keep your digestive system healthy.

- **Lignans** are found in the cell walls of plants and have hormone-like properties. Flax and soy are particularly rich in lignans and may help to reduce the risk of cardiovascular disease.

✔ **Carotenoids** are related to vitamin A and are found in red, yellow, and orange pigments. Examples include beta-carotene, lycopene, and lutein. The carotenoids may help to keep your vision healthy, bolster your immune system, and reduce your risk of cardiovascular disease and some cancers.

✔ **Phytosterols** are the plant equivalent of cholesterol. However, unlike the cholesterol found in animal products, phytosterols are good for you. Some phytosterols, such as *beta-sitosterol,* help to reduce the symptoms of an enlarged prostate and are effective for keeping your cholesterol levels in check.

Not every superfood fruit or veggie has all the phytochemicals you need. Eat a variety of superfoods to be sure you get all the different phytochemicals.

Creating a Healthy, Balanced Superfoods Diet

Creating a healthy diet requires a little planning, so start by determining how many calories you (and your family members) need. Knowing how many calo-ries you need helps you determine how much and which kinds of foods you should eat. Superfoods have excellent nutrient-to-calorie ratios when com-pared to other foods.

If you need to lose some weight, cut back on calories by choosing more foods that are high in fiber and low in fat and sugar, which describes many super-foods. If you want to gain weight, add more energy-dense foods like olive oil, nuts, and seeds to your diet so you can gain weight without losing out on valuable nutrients.

You can find books and Web sites that list the calorie counts for many foods. The United States Department of Agriculture (USDA) has a very large database of nutrition information for just about every food you can think of at www. usda.gov. Simply click Food and Nutrition from the menu on the left and then click What's in the Foods You Eat – Search Tool.

Forgoing fad diets

Fad diets come and go quickly, mostly because, in the end, they're not particularly successful. The typical fad diet requires you to restrict specific foods (sometimes most or all of certain food groups) while claiming that you don't need to watch calories, exercise, or do anything else — but you may need to buy expensive diet pills. Don't fall for these diet claims; they don't work in the long run. Fad diets may help with quick weight loss, but to lose weight and keep it off, you need to eat less, eat right, and exercise more. There aren't any exceptions.

The USDA also has created a food pyramid that helps guide your dietary choices. If counting every calorie seems tedious, you may want to keep track of the number of servings you have of each of the food groups instead.

How do you fit all those servings into your day? Planning your meals and your daily menus makes eating a healthful diet much easier. Plus it makes grocery shopping less of a chore. By planning your meals for a week, you can make a shopping list and buy all the foods and ingredients you'll need at one time. You can even prepare a lot of your meals ahead of time to make eating healthfully easier if you have a hectic schedule. (See Chapter 15 for more on storing and freezing your superfoods.)

Determining how many calories you need

Calories (sometimes called *kilocalories*) measure the amount of energy available in the foods you eat. The number of calories you need every day depends on how old you are, how big you are, whether you're male or female, how active you are, and whether you're pregnant or nursing. When you get the right number of calories every day, you'll be at a healthful weight. If you don't eat enough calories, you'll become underweight. And if you get too many, you'll become overweight and possibly obese. Being overweight or obese increases your risk of cardiovascular disease, diabetes, and some cancers.

 You can go online and find calculators to help you estimate how many calories you need every day to maintain, gain, or lose weight. Check out www.bmi-calculator.net or www.nutritiondata.com for easy-to-use calculators. Or you can calculate your calorie needs with two formulas. The first one calculates how many calories you need just to be awake and breathing. The second formula factors in your activity level:

Basal Metabolic Rate (BMR) Formula

Women: BMR = 655 + (4.35 × weight in pounds) + (4.7 × height in inches) − (4.7 × age in years)

Men: BMR = 66 + (6.23 × weight in pounds) + (12.7 × height in inches) − (6.8 × age in years)

Harris Benedict Formula

If you're sedentary (little or no exercise): Calorie Calculation = BMR × 1.2

If you're lightly active (light exercise/sports 1–3 days/week): Calorie Calculation = BMR × 1.375

If you're moderately active (moderate exercise/sports 3–5 days/week): Calorie Calculation = BMR × 1.55

If you're very active (hard exercise/sports 6–7 days a week): Calorie Calculation = BMR × 1.725

If you're extra active (very hard exercise/sports and physical job or double training): Calorie Calculation = BMR × 1.9

For example, a 35-year-old, moderately active woman who is 5'5" tall and weighs 125 pounds has a BMR of 655 + (4.35 × 125) + (4.7 × 65) − (4.7 × 35), or 1,340 calories. Because she's moderately active, we multiply 1,340 × 1.55 for a grand total of 2,077, which is the number of calories she needs every day to maintain her weight.

We include nutrition information for all our superfoods, including calorie counts, so you'll know how the superfoods fit into your daily intake of calories. Most of our superfoods are low in calories, and the ones that are more *energy dense* (higher in calories) are very rich in nutrients so you only need to eat a little bit to reap their rewards.

Following the food pyramid with superfoods

The USDA created its food pyramid to help Americans understand how many servings of healthful foods they need every day. You can find more information on the food pyramid at www.mypyramid.gov, but here's the general idea:

- ✔ **Breads and cereals:** Six to eleven servings every day. At least half of your servings from this group should be whole-grain. Choose bread, plain cereals, and pasta. Avoid pastries and sugary cereals.

- ✔ **Fruits and vegetables:** At least 2 cups of fruit and 2¹/₂ cups of vegetables. Eat fresh fruits and vegetables whenever possible, and remember that cooking methods matter — steaming is better than boiling.

- ✔ **Dairy products and calcium:** Three servings every day. Choose low-fat milk, cheese, or yogurt.

- ✔ **Meats and proteins:** Two or three servings each day. Choose fish, poultry, eggs, lean meats, legumes, nuts, and seeds. Cut back on fatty red meat and avoid deep-fried meat.

- ✔ **Fats and oils:** Two servings of fats and oils daily, which should come from fish, nuts, seeds, or vegetable oils.

- ✔ **Discretionary calories:** The pyramid leaves just a little room for treats — usually about 100 to 150 calories or so per day.

Here's how you can fit superfoods into the USDA pyramid:

- ✔ **Breads and cereals:** At least half of your servings from this group should be whole-grain. Superfood grains include oats and quinoa (see Chapter 8). Both grains make great breakfast cereals, and quinoa can be eaten as a side dish. Oats can be added to bread and other baked goods, and sometimes oats can be used in place of flour in cooking (see Chapters 16–19 for some ideas).

- ✔ **Fruits and vegetables:** We think this is the most important group because fruits and vegetables are packed with nutrition and fiber, and most people don't eat enough of them. Superfood fruits include oranges, bananas, strawberries, blueberries, cherries, cranberries, and pomegranate (see Chapter 4). All these fruits can be enjoyed as fresh snacks or added to healthful foods. Superfoods vegetables include spinach, broccoli, kale, tomatoes, avocadoes, beets, and carrots (see Chapter 5). They're all terrific in salads, sides, and some main dishes.

- ✔ **Dairy products and calcium:** We didn't include any dairy products in our list of superfoods; however, many of our superfoods go great with non-fat yogurt (think of a berry and nut parfait). Non-fat yogurt is a great source of calcium and contains beneficial bacteria that are good for your health. Calcium is very important for good health, and superfoods sources of calcium include spinach, broccoli, and kale (see Chapter 5); sardines (see Chapter 7); soy (see Chapter 8); and almonds and Brazil nuts (see Chapter 6).

- ✔ **Meats and proteins:** Salmon, tuna, sardines, and trout are rich in omega-3 fatty acids and low in saturated fat, so they're terrific as protein sources (see Chapter 7). Dry beans, soy, and lentils are high-quality plant proteins that can be used as substitutes for high-fat red meats (see Chapter 8). Nuts and seeds make great protein- and fiber-rich snacks (see Chapter 6).

✔ **Fats and oils:** Olive oil is rich in monounsaturated fatty acids that are good for your health (see Chapter 9). Flax oil is good for you, too (see Chapter 6). These oils are much healthier than the saturated fats found in red meat and dairy products. Olive oil is good for cooking or for making salad dressings. You don't want to cook with flax oil, but it makes a great supplemental oil or topping for salads and vegetables.

✔ **Discretionary calories:** Depending on how many calories you can have each day, you'll probably want to save a few for snacks and tasty treats. We suggest a little dark chocolate or a small glass of wine because of their antioxidant properties (see Chapter 9).

Planning superfood meals and menus

The first step in planning healthful meals is to go for a balance of carbohydrates, proteins, and good fats, while reducing sugar, excess sodium, and bad fats. You can accomplish that by following the food pyramid serving suggestions.

The second step is to find places to fit the superfoods into your menu. Superfoods vegetables make great side dishes or salads. The fruits and nuts are perfect for snacks or dessert. The superfoods fish and legumes fit nicely into any dinner. Oats are great for breakfast, and there's even room for a small glass of red wine with dinner or a piece of dark chocolate later on.

So what does a superfood menu look like? We suggest you start out by focusing on a healthful, balanced diet that includes two superfoods each day. Your day could look something like this:

✔ **Breakfast:** Oatmeal with low-fat milk, raisins, and honey; one slice of toast with peanut butter; and coffee. Oatmeal counts as your first superfood of the day.

✔ **Mid-morning snack:** Celery sticks with veggie dip.

✔ **Lunch:** Chicken sandwich with light mayonnaise, one slice of cheese, and lettuce on whole-grain bread, and a small green salad with no more than 2 tablespoons of salad dressing.

✔ **Mid-afternoon snack:** Six crackers with thin slices of cheese, one sliced pear, and a diet soft drink.

✔ **Dinner:** Roast beef, a baked potato with light sour cream, and a side of steamed broccoli with a dab of butter or non-trans-fat margarine. Broccoli is your second superfood for the day.

✔ **Evening snack:** One cup of flavored yogurt.

As you can see, a daily menu like this has plenty of food and flavor without sacrificing good nutrition. And it's easy to add even more superfoods. The following meal plan incorporates five:

- **Breakfast:** Oatmeal with low-fat milk, blueberries, and honey; one slice of toast with peanut butter; and coffee. Oatmeal is your first superfood, and blueberries are your second.

- **Mid-morning snack:** One apple with one slice of cheddar cheese and water. The apple is your third superfood.

- **Lunch:** Bowl of low-sodium chicken noodle soup, one whole-grain roll, and a green salad with no more than 2 tablespoons salad dressing.

- **Mid-afternoon snack:** A single-serving bag of almonds. Almonds are your fourth superfood.

- **Dinner:** Baked salmon with mashed potatoes and green beans. Salmon is your fifth superfood for the day.

- **Evening snack:** One cup of flavored yogurt.

These are just two examples of superfoods menus — throughout the book, we describe more ways to fit superfoods into your day. Enjoying a superfoods diet is easy and delicious.

Taking the First Steps toward a Healthier You with Superfoods

Now that you're armed with nutrition information and you know how to plan your meals, it's time to get started on your superfoods diet. In the following chapters, we tell you more about superfoods, how to prepare them, and how to fit each of them into your superfoods diet. Here's your game plan:

- **Read the rest of this book.** We don't mind if you jump around the book and read whichever chapters interest you the most first. The book contains a lot of information on superfoods, and we know you'll discover a lot.

- **Start with two superfoods each day and increase the number as you feel comfortable.** We've mentioned a few superfoods in this chapter (or you can look ahead for more), so you can get started with your superfoods regimen right away.

- **Reduce the amount of foods you eat that are bad for your health.** That includes the fatty red meats, deep-fried foods, sugary foods, greasy snack foods, and foods that are heavily processed. Replace those bad foods with good foods like fresh fruits and vegetables, whole grains, lean meats, nuts, seeds, legumes, and low-fat dairy products.

✔ **Keep a food diary to help you keep track of your superfoods diet.** Writing down the foods you eat and the beverages you drink every day improves your chances of turning your new dietary changes into a permanent lifestyle. You really don't need anything fancy; a small notebook will do. At the end of every day, you can see whether your food choices were good or bad and how many superfoods you ate.

✔ **Exercise.** The American Heart Association recommends a minimum of 30 minutes of exercise five days a week. Exercise works along with superfoods to help you manage your weight and promote a healthy heart.

✔ **Get your family and friends involved.** It's much easier to accomplish diet and exercise goals when you do it with a partner. Lead by example and rope some friends or family members into a healthy lifestyle.

If at first you don't succeed . . . don't give up! Rome wasn't built in a day and you don't have to change your diet overnight. It's okay if you slip up — just start again and continue to make healthier food choices and add more superfoods. Ultimately, your superfoods diet will last a lifetime (and a long one at that!).

Chapter 2

Appreciating the Ageless Wonders of Superfoods

In This Chapter

▶ Discovering the healthy benefits of superfoods

▶ Unlocking anti-aging abilities

▶ Starting off on the right foot — superfoods for children

People today typically eat for pleasure rather than for good nutrition. Unfortunately, there just aren't many health benefits in most of the foods we eat for pleasure. If eating a candy bar could decrease your blood pressure or reduce your risk for cancer, we'd have one heck of a healthy population — but this just isn't the case.

One of the reasons people don't choose healthier food is because they haven't been educated on the health benefits of eating the good stuff. But read on, because in this chapter we tell you how the foods you and your kids eat can affect — and even improve — your health, perhaps resulting in fewer visits to the doctor. Of course, we aren't suggesting that doctors are bad guys, but if reducing your number of doctor visits each year simply by eating more healthfully is possible, why not?

Boosting Your Immune System

As you may expect, superfoods are good immune-system boosters, helping your body fight and prevent various diseases. Research on the abilities of certain foods to strengthen immune function, fight against heart disease, prevent cancer, and lower the risk of other inflammatory diseases has been consistently increasing. Of course, cancer is much less common than colds and minor infections. Fortunately, superfoods can help with these everyday ailments, too. Here are two good examples:

✔ **Resveratrol,** a compound found in red wine, has been shown to be quite beneficial. It has antiviral properties and can help prevent common cold viruses from taking hold in your body. It's also being studied extensively in anti-aging medicine, and early results are pointing at a breakthrough in this area (see Chapter 9 and the section "Aging Beautifully" later in this chapter for more info).

✔ **Garlic** has been used as a natural antibiotic for more than a century. Louis Pasteur studied the use of garlic as an antibiotic and found that it killed bacteria in the lab. (See Chapters 9 and 20 for more on garlic's superfood qualities.)

If you're on any medications, see your doctor before you add high doses of garlic to your regimen. Garlic can interfere with certain medication functions.

Superfoods have some great properties to help the body's immune system. However, if you're thinking of taking any superfood supplements, talk to your doctor first. Supplements, even those with superfood properties, can interact negatively with certain medications, so it's vital to discuss diet and supplements with your physician. See Chapters 3 and 21 for details on dietary supplements.

Helping Your Heart

Your heart pumps about 2,000 gallons of blood throughout your whole body every day, but most people don't appreciate that workload. You don't have to consciously think about your heartbeat, so it's easy to take your heart for granted. Unfortunately, sometimes it takes a serious medical condition to become aware of your heart — by which time you may already have heart disease.

Heart disease is still the leading cause of death in both men and women, so reducing risks should be a priority for both genders. Superfoods can help by tackling cholesterol and triglycerides, believed to be major risk factors for cardiovascular disease. (Not sure what cholesterol and triglycerides are? Check out the nearby sidebar.)

The American Heart Association recommends that everyone 20 years of age and older have a *fasting cholesterol profile* test every five years. This test measures your total cholesterol and triglyceride levels to keep an eye on your risk for cardiovascular disease. If you have any underlying health conditions, such as hypothyroidism, diabetes, liver disease, or other cardiovascular risks, your doctor may want to run this profile more frequently. Once patients reach the age of 40, most doctors check their cholesterol yearly.

Cholesterol and triglycerides

Cholesterol is a fat-like substance that's essential for normal body function. It plays a role in producing cell membranes and hormones. *Triglycerides* are a type of fat that makes up one portion of the cholesterol.

Cholesterol is found in different forms in your body. One form is "good" cholesterol, called high density lipoprotein (HDL), and the other is "bad" cholesterol, called low density lipoprotein (LDL). These lipoproteins are actually protein molecules that carry cholesterol through your bloodstream. LDL, the bad form, carries cholesterol from the liver, where it's made, to the rest of your body. HDL, the good form, carries cholesterol back to the liver, where it's removed from your body.

You need to know your ratio of HDL to LDL to determine just what harm cholesterol may be doing to your heart (your doctor can draw your blood and perform a *fasting cholesterol profile* test to determine your ratio). You want to have higher levels of HDL and lower levels of LDL, because that means your body is getting rid of extra cholesterol. When your blood has too much LDL and too little HDL, the cholesterol may combine with other substances to form *plaques* on the walls of your arteries. Plaques make your arteries narrow and less flexible, which leads to a condition called *atherosclerosis*.

Atherosclerosis reduces blood flow, often leading to strokes and heart attacks.

About ²/₃ of the cholesterol in your body is produced in your liver, and the rest comes from the foods you eat. Your body needs cholesterol for certain functions; in most cases, the liver produces what the body will use and doesn't need extra. The balance between good cholesterol and bad is often determined by the food choices you make. Foods high in dietary cholesterol and saturated fats increase your bad cholesterol and decrease your good cholesterol. To make matters worse, some people inherit genes that actually cause the body to make more bad cholesterol and less of the good kind. Unhealthy levels of cholesterol can build up quickly in people who inherit this condition of over-production.

When you consume more calories than you need, your body turns the extra calories into triglycerides that are stored in your fat cells for later use. Triglycerides are grouped in with the LDL as bad cholesterol because high levels of triglycerides are thought to lead to plaque build-up in the arteries. No one knows exactly how triglycerides are involved in plaque formation, but high levels have been consistently linked to heart disease. Researchers are continually trying to discover exactly how elevated triglycerides affect the body.

Superfoods work to keep your heart healthy and improve your ticker's longevity without the potential side effects or additional expense of cholesterol-lowering prescription medications. They can really make a difference in your heart's health. Here's how:

- ✔ Eating superfoods means you're improving your overall diet and getting the vitamins and minerals you need every day — without extra calories. Too many extra calories cause elevations in triglycerides (see sidebar) and an increased risk for heart disease.

- ✔ Some superfoods, such as colorful fruits and vegetables (see Chapters 4 and 5 for foods that fill the bill), contain natural disease-fighting substances called *flavonoids*. These can reduce inflammation of your arteries, decrease your cholesterol, lower your blood pressure, and stimulate antioxidant activity. Antioxidants repair damage done to the cells in your body by smoking, pollution, poisons, fried foods, and also as a by-product of normal metabolism.

✔ Fish, nuts, and seeds all contain healthful polyunsaturated fatty acids that keep your cholesterol in check. Fish oil (omega-3 fatty acids) is particularly super because it also helps regulate your heartbeat and your blood pressure. (See Chapter 6 for the lowdown on nuts and seeds, Chapter 21 for info on omega-3 fatty acids, and Chapter 7 for more fish facts.)

✔ Fruits, vegetables, and oatmeal (see Chapters 8 and 20 for more on this powerful grain) all contain dietary fiber that lowers cholesterol and helps keep you feeling full, which can prevent overeating, a risk factor for heart disease.

Losing Weight

More than 70 percent of the United States' adult population is overweight, and a third of that population is obese. Overweight is defined as having a *body mass index* (BMI) over 25. Adults with a BMI over 30 are considered *obese*. (The "Body Mass Index" sidebar tells you how to calculate your BMI.) Obesity is the second most preventable health risk, just behind smoking. It's a problem worldwide and one that just keeps getting bigger (no pun intended).

Body Mass Index

Body Mass Index (BMI) is an indirect way of calculating your percentage of body fat. Calculating BMI is easier and less expensive than direct-measurement tests, and, according to the Centers for Disease Control and Prevention (CDC), BMI is an accurate reflection of the results of direct body-fat measurement. The BMI formula for adults is:

Your weight in pounds divided by your height in inches squared, times 703.

So, if you weigh 150 pounds and you're 5 feet 5 inches tall, your BMI formula looks like this:

$$150 \div 65^2 \times 703 = 24.96$$

The CDC Web site has BMI calculators for adults, children, and teenagers. You can check them out at www.cdc.gov/nccdphp/dnpa/healthyweight/assessing/bmi/index.htm.

Another problem is how quickly this overweight epidemic has spread to children. The World Health Organization estimates that 20 million children under the age of five are obese. Children are being diagnosed with high cholesterol, high blood pressure, and diabetes — all previously thought to be exclusively the problems of adults — at alarming rates. Why is this happening?

As with heart disease, poor eating and physical inactivity are largely responsible for weight gain. Weight loss isn't easy, but for many people it's necessary to restore and maintain good health. Don't worry; we help you choose the superfoods that, along with a healthful diet and exercise plan, can help you lose the extra weight. Some superfoods that fill this bill include omega-3 fatty acids (see Chapters 7 and 21), green tea (see Chapters 9 and 21), dark chocolate (yes, dark chocolate — see Chapter 9), and *chia* (an edible seed that absorbs water and keeps you feeling full for hours; see Chapter 10).

Protecting Against Cancer

When people are asked what health condition they fear the most, cancer is the number one answer. This is a justifiable fear as cancer is the second leading cause of death in the United States, just behind heart disease. Although many people believe that cancer is an uncontrollable health condition, evidence suggests otherwise, and some of the superfoods may help to prevent cancer and improve the well-being of cancer patients.

We've seen success story after success story where people defied their prognoses and beat cancer, and we think that eating healthy foods had a lot to do with it. The role of nutrition in the prevention of cancer has been studied for many years. The largest cancer research organization in the United Kingdom, World Cancer Research Fund (WCRF), supports the notion that between 35 and 70 percent of cancer is related to eating an unhealthy diet. A healthy diet rich in superfoods, on the other hand, may decrease your risk of many cancers.

Many superfoods have cancer-fighting properties. In general, you should seek those foods with the highest amounts of phytochemicals, fiber, and antioxidants. For example:

- Lycopene, a phytochemical found in tomatoes, is being studied for its reduction of risk for prostate cancer. According to the American Cancer Society, foods rich in lycopene may lower the risk of other cancers as well; however, more research is needed. See Chapters 5 and 20 for more on tomatoes.

- Berries (see Chapters 4 and 20) contain phytochemicals that have been shown to help fight the development of cancer. These phytochemicals trigger antioxidant reactions that neutralize damage done to your cells.

✔ Red wine contains two polyphenols called catechins and resveratrol, both of which provide cancer protection by inhibiting the growth of cancer cells. See Chapter 9 for more info on the wonders of wine.

✔ Broccoli (see Chapter 5) contains a chemical that has been found to slow down the progression of cancer cells, especially hormone-sensitive cancers such as breast and ovarian cancer.

✔ A lot of money has been spent on research to explore the cancer-fighting properties of garlic and garlic extracts. Several studies already support the theory that garlic can reduce the risk of cancer, and more studies are underway to explore exactly how garlic functions in cancer protection. See Chapters 9 and 20 for the lowdown on garlic.

✔ Several beans (legumes) are great sources of fiber, which has been proven to help reduce inflammation in the colon and has been associated with a reduction of colon cancer. See Chapter 8 for more info on legumes.

Improving Digestion

Most people suffer digestive stress at one time or another. For example, constipation is common and can lead to abdominal bloating, hemorrhoids, and unnecessary pain. Indigestion or acid reflux (heartburn) is a common cause of emergency department visits and can lead to damage in the esophagus if not treated. Regularity of the digestive system is important for the proper metabolism of the foods you eat so they can be utilized by the body.

One way to help your digestive system is to eat foods with lots of fiber. The average diet consists of about 10 grams of fiber a day — far less than the 25 to 40 grams per day that your body needs. Boost your fiber intake by adding superfood fruits, vegetables, nuts, grains, and legumes to your diet. The following list contains just a few superfoods that are high in fiber (see the accompanying chapter cross references for more details on the benefits they have to offer):

✔ Almonds (Chapters 6 and 20)

✔ Apples (Chapter 4)

✔ Avocados (Chapter 5)

✔ Black beans (Chapter 8)

✔ Broccoli (Chapter 5)

✔ Chia (Chapters 10 and 20)

✔ Lentils (Chapter 8)

A fiber primer

If you aren't sure what fiber is and why it's good for you, you're not alone. Fiber is the part of plant foods (fruits, vegetables, grains) that can't be broken down by your digestive system. Fiber is important for your health — it keeps your digestive system healthy and helps to control blood sugar levels.

There are two types of fiber:

✔ **Insoluble fiber:** This type of fiber doesn't dissolve in water and cannot be digested. It absorbs water and bulks the stool to help regulate bowel movements. Insoluble fiber is found in grains and some vegetables.

✔ **Soluble fiber:** This type of fiber dissolves in water, forming a gel-like substance that moves through the intestines. Found in fruits, vegetables, and legumes, soluble fiber is associated with lowering cholesterol and controlling blood sugar.

A food is considered to have a high fiber content when it has more than five grams of fiber per serving.

✔ Lima beans (Chapter 8)

✔ Oatmeal (Chapters 8 and 20)

✔ Quinoa (Chapter 8)

✔ Blueberries (Chapter 4)

✔ Soy beans (Chapter 8)

 Water isn't on our list of superfoods, but it's a great addition to your diet to help some of the super-fiber foods work better. Drinking half your body weight (in ounces) of water each day helps counter the fluids that fiber absorbs. If you weigh 120 pounds, for example, you should aim to drink 60 ounces of water a day.

 Good digestive health is very important for the body to absorb nutrients and water, so make sure you're getting your daily fiber and alert your doctor with any concerns.

Easing Inflammation

When it comes to staying healthy, your body is always in a tug-of-war with detriments like pollution, unhealthy foods, smoke, too much alcohol, excessive sunlight, and even the side effects of fighting infections and digesting high-fat meals. Exposure to these things causes cell damage and *inflammation* (the body's response to this damage, such as tissue swelling, redness, and triggering of the immune system). *Chronic inflammation,* or inflammation that happens over and over again, can lead to problems in many areas of the body, such as the joints, the heart, the colon, and even the skin.

Your body works hard to fight inflammation and cell damage. You can give your body an edge in this tug-of-war by eating superfoods rich in antioxidants and prostaglandins, which we discuss in the following sections.

The role of antioxidants

Antioxidants are natural substances, such as the compounds that give fruits and vegetables their colors, and vitamins like C and E, which fight cell damage. They work to fight inflammation by neutralizing free radicals in the body. *Free radicals* are unstable molecules that can travel throughout the body trying to take particles from healthy cells — a process that creates more free radicals. Free radicals damage cells, causing inflammation and starting a chain reaction in tissues as more and more cells become affected.

Superfoods are packed with antioxidants that move through the body and stop the free radicals so they don't damage healthy cells. Many of the super-foods that we discuss in this book have antioxidant properties. Here are some of the most powerful ones (see the chapters referenced for more specifics):

- Acai berries (Chapter 10)
- Blueberries (Chapters 4 and 20)
- Broccoli (Chapter 5)
- Cranberries (Chapter 4)
- Green tea (Chapters 9 and 21)
- Pomegranate (Chapter 4)
- Spinach (Chapters 5 and 20)

Fats and inflammation

Your body makes chemicals called *prostaglandins* that contribute to starting or stopping inflammation reactions in your body (depending on the type of prostaglandins). Have you ever taken aspirin or ibuprofen for a headache? These medicines stop inflammation by blocking the prostaglandins. That's great, but sometimes they have rather unpleasant side effects; for example, some people experience an upset stomach when they take aspirin or ibuprofen.

Some foods can increase the amount of inflammatory prostaglandins (the bad ones) and decrease the amount of anti-inflammatory prostaglandins (the good ones) in your body. Eating these foods increases inflammation in your body. Eating a diet high in saturated fat (a type of fat found in red meat; see the sidebar "Not all fats are alike" for more info) is a major cause of this prostaglandin imbalance and the resulting inflammation. Fortunately, there are superfoods that combat that inflammation.

Unlike saturated fats, unsaturated fats are actually good for the body. They come in two forms: polyunsaturated and monounsaturated (see the nearby sidebar for details on the differences).

A type of polyunsaturated fat known as omega-3 fatty acids is especially good for you. Omega-3s have been researched extensively and found to reduce inflammation. This means that eating foods rich in omega-3 fatty acids can help prevent heart disease, cancer, and arthritis.

Not all fats are alike

While fats have generally gotten a bad reputation, not all fats are bad. Knowing the difference between good fats and bad fats can have a significant impact on your health.

Saturated fats get their name from being saturated with hydrogen atoms. They can cause an unhealthy build-up of cholesterol (LDL, the bad cholesterol) and triglycerides in the body if consumed in excess — not a good thing. Saturated fats are found in foods from animal sources, such as meat and dairy products. Baked, fried, and processed foods are unfortunately also big donors of this unhealthy fat. The American Heart Association recommends that saturated fats comprise no more than 7 percent of your daily caloric intake.

Trans fats can be found in processed foods, some stick margarines, and baked goods. Trans fats are created by a process called *hydrogenation*, whereby the polyunsaturated fats in vegetable oils are structurally altered. This alteration makes the oil more solid (kind of like saturated fats — think of butter that stays fairly solid at room temperature) and helps to slow down spoilage of the oil.

Unfortunately, it also turns healthy vegetable oils into unhealthy trans fats that are even worse for your heart and your health than saturated fats. Why? Because after being "partially hydrogenated," the trans fats are more like saturated fats and less like the healthy polyunsaturated fats.

Unsaturated fats, on the other hand, are actually beneficial to your health. Polyunsaturated fats are simple fats with many (poly) double carbon bonds, while monounsaturated fats are simple fats with only one double carbon bond. You can feel good about eating these kinds of fat. Unlike saturated fats that increase bad cholesterol, unsaturated fats actually raise the good cholesterol and lower the bad. Monounsaturated fats are found in olive oil, nuts, and avocados. Polyunsaturated fats are found in canola oil, soy, nuts, seeds, fish, and seafood. Omega-3 fatty acids are one form of polyunsaturated fats that are particularly good for you because they fight inflammation in your body. You'll find these fats in fish, seafood, soy, canola oil, flax, chia, walnuts, and pumpkin seeds.

You have to get these fats from the foods you eat; your body can't produce them. So, if you don't get enough from your diet, it's important to take a good-quality supplement. (See Chapter 7 for more on superfoods high in omega-3 fatty acids, and Chapters 3 and 21 for info on using supplements.)

Monounsaturated fat is also good for you. It's the fat found in olive oil, and it may be one big reason why people who eat Mediterranean diets tend to be very healthy.

The following superfoods are packed with good poly- and monounsaturated fats:

- ✔ Fish and seafood contain lots of omega-3 fats (see Chapter 7).

- ✔ Chia, walnuts, and flax seeds are great plant sources of omega-3s (see Chapters 10 and 20 for more on chia and Chapter 6 for the lowdown on nuts and seeds).

- ✔ Avocados and olive oil are healthy monounsaturated fats (see Chapter 5 for a discussion of avocados, and Chapters 9 and 20 for details on olive oil).

These are just a few of the many superfood options that can help pump up your body's anti-inflammatory defense system. See the chapters in Part II to find out more specifics, including the recommended servings per day.

Aging Beautifully

Superfoods do a lot of things, but trying to turn a frog into a prince might be pushing it. Offering some benefits that can help you live a longer and more vigorous life, however, is definitely within their call of duty.

Eating superfoods helps you stay youthful, and the earlier you start with superfoods, the more age-defying benefits you can gain. Of course, these foods need to be a piece of the whole puzzle, not the sole solution for beautiful skin and a healthy body. Don't forget about smart lifestyle choices — like exercising regularly, giving up smoking, and so on — too.

Keeping that youthful glow

The health and beauty sections of every store from Wal-Mart to Macy's are stuffed with creams, lotions, cleansers, moisturizers, and make-up designed to minimize the signs of aging. But a diet that includes superfoods can do just as much — and even more — to keep your skin healthy and young-looking.

The skin deals with so many different factors — sun, pollution, extreme weather, and other irritants — that it needs a continual supply of antioxidants to help protect it. Fortunately, superfoods are chock-full of many of the main nutrients your skin needs, including:

- **Vitamins A, E, and C:** These are all common additions to popular skin creams because they're helpful in protecting the skin and vital in repairing damaged skin. Common foods that contain high levels of these vitamins include carrots (vitamin A); nuts and seeds (vitamin E); spinach (vitamins A and E); and broccoli, strawberries, and oranges (vitamin C). See Chapter 4 for more on the benefits of strawberries and oranges; Chapter 5 for details on carrots, broccoli, and spinach; and Chapter 6 for the lowdown on nuts and seeds.

- **Zinc and selenium:** Zinc, which is active in the synthesis of collagen, is another common addition to sunscreens and skin lotions. Pumpkin seeds (see Chapter 6) are an excellent source of zinc, as are nuts and beans. Selenium exhibits antioxidant effects that have been found to reduce skin cancer. Selenium is found in fish and nuts (especially Brazil nuts — see Chapter 6).

- **Bioflavonoids:** Sometimes known as "vitamin P" because of their many benefits, *bioflavonoids* aren't really vitamins. They're the pigments found in the skins of colorful fruits and vegetables. These pigments contain concentrated antioxidants that actually are more powerful than vitamins. They help increase vitamin C levels and reduce destruction of collagen in the skin.

- **Alpha-lipoic acid (ALA):** This is a fatty acid made by the body and found in foods such as broccoli and spinach. Although the body produces ALA, it doesn't make nearly enough to be helpful for fighting disease and inflammation. Plus, your body produces less as you age, so making sure you get enough from your diet becomes even more important the older you get. Alpha-lipoic acid not only has antioxidant properties, but also can help recycle some vitamins and other antioxidants.

Pumping up your pep

Gaining some super sensations from what you eat and drink is a common goal. How often have you told co-workers you need coffee or chocolate or an "energy" drink to get you through the slumps in your day? The problem with artificial stimulants is that they often pose unwanted dangers to your body. Plus, many of these options are high in sugar and artificial additives. A better option: Go natural and use superfoods to put some pep in your step.

Superfood supplements

Superfood supplements are really exploding onto the scene, and many manufacturers claim they can get more of some of the superfood qualities in supplements than you can get by eating healthful foods. Superfoods supplements give your nutrition a boost by concentrating some of the nutrients, but they shouldn't replace the healthy foods in your diet. You need to continue to eat wholesome foods that provide you with fiber, protein, and other nutrients that build your body and keep you strong. Eating a junk food diet is unhealthy no matter what supplements you take.

Superfood supplements are great for those times when you're under a lot of stress, trying to lose weight, or fighting infections, or if you're a picky eater. But your best option still is to get the energy-building properties you need from the food you eat, rather than solely from a supplement bottle. See Chapter 3 to find out more about supplements' benefits and limitations.

Getting a natural boost of energy is important not only for getting through your daily routine, but also for summoning extra energy to tackle your exercise program or other activities. When you use the right foods and eat small meals throughout the day, you can really ramp up your metabolism and get that extra energy you need.

If you're on the go and can't find the time to grab a healthy meal, these superfoods can be a great option:

- ✓ **Goji berries:** Rich in antioxidants, goji berries (see Chapter 10) have been used in Chinese medicine for years. They've also been found to help boost energy and enhance your mood.

- ✓ **Green tea:** This is another superfood that has been used for hundreds of years. The *American Journal of Clinical Nutrition* found that green tea's effect on energy was similar to that of caffeine. (Check out Chapter 9 for more on green tea and Chapter 21 for info on green tea extract.)

- ✓ **Chia seed:** The Aztecs used chia seeds to prepare for battles and long explorations. The seeds can absorb ten times their weight and are slow to digest, offering sustained energy for several hours. Chia seeds can be added to protein shakes or other meals to help give you that sustained energy throughout the day. (See Chapters 10 and 20 for more on chia.)

- ✓ **Quinoa:** This protein-rich seed, though considered a grain, is actually a leafy plant that's related to spinach and beets, and it can give you a power punch. Much as Aztecs used chia, the Incas used quinoa as a source of energy for their battles. (See Chapter 8 for more on quinoa.)

Seeing — and believing

Many bodily functions change with age, and vision is no exception. Many people develop the need for some type of visual correction as they grow older. Just like other age-related conditions that can be alleviated by super-foods, the eyes can be aided by the following superfood constituents:

- ✔ **Beta carotene:** You've probably heard that eating carrots is supposed to help improve your vision and reduce your risk for *macular degeneration,* a progressive disease of the retina that affects the light-sensing cells, causing blurring or blind spots in your central vision. That's because carrots (see Chapter 5) contain a lot of beta carotene, a precursor to vitamin A. Beta carotene is virtually a staple ingredient in vision-related nutritional supplements.

- ✔ **Acanthocyanins:** These are bioflavonoids that give color to the skin of fruits and veggies. Their antioxidant properties help protect not only your eyes, but other organ systems as well.

- ✔ **Lutein:** Lutein is concentrated in your retinas. Carrots have high levels of lutein. Other good sources are broccoli, spinach, and orange and yellow fruits. Kale not only has lutein but also is a great source of vitamin A. (See Chapter 5 for more on the benefits of broccoli, spinach, carrots, and kale.)

- ✔ **Omega-3 fatty acids:** Omega-3s protect the light-sensing cells in your eyes. One Harvard study found that people who eat fish at least twice a week cut their risk of developing age-related macular degeneration in half. Other studies found that omega-3s also may be helpful in reducing cataracts. (See Chapter 7 for more on omega-3 fatty acids.)

Understanding the Benefits of Superfoods for Your Children

The earlier you incorporate superfoods into your diet, the sooner you can benefit from all the advantages superfoods offer. And this is true for your children, too. Get them started eating superfoods at a young age, and you'll be instilling healthy habits that can serve them for a (perhaps longer) lifetime. Not only that, but you'll also be helping their immune systems, promoting strong bones and teeth, and helping them maintain a healthy weight, at a time when their young bodies can use all the help they can get.

Turn to Chapter 12 for advice on making superfoods kid-friendly. It's not as hard as you may think!

Protecting kids' immune systems

The immune system is a collection of systems and reactions in the body that act as its defense mechanism against any factors that may attempt to make the body weak or ill. Foes include everything from bacteria and viruses to inflammation and cancer. It's a tough job, considering how many different organisms can cause disease. Getting the immune system bulked up, armed, and ready for battle is important at all ages of life.

Setting the stage for a healthy immune system starts at birth. Mothers often breast-feed their infants to pass along *antibodies* (protective immune-system cells) until the baby's body can produce its own. As children grow, getting them to eat the recommended five servings of fruits and vegetables each day gives their bodies antioxidants to protect against all kinds of cell damage, and reduces their risk of cancer in the future. Because they're naturally sweet, fruits are a logical substitute for high-sugar snacks like cookies.

Sugar-dense snacks can actually weaken the immune system. They've also been found to increase inflammation in the body.

Once your children are over the age of 3 (due to the risk of allergies), you can grind walnuts, pecans, or almonds and sprinkle them on other foods like cereals, eggs, or sandwiches. You can do the same with chia and berries, too. Often, your child won't even taste the difference.

Garlic has great antibiotic activity. Not only does it boost the immune system to fight against the common cold, but also strong evidence exists that garlic plays a role in reducing your risk for cancer. (See Chapters 9 and 20 for more on the wonders of garlic.) Because garlic has such a strong taste, you may need to introduce it to your children in graduated amounts — although some kids love the taste, especially as they get older.

If your child absolutely refuses to eat anything with garlic in it, you can try having her take an odorless garlic supplement.

Building strong bones and teeth

The bones in your child's body need a rich source of nutrients for a good long time; the most important period of bone growth occurs before the age of

35. Children who eat foods that help build the strongest frame early on have a lower risk of weak bones as they age. Teeth also need certain minerals to become strong and to reduce the risk of cavities.

Diets high in caffeinated and carbonated drinks are major contributors to decreased bone strength, which can lead to fractures and fragile bones.

The most important factor for building strong bones and teeth is a calcium-rich diet. Dairy is the number one calcium contributor, but there are other great superfood options, such as soy milk or orange juice fortified with calcium. Many green leafy vegetables, such as broccoli and spinach, and the legume family are also excellent sources of calcium.

Children between the ages of 2 and 8 should get at least the equivalent of 2 cups of milk a day. Children ages 9 and older should consume 3 cups or more a day.

Milk has been thought of as the gold standard, but you can actually get more calcium by adding yogurt into a kid's daily meal plan. Most children like yogurt, and choosing yogurts packed with fruit — or adding your own — gives your child a double nutritional punch.

Some children get accustomed to consuming a few foods and put up quite a struggle when faced with change. If your kids are picky eaters, you may want to consider supplemental nutrients to ensure they're getting all they need. See Chapter 3 for more information on superfood supplements, and Chapter 12 for tips on working with picky eaters.

Figuring out the fluoride question

In 1930, fluoride was found to be important in the development of teeth and reduction of disease. Check with your pediatrician to see whether your child requires fluoride supplementation. Fluoride is often found in municipal water supplies — call your local water company to find out how much fluoride your tap water contains.

Most foods have some fluoride, but often not enough to make a difference. You can get higher concentrations of fluoride in citrus fruits and lettuce, but your children still need other sources for growing teeth. Using toothpaste with fluoride and fluorinated water are good alternatives to supplements. If you find that your water source doesn't have enough fluoride (0.7 to 1.2 parts per million, or ppm), your doctor or dentist may prescribe drops or tablets. If you have any questions about fluoride, ask your doctor or dentist for some guidance.

Helping maintain a healthy weight

Childhood obesity is rising at a staggering rate, and poor diet and decreasing activity levels are the main causes. Replacing highly processed junk foods (that are full of refined sugar, saturated fats, and calories) with superfoods can be one huge step towards slowing down this problem.

Getting your children to eat superfoods at a young age will help them grow into lean and healthy adolescents and adults. Add extra superfood vegetables at mealtimes to keep them feeling full without adding lots of calories. Serve superfood fruits and berries as sweet desserts instead of cookies, cake, and ice cream. Nuts and seeds make nutritious between-meal snacks.

The early years of life are some of the most important for the growth and development that will carry your children into adulthood. Staying at a healthy weight by eating superfoods will not only reduce their risk of obesity-related diseases such as diabetes and heart disease, but the antioxidants and other helpful nutrients will help prevent other diseases as well.

Chapter 3

Supplementing Superfoods

In This Chapter

▶ Understanding how dietary supplements work

▶ Evaluating the pros and cons of taking supplements

▶ Knowing what to look for and where to find it

*Y*our body doesn't make many of the essential nutrients it needs, so you must get most of them from your diet. But what happens if you don't get all of those needed nutrients even from a diet rich in superfoods? Maybe you don't eat as many servings of fruits and vegetables as you need every day, or maybe you don't eat the most nutritious foods. In either case, you may need more nutrients than your diet provides, and you may want to consider using dietary supplements.

Let's be clear: Supplements are no substitute for real food, superfoods, or a healthy, balanced diet — and they aren't appropriate for everyone. They shouldn't be used as meal replacements. Supplements can be packed with vitamins, minerals, and antioxidants, but they don't contain natural sources of fiber, carbohydrates, and proteins necessary for bodily functions. Used judiciously, however, they may help you to fill in the gaps in an otherwise superfood-rich diet.

In this chapter, we take the mystery out of supplements. We explain their benefits and their potential hazards, and give you some guidance to help you decide whether they're right for you. And we offer tips on what to look for — and where to look — when choosing the supplements you want.

Understanding How Dietary Supplements Work

Federal law defines a dietary supplement as "a product (other than tobacco) that is intended to supplement the diet that bears or contains one or more of the following dietary ingredients: a vitamin; a mineral; an herb or other botanical; an amino acid; a dietary substance for use by man to supplement the diet by increasing the total daily intake; or a concentrate, metabolite, constituent, extract, or combinations" of these ingredients. The law also specifies that a supplement must be in the form of a pill, tablet, capsule, or liquid, must not be intended to replace food, and must be labeled as a "dietary supplement." Beyond that, though, manufacturers have a lot of leeway in how they make and market their supplements.

That doesn't mean supplements are bad. In fact, some of them go beyond mere supplementation and may help to prevent — or, in some cases, even treat — certain diseases. However, your body isn't nearly as efficient in absorbing nutrients from supplements as it is in absorbing nutrients from food. So supplements can't take the place of a healthy, balanced diet (liberally dosed with superfoods, of course).

Exploring the difference between foods and supplements

The main difference between vitamins and minerals found in the foods you eat and the nutrients found in dietary supplements is how your body absorbs and uses them. This activity is known as *bioavailability:* the rate at which a substance is absorbed and made available to your body. Nutrients are broken down in the stomach and passed into the small intestine, where they're absorbed and then metabolized by the liver or kidneys. From there, the nutrients are delivered to different parts of your body. It's a long journey, and the body has plenty of opportunities to alter the way the supplements end up being used.

Studies have shown that many dietary supplements aren't absorbed as well as the nutrients in the foods you eat (although, as with every rule, there are exceptions — folic acid, for example, is actually better absorbed than its natural form, folate). Because of the difference in absorption rates, you may have to take six or even a dozen capsules a day to get the same amount of nutrients you'd get from eating a healthy diet. (And that's assuming your body absorbs all the nutrients in the capsules, which doesn't usually happen.)

Nutrition + Pharmaceutical = Neutraceutical

Dr. Stephen L. DeFelice coined the term *neutraceutical* to refer to foods or dietary supplements that have health and medical benefits and may prevent or actually treat disease. According to Dr. DeFelice, an orange is a neutraceutical because it contains enough vitamin C to treat scurvy. Of course, a vitamin C tablet would also treat scurvy and would fit this definition as well.

How much of what do I need and when?

The Food and Nutrition Board of the National Academy of Sciences created the *Recommended Daily Allowances* (RDA) of certain nutrients in 1941 for the purpose of evaluating nutritional intakes of large populations of people. This information was used to prevent nutritional deficiencies by establishing guidelines for nutritional labeling and for setting standards for food assistance programs. The U.S. Food and Drug Administration (FDA) established the *US RDA* for protein, vitamins, and some minerals in 1973. The US RDA had only one value for each nutrient and didn't differentiate for gender or age.

The RDAs were useful for large groups of people, but they weren't intended to be used for the assessment of any one person's diet. So, in the 1990s, the board created the *Dietary Reference Intakes* (DRIs). The DRIs include four different nutritional measurements and can be used to create meal plans and diets for an individual. The four measurements are

✔ **RDAs:** Were slightly redefined

✔ **Estimated Average Requirement (EAR):** Represents the amount of a nutrient that meets the needs of half of the population and is based on strong scientific evidence

✔ **Adequate Intake (AI):** Similar to the EAR but is more of an estimate for nutrients that don't have quite as much research available

✔ **Tolerable Upper Intake Level (UL):** The highest amount of a nutrient that can be safely consumed on a daily basis

Even though the US RDAs aren't used anymore, those values became the basis for the Daily Values you see on current Nutrition Facts labels and don't always correlate with the DRIs. Although the food labels serve as a terrific guide, it's important to know that any one individual's nutritional needs may vary.

Most manufacturers attempt to make capsules and pills so that they dissolve in the right spots, therefore maximizing absorption and improving bioavailability. Still, many pills and capsules have low bioavailability (which is one reason that getting your nutrition from food is often a better option).

Supplements are most useful when they provide the same nutritional value as a large quantity of food — especially when it's virtually impossible for you to eat that much of a particular food or food group on a regular basis. That's why fiber supplements are so popular; because foods that have a lot of fiber are quite filling, many people find it impossible to get their recommended daily intake through diet alone.

Getting the nutrients you need

How do you know how much of each nutrient you need? The Food and Nutrition Board of the Institute of Medicine determined dietary reference intakes (DRIs) for all the vitamins and minerals for the average person. Dietary supplements are intended to add any nutrients that your body may be lacking. The chart in Table

3-1 shows DRIs for vitamins and minerals, particular foods you'd need to eat to get your DRI (note that in many cases superfoods fill the bill!), and whether supplements for that particular nutrient may be a good idea for the average person.

The supplement recommendations in Table 3-1 are for the average person with no medical or lifestyle considerations that may warrant additional supplements. See the section "Determining Whether You Need Supplements," later in this chapter, for more info.

Table 3-1	Dietary Reference Intakes (DRIs) for Specific Vitamins and Minerals		
Nutrient	**DRIs**	**Foods**	**Supplement?**
Vitamin A	Men 3,000 IU/day Women 2,300 IU/day	Orange and yellow vegetables	No
Vitamin D	200–600 IU/day	Fortified milk	Yes
Vitamin E	22.5 IU	Nuts and seeds	No
Vitamin K	Men 120 mcg/day Women 90 mcg/day	Green leafy vegetables	No
Vitamin C	Men 90 mg/day Women 75 mg/day	Fruits, berries, and vegetables	Yes
Thiamin (B1)	Men 1.2 mg/day Women 1.1 mg/day	5-ounce pork chop	No
Riboflavin (B2)	Men 1.3 mg/day Women 1.1 mg/day	Vegetables, meats, and dairy	No
Niacin (B3)	Men 16 mg/day Women 14 mg/day	Meats, fish, legumes, and nuts	No
Pyridoxine (B6)	1.3 mg/day	Beans, meat, poultry, fish	No
Folate	400 mcg/day	Fruits and leafy green vegetables	Yes
Cobalamin (B12)	2.4 mcg/day	Meats, poultry, fish, dairy, and eggs	No
Calcium	1,000 mg/day	Dairy and green leafy vegetables	Yes

Nutrient	DRIs	Foods	Supplement?
Magnesium	Men 420 mg/day Women 320 mg/day	Green vegetables, nuts, seeds, and grains	No
Chromium	Men 35 mcg/day Women 25 mcg/day	Meats, grains, fruits, and vegetables	No
Iron	Men 8 mg/day Women 18 mg/day	Meat, poultry, legumes, and oats	No
Selenium	55 mcg/day	Meats, poultry, fish, nuts, and grains	No
Zinc	Men 11 mg/day Women 8 mg/day	Meats, poultry, fish, nuts, and grains	No
Potassium	4,700 mg/day	Fruits and vegetables	No
Sodium	1,500 mg/day	Processed foods	No

Heeding a few precautions

For the most part, dietary supplements are very safe. However, taking large doses of dietary supplements without medical guidance isn't a good idea. Believe it or not, it's possible to overdose on vitamins and minerals. Table 3-2 shows how taking too much of certain nutrients can harm your health.

Table 3-2	How Overdoses of Certain Nutrients Can Affect Your Health
Too Much of This Nutrient	*Can Cause These Effects*
Niacin (B3)	Flushing of skin, gastrointestinal upset
Pyridoxine (B6)	Nerve pain and numbness of the extremities
Vitamin C	Gastrointestinal upset and kidney stones

(continued)

Table 3-2 *(continued)*

Too Much of This Nutrient	Can Cause These Effects
Iodine	Increase thyroid-stimulating hormones
Iron	Gastrointestinal upset, bowel irregularity, black stools, decreased absorption of other minerals, headaches, arthritis
Magnesium	Muscle weakness, respiratory distress
Zinc	Reduced benefits of vitamin D

In addition, some dietary supplement companies make false or misleading claims for their products. Remember, dietary supplements are only loosely regulated, and the claims they make aren't evaluated by the Food and Drug Administration (FDA) or any other agency. Dietary supplements do not have to be tested to prove they are beneficial or safe before they're sold.

Here are some things to be wary of when you're shopping for supplements:

- **Outlandish claims:** Be alert to over-the-top claims you see in advertisements or on labels. Phrases like "miracle cure," "medical breakthrough," or "newest discovery" should raise red flags for you and encourage you to do more research before you buy. You can (and should) ask your doctor about any supplements you're thinking of taking.

- **Poor manufacturing:** Remember that the supplement industry is not tightly regulated, so to avoid poor manufacturing, look for nationally known brands with label statements about testing and certification. If you're not sure whether a supplement is tested and certified, call the company and ask for a certificate of analysis showing that they have properly formulated the supplement. See the later section "Knowing What to Look For" for info on researching products and manufacturers.

- **Unstated health interactions:** Many labels don't warn you of potential health risks or interactions with other supplements or medications. That's why you should always consult your doctor before you begin taking any supplements.

Consulting your doctor before taking any supplements is particularly important if you're about to undergo any medical procedures, because some nutrients can affect bleeding and how your body reacts to anesthesia. To be safe, bring your supplements with you so your doctor can read the labels and identify any potential concerns.

Determining Whether You Need Supplements

It's amazing how easy it is to be convinced to take an herb or vitamin based on a recommendation from a friend, colleague, or your doctor. After all, everyone wants to feel better and remain healthier. If someone says that he or she takes 10,000 milligrams of vitamin C and feels capable of moving a mountain, it's human nature to think, "Well, I should give it a try, too!"

The truth is that in some instances it makes sense to get additional nutrients through supplements. But in other cases, taking supplements can actually aggravate an existing health problem.

When supplements make sense

Some medical conditions and lifestyle factors can be alleviated by increasing your intake of certain nutrients. Here are some common situations that may call for higher-than-normal nutrient intake levels:

✔ **Smoking:** Smokers are thought to need an almost 50 percent higher intake of daily nutrients than non-smokers. Cigarettes (and even pipe and chewing tobacco) are loaded with chemicals that react badly with the body. These chemicals can cause inflammation and disease, but the effects can be mitigated by consuming higher doses of certain nutrients, like vitamin C.

✔ **Disease:** Several diseases can harm your body's ability to absorb and use nutrients, so you may need supplements to counter these effects. For example, gastrointestinal ailments may decrease nutrient absorption, and you may need to take supplements intravenously (under a doctor's supervision, of course). Inflammatory conditions may require more antioxidants to help reduce swelling. Some nutrients (many of them found in the superfoods we cover throughout this book) can help slow the progress of cancer and other diseases as well as increase overall well- being.

✔ **Medications:** Certain medication classes can interfere with absorption of vitamins and minerals by disrupting either the transport or metabolism of certain nutrients. Anti-seizure medications, oral contraceptives, anti-inflammatories, and chemotherapy drugs are among those known to interfere with nutrient absorption.

✔ **Occupational exposures:** People who are exposed to chemicals in their work environment often have higher rates of vitamin deficiency. Toxic levels of metals (see the "Seeing secrets held by hair" section later in this chapter) can cause deficiencies in both minerals and vitamins.

✔ **Malnourishment:** If you don't eat enough fruits and vegetables or if your diet is high in trans fats, sugar, and other highly processed foods, you'll probably need to take daily supplements until you get established on a proper diet. People with anorexia or bulimia also fall into this category.

Vegetarians and vegans don't necessarily fall into the malnourished category, but they do have some special needs based on their food intake. If you don't eat meat or any animal products, you may need to consider supplementing your intake of vitamin B12, iron, calcium, vitamin D, and zinc.

✔ **Alcohol or other drugs:** Most drugs, including alcohol, cause a depletion of important vitamins and minerals. Alcohol can cause irritation of the stomach, which effects nutrient absorption. In addition, the empty calories from alcohol often replace healthy food intake, which can make vitamin and mineral deficiencies worse.

✔ **Age:** You can use more of certain nutrients as you get older. Studies have shown that people over age 60 can use almost 30 percent more B6, and vitamin D and calcium also should be taken in higher quantities. As always, make sure you discuss supplements with your doctor before you start taking them.

✔ **Pregnancy:** This is an important time to get some extra nutrition. The female body shares nutrients with the fetus, so needing more than usual makes sense. Folate is particularly important for healthy fetus development.

Although supplements can provide moderate amounts of various nutrients, the best way for your body to utilize nutrients is through a balanced, healthy diet with superfood additions. This, along with a healthy lifestyle, keeps your body in the best position to remain disease free.

When supplements don't make sense

Supplements can be beneficial, but they aren't right for everybody all the time. Hard as it may be to believe, in some situations, supplements do more harm than good. Some vitamins, when taken in excess, can interfere with medications and can also cause some general symptoms of malaise (see Table 3-2, earlier in this chapter, for more details on the effects of overdosing).

If you take any medications, you should check with your doctor to make sure the supplements you plan to take won't affect the potency or effect of your medications. Following are a few medical conditions that can be aggravated by dietary supplements:

✔ Cancer

✔ Diabetes

✔ Heart disease

✔ Epilepsy or seizure disorder

✔ Enlarged prostate

✔ Thinning of the blood that could lead to bleeding of the gums or nose or blood in the stool

✔ Cardiovascular disease (including high blood pressure)

✔ Hormone imbalance

✔ Parkinson's disease

Some dietary supplements can slow down or speed up metabolism of prescription medications, so you should have your doctor review your supplements to make sure there are no interactions. Here are some that warrant medical clearance before you take any supplements:

✔ Blood thinners

✔ Anti-seizure medications

✔ Blood pressure medications

✔ Diabetes medications

✔ Psychiatric medications (including antidepressants)

Testing for Your Supplement Needs

You can have your nutrient levels tested to see whether you need supplements. Your doctor may be able to order blood or hair tests that can reveal deficiencies or excesses of certain nutrients or exposure to substances that may indicate the need for supplements.

The role of nutrients in health is well-established, but regular testing is still not common practice and insurance companies are slow to respond to the demands of consumers. Some insurance companies cover a portion or all of the costs for vitamin and mineral testing, but it depends on the company and selected plan, so check first.

Some symptoms, such as fatigue, weight gain or weight loss, headaches, and joint pain, may indicate a serious health problem. But they also could be caused by nutritional deficiencies or overabundance of certain nutrients. If your doctor doesn't find any medical explanation for such symptoms, you may want to explore nutrition as a possible solution.

Nutritional testing labs

Several U.S. labs specialize in nutritional testing. Spectracell offers a variety of tests. They can assess the function and the deficiency of many vitamins, minerals, and amino acids; they also offer a test for antioxidant function and actually can test for a few specific antioxidants. Other labs like this exist, and your physician may be able to direct you to such reputable sites.

Direct Laboratory Services is one of numerous online labs that offer several different lab packages to assess vitamin levels, including imbalances and abundances, and give concise recommendations to restore healthy levels. Most online labs will send you kits that you can do at home; some require you to have blood drawn at your doctor's office or local blood-drawing station.

Doing blood analysis

Wouldn't it be nice if you could have your blood drawn and end up with a printout of exactly what you need, don't need, and have the right amount of? Fine-tuning nutritional needs with simple blood tests is a process that's well underway. If your doctor suspects nutritional deficiencies based on your symptoms and medical history, blood tests can offer concrete data to help determine which dietary changes or supplements make sense.

Blood testing is one way to determine what your body needs — and what you may not be getting from your diet. Some blood tests give you a specific breakdown of nutrient levels, such as the amounts of vitamins, minerals, amino acids, and fatty acids your body contains. This direct testing helps identify deficiencies or abundances in your nutritional make-up.

Routine medical blood tests can indirectly reveal nutritional issues, even though they aren't testing for any specific deficiencies. When regular blood tests show values that are out of normal ranges, doctors often look for various diseases as the cause. But sometimes these same results can be caused not by disease, but by nutrient imbalances. Additional testing for specific vitamin and mineral levels can be very helpful — and may lead to much different treatment options.

This area of blood testing is growing because knowing how well your body is doing nutritionally can allow you to maximize diet and supplementation. If you aren't a big fan of having your blood drawn, you can always seek other testing modalities, such as hair and saliva. Saliva testing is very reliable for evaluating hormones and is starting to be used for vitamins and minerals. This may become an important test option because it's less invasive than other types of testing.

These tests are becoming a very important tool as doctors are finding how important the use of dietary and nutritional therapy can be. Testing can range from $100 to $1,000, depending on how much data you're trying to collect. In the future, this type of testing may become a part of annual blood testing, but for now it's not a bad investment to get some form of testing done, either yearly or when you're not feeling well.

Seeing secrets held by hair

If you watch crime shows on television, such as *CSI* or *Forensic Files*, you know that your hair can reveal a lot about your body. Hair analysis is the Environmental Protection Agency's test of choice for determining exposure to toxic metals and levels of trace minerals because the mineral content in your hair accurately reflects the amount of that mineral in your entire body. These days, hair is regularly tested to determine levels of minerals, metals, and other substances, including vitamins and even poisons.

Most chiropractors and homeopathic physicians offer hair testing or other similar tests, and more conventional doctors are discovering the benefits of hair testing. If your doctor doesn't do this type of testing, he or she should be able to recommend a lab or clinic that does.

Hair analysis can differ from lab to lab, raising questions about the accuracy of the results. If you choose to have your hair tested to determine whether you need supplements, and if so, which ones, be sure to have the test done by a reputable lab.

Several body functions can be affected by heavy metals and minerals, including hormone function, blood sugar control, and other metabolic pathways. Common metals that can interfere with metabolism, vitamin and mineral balances, and organ function at high levels include the following:

- ✔ **Lead:** High levels of lead can cause severe problems with nerve function, reproduction, and kidney function. Lead poisoning once was fairly common because of the prevalence of lead in paint, although that's less of a concern today. Still, lead levels need to be monitored and considered in health evaluations. Furthermore, levels that were once considered safe are now often associated with symptoms of lead poisoning.

- ✔ **Mercury:** Mercury can accumulate in your body and cause problems with your liver, gastrointestinal tract, and central nervous system. The most common way to ingest potentially harmful levels of mercury is through eating fish from mercury-contaminated waters (see Chapter 7 for more on mercury in fish).

✔ **Aluminum:** Dietary aluminum is very common, but mostly in such small quantities that it's irrelevant. However, people who have kidney disease or other conditions that prevent their bodies from excreting aluminum can accumulate high levels of this metal and develop symptoms. Some of these symptoms mimic those of Alzheimer's disease, such as memory loss and mental confusion.

Some urban water supplies have higher amounts of aluminum; check with your local water company to see whether your water has high aluminum levels. Aluminum is also a common addition to antacids, so you should take them sparingly.

✔ **Cadmium:** This metal is mostly found in industrial work areas. It is highly toxic and has led to disease and death in welders. Some paints also contain cadmium.

Hair analysis is a good option, even if you're feeling fine. If you discover imbalances in your nutrient levels before you have symptoms, you can adjust your diet (and perhaps use — or stop using — supplements) to correct them.

Considering Your Intake Options

There are some important differences in the way supplements are made and how they're consumed. One of the main objectives of nutritional companies is to find the best ways to get nutrients into your cells. In the search for maximum absorption, manufacturers have begun to move away from pills and capsules in favor of other forms, such as liquids, dissolving tabs, and injections. Snack bars and healthy drinks also are great alternatives because they get you closer to real, whole foods. They're a good choice when you're on the go and just don't have time for a traditional meal.

Taking tablets, capsules, or liquids

Most people assume that all supplements are created equal, but this is far from the truth. Manufacturing processes can affect how well your body absorbs the nutrients, and with the loose regulations currently in place, manufacturers can easily produce supplements that give you little or no actual benefit. Turn to "Knowing What to Look For," later in this chapter, for more on researching products and manufacturers. Here's a quick look at some things to think about when you're deciding whether to take supplemental tablets, capsules, or liquids:

- ✔ **Tablets** are made by mixing organic or inorganic materials and then using machines to compress them into shape. Manufacturers use different types of materials to hold the supplements together, and those materials can affect how efficiently your body absorbs the nutrients you're after. Even the process used to compress the pills can affect absorption.

- ✔ **Capsules** are gelatin containers that commonly dissolve faster than tablets. However, capsules often have significant amounts of filler material, and the kind of filler varies depending on the manufacturer. These fillers can affect absorption, too.

- ✔ **Liquids** generally claim to have better absorption rates than tablets or capsules. However, as with tablets and capsules, liquid supplements contain other substances that may inhibit the release of the actual nutrient into your system. Taste is a factor, too; you're unlikely to take a liquid supplement regularly if the taste makes you gag.

Different supplements come in different forms. For example, you may have a tablet of vitamin E and a capsule for fish oils. You may also have to consider the size of the tablet or capsule, because often people complain that supplements are too big to swallow. Liquids are nice because there's no problem with swallowing, and you often can dilute liquid supplements in water or other drinks to offset taste.

Reputable companies use the right materials and tested delivery methods to give you the best availability of the nutrient. Don't spend too much time investigating the actual delivery form; instead, spend that time looking into the company making the supplement.

Superfood bars and drinks

Some great snack bars and drinks are available that are loaded with superfoods and are definitely a decent alternative to more common supplements. Be careful, though; some of these products contain additives and calories that you won't get in simple supplements.

Raw bars are functional foods in the shape of a convenient-to-eat snack bar. These bars tend to be loaded with superfoods, and they don't have unhealthy additives like refined sugars or trans fats. Raw bars are made to be closest to eating a real meal and can be found with many super-duper superfoods (see Chapter 20).

Raw bars are available in several brands. Our favorites include Raw Revolution (www.rawindulgence.com) and Organic Pure (www.thepurebar.com).

If you aren't a snack bar fan, how about a delicious superfood drink? Many healthy drinks use superfood berries like strawberries or acai berries, often with the addition of green tea. You can get these in ready-to-drink or -mix forms. Some superfood drinks even contain important greens like broccoli and spinach, as well as grasses and other vitamins.

We recommend Go Greens superfoods drink (www.togobrands.com), Dr. Schulze's Super Food Plus (www.dr-schulze.com), and Vibe Neutraceutical Concentrate (www.eniva.com). If you can't find these products or don't want to order them online, V8 (the low-sodium variety) and V8 Fusion are good alternatives.

Like any other supplement, snack bars and drinks are no substitute for healthy meals. Use them to fill in the gaps between meals rather than to replace meals.

Knowing What to Look For

Once you've decided you want to supplement your diet, the sheer volume of supplement options and brands can be bewildering. Are store or generic brands as good as national brands? How can you be sure a given supplement is actually effective? What should you look for?

Here are some tips to make your search a little less daunting:

- ✔ **Ask your doctor, family, and friends for recommendations.** If people you trust are happy with the supplements they take or recommend, this is a good starting point for your own purchase.

- ✔ **Ask your doctor if a quality generic or store brand is available.** Your doctor may know of quality generic or store brands that are significantly cheaper than big-name brands but just as effective.

- ✔ **Do some research online.** The Internet makes it easy to find information about dietary supplements. Search by brand name, ingredient, or nutrient, and be sure to evaluate both negative and positive information. A simple search of a manufacturer's name can turn up review sites where consumers share their experiences with a particular product.

  You also can check out manufacturers at www.consumerlab.com. This site lists products that have been tested and certified, so you know that they contain the stated amounts of nutrients and that they're safe.

  Online communities and blogs can also be great sources of information on supplements, including reputable products. Check out www.supplementinfo.org or www.ods.od.nih.gov, or type "dietary supplement blog," or "healthy supplement blog" into your browser's search engine.

✔ **Look for food-base supplements.** *Food base* is concentrated plant material to which vitamins and minerals are added. Supplements with a food base contain enzymes and nutrients that boost absorption of the vitamins and minerals. This is probably the best type of supplement you can buy, but the tablets are larger, and you may have to take more of them.

✔ **Check the expiration date.** Supplements typically have a long *shelf life* — the length of time they can be stored and remain safe, effective, and usable — but you should always check the expiration date before you buy. There's no point in buying 500 multivitamins that expire in six months.

Although many manufacturers claim that synthetic vitamins are chemically identical to the real thing, your body knows the difference between synthetic and natural vitamins. Numerous studies have shown that the human body uses natural vitamins more effectively and more efficiently than synthetic versions. This is another reason why supplements can only complement your diet; they can't take the place of real foods — or superfoods.

Knowing Where to Look

Virtually every grocery store has a selection of vitamins and more popular dietary supplements on its shelves. But that doesn't mean you'll get the best product or the best price. Discount retailers like Wal-Mart and Target typically have a larger selection of supplements, including both national brands and their own store brands. And many cities large enough to have a mall also boast a health store of some sort.

No matter where you live, you can go online to order supplements from reputable manufacturers. Larger stores usually get volume discounts that can be passed on to the consumer, so you're likely to find better prices at big-box stores. Online stores have less overhead, which can also lead to lower costs. One option is to research supplement manufacturers and prices online, and then check your local brick-and-mortar stores to see whether they offer similar or better prices. Two of our favorite sites are www.wholefoodsmarket. com and www.organicstorelocator.com. You can order directly from the Whole Foods site; the second site directs you to organic and homeopathic stores near you, and some of these allow you to place orders online.

Part II

From Apples to Wheat Grass: A Look at the Superfoods

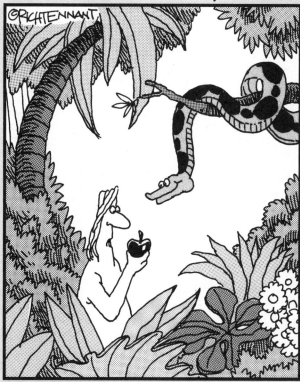

The 5th Wave By Rich Tennant

@RICHTENNANT

"This isn't some sort of fad diet, is it?"

In this part . . .

Fruits, veggies, nuts, seafood, grains, and even herbs can pack a superfood punch, boosting your overall health and well-being. In this part, we take a closer look at each of the superfoods, identifying what makes them so super and showing you how to integrate them into your eating regimen. We also offer tips on selecting, storing, and preparing each of these superfoods.

We even explore some exotic superfoods that are common in many parts of the world, but not so well-known in Western countries.

Chapter 4

Getting Fruitful and Reaping the Rewards

Fruits and berries are sweet and delicious, so they're very easy to incorporate into your healthy new superfoods diet. The word *fruitful* means "beneficial" and "abundant," two words that make it easy to remember why you need fruits every day and how many you should eat.

Fruits and berries are beneficial for your health because they're rich in nutrients and fiber. They also have natural compounds called *flavonoids* that offer special health properties. Flavonoids are a specific form of *phytochemicals* found in the pigments that give fruits their colors. In nature, flavonoids and other phytochemicals protect the fruit; when you eat them, they protect *you* by working as antioxidants to prevent cell damage throughout your body — inside and out.

Fruits can also be an excellent source of fiber, providing a significant percentage of the recommended daily allowance. Most men need at least 38 grams of fiber a day, and most women need at least 25 grams.

How much fruit should you eat every day? Think "abundant," as in a large amount. Experts recommend eating four servings (or 2 cups) of fruits every day, with a typical serving being one piece of fruit, $^3/_4$ cup of fruit juice, or $^1/_2$ cup of chopped fruits or berries.

Not all your fruit servings need to be superfood fruits. While some fruits are better than others, we really can't think of any fruits that are bad for your health.

All fruits are healthful, but some special fruits and berries are stars in the superfoods world. We recommend adding at least one superfood fruit to your daily fruit intake. In this chapter, we explore the special health benefits of eight great fruits, and we tell you how to go about selecting, storing, and serving them.

Keep a bowl of fresh fruit on your kitchen counter where everyone can grab an apple, banana, or orange for a delicious and healthy treat.

Biting into the Amazing Apple

Does eating an apple a day really keep the doctor away? It actually might: Apples are low in calories and rich in nutrients and fiber.

Apples come in many varieties, so you can easily choose flavors and textures to suit your taste or cooking needs. The traditional, deep-hued Red Delicious apple is a perennial favorite, although many people prefer the flavor and texture of the newer varieties of sweet-tangy, crisp, bi-colored apples. Like something even more tart? Light green Granny Smith apples fill the bill and are great for cooking.

Put the health benefits of the amazing apple to work for you by adding this superfood fruit to your daily diet at least five times each week.

Appreciating the benefits of apples

The most potent flavonoid found in apples is *quercetin,* which is also a powerful antioxidant. Apples are an excellent source of fiber, too — one apple (with the skin) contains about five grams of fiber.

Much of the apple's fiber and phytochemicals are found in the colorful exterior, so get into the habit of eating both the flesh and the skin.

The nutrients, fiber, and flavonoids in apples work to keep you healthy in several ways. In fact, research shows several benefits of eating apples.

- ✔ **They fight high blood pressure.** According to *The Journal of Nutrition* in 2007, quercetin helps to lower blood pressure in humans.

- ✔ **They're good for your lungs.** The flavonoids work like antihistamines and anti-inflammatory agents to reduce the severity of asthma attacks and allergic symptoms. A 2001 study in *The American Journal of Respiratory and Critical Care Medicine* shows that people who eat five or more apples each week have a decreased risk of chronic lung disease.

✔ **They protect you from cancer.** The journal *Prostate* reported in 2008 that, in laboratory tests, quercetin slows the growth of cancerous cells without harming prostate cells. The American Cancer Society suggests that eating a diet rich in fruits like apples may help to prevent a variety of cancers.

✔ **They keep your mind sharp and clear.** Older people who eat more apples and drink apple juice may have stronger brain function. According to *The Journal of Alzheimer's Disease* in 2006, flavonoids help protect your brain from free-radical damage.

✔ **They help you lose weight.** Because apples are rich in fiber, they keep you feeling full longer so you're less likely to snack on high-calorie snack foods. (An apple has only about 90 calories.) Their sweet, juicy flavor and crunchy texture make fresh apples a healthy dessert or afternoon snack.

✔ **They help maintain a healthy digestive system and regulate cholesterol levels.** These benefits can also be credited to the high fiber content of apples.

✔ **They help fight viral infections, like colds and flu, plus they keep connective tissue healthy.** One apple contains about 8 milligrams of vitamin C (about 8 percent of the daily requirement).

Choosing, storing, and using apples

Apples are easy to find in every grocery store and even in many convenience stores. Look for apples that have shiny, smooth skins free from blemishes and punctures. During the fall months, look for local orchards or festivals that offer super-fresh apples, apple juice, and homemade applesauce.

Most of the apples you buy in the store have been covered with a clear, edible wax that helps to protect them during shipping. The wax helps keep moisture in the apples so they stay fresh and crisp all the way from the orchard to your table. You don't need to remove the wax, but you should still wash apples before eating them.

Which apples are best for what?

Some apples are best for eating and some are better for cooking. Here's a short list of some of the common apples and their best uses:

✔ For eating: Red Delicious, Gala, and Fuji

✔ For baking: Granny Smith, Golden Delicious, and Rome

✔ For applesauce: Cortland, Macintosh, and Jonathan

For convenience, you can keep a few apples in a fruit bowl on your kitchen counter. However, apples stay fresher longer in cool air, so it's best to store them in the refrigerator in a paper bag that is loosely closed.

Apples give off a gas called *ethylene* that actually makes some fruits (such as bananas, pears, peaches, and plums) ripen faster. This same gas can cause damage to some vegetables such as leafy greens, broccoli, cauliflower, and cucumbers. Keep an apple with green bananas to make them ripen more quickly, but keep apples away from the vegetable bin in your fridge.

Apples are quite versatile. An apple makes a great snack on its own or with a handful of healthful nuts, or you can slice it and spread peanut butter on each slice. Serve Granny Smith slices with blue cheese or brie and a glass of red wine. If you're looking for a delicious dessert, slice up a Granny Smith and top with a light drizzle of caramel sauce and some chopped pecans. During cooler weather, try some hot apple cider mulled with cinnamon and other spices to warm you up.

Peeling the Benefits of Bananas

Bananas are one of the most popular and least expensive fruits to add to your diet. As such, they're an economical way to help meet your daily fruit and vegetable requirements.

More than just a naturally sweet snack and versatile ingredient, the banana is also a superfood — thanks to its nutrients, phytochemicals, and fiber. You need to eat at least 2 cups of fruits every day, and eating a large banana satisfies half of that daily need. We suggest you eat a banana two or three days each week.

One banana contains more than 450 milligrams of potassium, a mineral that's important for keeping your body fluids in balance, which in turn keeps your blood pressure at healthy levels. Experts agree that everyone needs about 4,700 milligrams of potassium every day. But bananas have many other benefits, too. Read on!

Eating bananas for more than just potassium

Bananas protect your heart because they contain potassium and dietary fiber, and they're low in sodium. However, bananas can do so much more. Eating bananas (along with other fruits and vegetables) is an important part of a healthful diet.

Eating bananas provides you with potassium, vitamins B6 and C, plenty of fiber, and some magnesium, all of which are essential for good health. Bananas have the following in their favor:

- ✔ **They lower your blood pressure.** Bananas are not only high in potassium, but also low in sodium, a combination that may reduce high blood pressure. This means your heart doesn't have to work so hard to pump blood throughout your body.

- ✔ **They're high in vitamin B6.** Your body needs B6 to produce red blood cells and to break down protein into components your body can use. Vitamin B6 also helps keep homocysteine levels in check. High homocysteine levels correlate to a higher risk of cardiovascular disease.

- ✔ **They have lots of dietary fiber.** Studies confirm that people who eat diets high in fiber have lower rates of cardiovascular disease. Fiber is also important for keeping the digestive tract healthy by keeping bowel movements regular.

- ✔ **They're rich in fructooligosaccharide (FOS), a natural substance that feeds the friendly bacteria that live in the colon.** These beneficial bacteria produce vitamins, enzymes, and other organic acids that help protect you from unfriendly bacteria. Bananas also contain a compound that combats the bacteria that causes stomach ulcers and works as a natural antacid.

- ✔ **They may help protect you from cancer.** A diet rich in fruits and vegetables has been associated with a reduced risk of several types of cancers, including a kidney cancer called *renal cell carcinoma.* Of all the fruits and vegetables studied, the *International Journal of Cancer* reported in 2005 that bananas have the strongest association for prevention of this disease. Bananas also contain plant *lectins,* proteins that survive digestion intact. Lectins are very biologically active and may fight cancer by killing cancerous cells and inhibiting tumor growth.

- ✔ **They may help protect your bones.** Bananas may help reduce calcium loss through the urine and improve your body's ability to absorb nutrients, including calcium and other minerals needed for strong bones.

Adding bananas to your superfoods diet

You can find bananas in the produce department of every grocery store and even on the shelves in many convenience stores. They're easy to store, easy to prepare, and easy to eat.

When bananas reach your grocery store, they may be more of a greenish tint and not fully ripe. That's okay; just take your bananas home and let them ripen on the counter at room temperature.

Cold slows down the ripening process, so don't put your bananas in the refrigerator until they are fully ripened, with yellow skin and brown spots.

The banana is a very versatile fruit. The simplest way to enjoy a banana is to simply peel one and eat it. Bananas are naturally sweet and don't need anything to dress them up. You can also slice a banana and add it to a bowl of oatmeal to double up on superfoods (see Chapter 8 for more about oatmeal).

You can even use bananas to top off a hot fudge sundae or a banana split, or make Bananas Foster (a dessert made with bananas, vanilla ice cream, and a sauce that includes butter, brown sugar, cinnamon, and dark rum). These treats are high in fat and calories, but it's okay to treat yourself occasionally. Really.

Bananas can also be used as an ingredient: You can add them to fruit salad or, when they get fully ripe, you can use them to make banana breads or muffins. Bananas also are the secret ingredient for making fruit smoothies. For richer and thicker smoothies, cut ripe bananas into one-inch chunks and freeze them. When it's time to make your smoothies, just pop four or five chunks into the blender with your other ingredients.

Picking Beautiful Blueberries

Blueberries burst with flavor and good health. They even came out on top for antioxidant activity when more than 40 commercially available fruits were tested. The dark blue pigment found in blueberries contains phenols called *anthocyanins* (flavonoids with powerful antioxidant capabilities). Consequently, they have many health benefits, so try to enjoy 3 or 4 cups of blueberries every week.

Tapping into the antioxidant power of blueberries

Blueberries are a significant source of vitamin C, manganese (an essential trace mineral important for many chemical reactions in your body), and fiber. Plus, like many superfood fruits, they're low in calories.

One cup of blueberries contains 14 milligrams of vitamin C, half a milligram of manganese, 4 grams of fiber, and only 84 calories. Blueberries help your body in several ways:

✔ **They keep your heart healthy.** The anthocyanins keep your blood vessels strong. According to the United States Department of Agriculture (USDA), the darker pigments in blueberries may lower cholesterol.

✔ **They help prevent cancer.** According to research published in 2008 in *The Journal of Agricultural and Food Chemistry,* antioxidants in blueberries may help to prevent colon cancer and ovarian cancer by promoting anti-cancer activity in your cells.

- ✔ **They keep your vision clear.** Blueberries contain natural compounds related to vitamin A called *lutein* that promote healthy night vision and prevent *macular degeneration* (an age-related eye disease that's the leading cause of vision loss in the elderly). The Age-Related Eye Disease Study conducted by the National Eye Institute in 2001 confirmed the effectiveness of lutein and other antioxidants.

- ✔ **They keep your mind sharp.** According to the Agency for Health Care Policy and Research, a substance in blueberries (as well as other berries) may help to protect you from some of the deleterious effects of Alzheimer's disease.

- ✔ **They prevent urinary tract infections.** The natural compounds in blueberries prevent bacteria from sticking to the walls of your bladder, which prevents urinary tract infections.

Purchasing, packing away, and preparing blueberries

Blueberries are usually easy to find in both the produce and freezer sections at your grocery store. Blueberries freeze very well, and they're good for you whether fresh or frozen.

During the summer months, you may be able to buy big, beautiful blueberries at farmers' markets, or you may find farms where you can pick your own.

Selecting blueberries is easy. Look for berries that are deep blue with little to no trace of green coloring; unlike many fruits, blueberries don't continue to ripen after they're picked. Healthy blueberries should be firm with a slight shimmer to the skin, and there should be no sign of mold.

Keep blueberries in your refrigerator. Don't wash them until you want to use them, because moisture hastens deterioration. Blueberries are delicate and quite perishable, so eat them within a few days or freeze them.

Blueberries freeze very well when you put them in sturdy plastic containers. Again, don't wash the berries before you freeze them because the water on the skins will make them tough. Instead, rinse the berries after they thaw.

Whether fresh or frozen, you can easily incorporate blueberries into your superfoods diet. Traditional uses of blueberries include baked goods such as pancakes and muffins because blueberries hold up well to heat.

If you buy premade baked goods, be sure they contain real blueberries, not the little blueberry-flavored sugar blobs commonly found in cheap baked goods.

Sprinkle some berries on your whole-grain cereal or oatmeal in the morning, or enjoy a bowl of blueberries with a little milk or cream and a few walnuts for breakfast.

Thawed berries can be used just like fresh ones. You can even add frozen blueberries and banana chunks, along with pomegranate or other juice, to your blender to make a tasty fruit smoothie.

Picking Cherries: The Dessert Topper

Cherries are another red-to-yellow superfood fruit rich in phytochemicals and nutrients. They're best known as the main ingredient in cherry pies and cobblers; however, they make a healthy and sweet treat when eaten alone.

There are two types of cherries: sweet and tart. Sweet cherries are delicious when eaten plain, while tart cherries are more likely to be used in baking or cooking. Tart cherries are usually processed right after harvesting, but you can find fresh sweet cherries in your local grocery store. We suggest you enjoy cherries at least twice a week.

Packing melatonin and phytochemicals

Cherries contain a hormone called *melatonin,* which is best known as a sleep inducer, but melatonin may also help to fight cancer and depression. Melatonin may work well in combination with the phytochemicals that are found in cherries. Additionally, cherries contain quercetin, a flavonoid best known as a natural antihistamine and anti-inflammatory agent.

Nutritionally, cherries are low in calories while providing substantial amounts of potassium (300 milligrams per cup), vitamin C (10 milligrams per cup), and fiber (4 grams per cup).

Eating cherries brings all sorts of health benefits, including the following:

- ✔ **Cherries are good for your heart.** Almost all superfoods are good for your heart, and cherries are no exception. The combination of phytochemicals and potassium helps keep your blood pressure regular, protect your body's good cholesterol, and keep your arteries healthy.

- ✔ **Cherries may help keep your brain healthy.** According to *The Journal of Agricultural and Food Chemistry* in 2005, the various phytochemicals found in cherries may have a beneficial effect on nerve cells, which may reduce the risk of Alzheimer's disease.

- ✔ **Cherries reduce your risk of cancer.** The cherry's coloring contains compounds that have been shown to have anti-cancer activity in the lab.

In 2004, the journal *Carcinogenesis* reported that *cyanidins,* which are anti-oxidants found in cherries, may help reduce the growth of cancer cells.

✔ **Cherries may help to relieve pain.** Many people suffer from pain and inflammation, and some of the superfoods may help alleviate that suffering. Cherries in particular contain many phytochemicals similar to those found in strawberries that act as anti-inflammatories — using the same mechanism painkillers like ibuprofen use, but without the adverse side effects.

✔ **Cherries may help you sleep.** Melatonin is the sleep hormone that your body naturally secretes in larger amounts at night. Eating cherries may help you to regulate your sleep, may reduce the effects of jet lag, and may be valuable for people who work night shifts and need to sleep during the day. Cherry extract is often used in natural, over-the-counter, sleep-aid supplements.

Culling, keeping, and enjoying cherries

You can find fresh cherries in the produce section of your grocery store. Choose cherries that are firm and plump, with healthy, shiny skins and green stems. Avoid cherries that have soft spots and discolorations. You can also find frozen, dried, or canned cherries, but watch out for added sugar.

Keep cherries in the refrigerator; warm temperatures cause them to spoil quickly. Only buy the amount of cherries you think you will eat within a week.

If you have more cherries than you can eat in a few days, you can freeze them. Simply rinse them and put them in sturdy plastic containers. When you're ready to serve your cherries, let them thaw partially for a nicer texture. You may also wish to remove the pits before freezing for easier serving later.

Cherries make a nice addition to garden salads and fruit salads. Simply rinse the cherries and remove the stems and pits. Cherries combine very well with almond flavorings.

Cherries are also available in a dried form that makes them very portable and easy to use. You can make your own trail mix by combining dried cherries, raisins, almonds, pecans, and your favorite whole-grain cereal.

Paying Homage to the Native Cranberry

Cranberries are very tart little red berries. They're related to blueberries, so they have many of the same properties. This berry is native to North America and was first discovered by Europeans in 1550. The Pilgrims used cranberries, and cranberry sauce is traditionally served in the United States at Thanksgiving alongside the turkey and stuffing. We think cranberries are great; however, their tartness makes them difficult to enjoy without adding extra sugar. Cranberry juice can be blended with other, sweeter juices, and cranberry extract is available as a dietary supplement. We suggest you eat cranberries or drink cranberry juice twice each week.

Blocking bacteria

Cranberries contain phytochemicals that help block bacterial growth, especially in the urinary tract. Cranberry juice has been a home remedy for prevention of bladder infections for many years.

One cup of cranberries also contains 13 milligrams of vitamin C that help keep your immune system and blood vessels strong. Cranberries are very low in calories with no fat and little natural sugar. Cranberries have other benefits, too.

- ✔ **They keep your heart healthy.** The phenols in cranberries help keep your arteries clear. According to *The British Journal of Nutrition* in 2008, cranberry juice may reduce the levels of LDL cholesterol, blood fats that may increase your risk of cardiovascular disease.

- ✔ **They treat and prevent bladder infections.** Bladder infections (also called *cystitis*) usually require antibiotic therapy; however, cranberries can speed the healing time and prevent future infections. *Hippuric acid,* a compound found in cranberries, keeps urine acidic and prevents bacteria from sticking to the walls of your bladder, so the bacteria can't catch on and proliferate.

- ✔ **They promote a healthy digestive tract.** Some of the phytochemicals found in cranberries fight off food-borne pathogens and may help keep you from getting sick at a picnic when someone leaves the potato salad out too long.

- ✔ **They fight cavities.** Cranberries' antibacterial properties extend to your mouth and may help to kill the bacteria that lead to tooth decay.

Buying, saving, and sweetening cranberries

Cranberries are available in fresh, dried, and canned form (the latter often has added sugar). Look for bags of fresh cranberries in the produce section of your local grocery store. They're available year-round and are especially popular in the autumn months. If they're on sale, buy an extra bag or two to pop into the freezer.

You can keep fresh cranberries in the refrigerator for a few days or in the freezer for two months if you use the bag you bought them in, which is vented, or up to one year if you use freezer bags. Keep dried cranberries in airtight containers. You can store cooked cranberries in the refrigerator for up to one month.

Unless you have a very strong taste for tart flavors, you probably won't be able to eat cranberries or drink the juice without the addition of sweeter flavors. For example, if you want to use cranberry juice to help prevent recurrent bladder infections, you can blend the cranberry juice with sweeter juices or with sparkling water. Drink at least 7 ounces of cranberry juice every day.

Be sure to buy 100 percent cranberry juice. Cranberry juice "cocktail" may not contain enough cranberry juice to be therapeutic.

You can make a simple cranberry sauce by combining a 12-ounce bag of cranberries with 1 cup of sugar and 1 cup of orange juice in a saucepan over medium heat for about 10 minutes, until the cranberries start to pop. We know that's a lot of sugar, so you may want to use 1 cup of sucralose instead.

Cranberries are often sold in dried form (like little red raisins) with a little sugar coating. You can use dried cranberries as a topping for salads, enjoy them as a snack alone, or mix them with other dried fruits and nuts.

Opting for Oranges

Sweet and juicy oranges are so popular that there's a color named for them. They're well-known for their vitamin C content, their beautiful color comes from many different beneficial phytochemicals, and the pulp contains lots of fiber.

Whether sliced or juiced, oranges can be a delicious part of your healthy superfoods diet. Calcium-fortified orange juice is also available as a healthy substitute for people who choose not to consume dairy products (and thus may not get enough calcium in their diets). We suggest you eat oranges at least five times each week.

Keeping healthy with vitamin C, folate, and phytochemicals

When you feel a cold coming on, do you run to the grocery store to stock up on orange juice? You should, because oranges are a great source of vitamin C — in fact, one orange contains 100 milligrams of vitamin C — well over 100 percent of the vitamin C you need for an entire day.

Oranges contain many phytochemicals, such as flavonoids and *polyphenols* (natural chemicals found in plants), that act like antioxidants to protect your body inside and out. *The Journal of the American College of Nutrition* reported in 2003 that drinking orange juice every day provides effective antioxidant protection.

Oranges also contain potassium, folate, and fiber, which keep your heart healthy. One medium orange has around 80 calories and 4 grams of fiber.

The benefits of oranges are truly impressive — especially when you see all the ways they help keep you healthy.

- ✔ **Oranges enhance your immune system.** Your body needs vitamin C for many processes, including a properly functioning immune system. And a healthy immune system is crucial for fighting off cold and flu viruses. But don't wait until you get sick to start eating oranges. Give your immune system a head start in fighting off viruses and infections by eating oranges year-round.

  Vitamin C alone — in the form of supplements, for example — doesn't appear to work as well as eating oranges. Unlike supplements, oranges have those phytochemicals that may work with the vitamin C to keep you healthy.

- ✔ **Oranges keep your skin smooth.** Your skin is attached to your body by connective tissue. Eating oranges provides vitamin C that helps to keep the connective tissue strong, which in turn helps to keep your skin looking younger.

- ✔ **Oranges prevent rheumatoid arthritis.** In 2003, *The American Journal of Epidemiology* published a study showing that women who ate the most oranges were at the lowest risk for rheumatoid arthritis.

- ✔ **Oranges may help to prevent certain cancers.** Oranges help protect you against lung cancer, and a study reported in 2008 in the journal *Nutrition and Cancer* reported that smokers who eat oranges are less likely to develop cancer of the esophagus (the tube that connects the mouth and stomach). Once again, the phytochemicals in oranges are to thank.

- ✔ **Oranges can protect unborn babies from spina bifida.** Oranges contain folate, a water-soluble B vitamin that prevents a defect from forming in an embryo that causes *spina bifida,* a potentially crippling spinal condition in which the spinal cord isn't properly enclosed.

- ✔ **Oranges help keep homocysteine levels low.** *Homocysteine* is an amino acid in your blood; high homocysteine levels have been linked to heart and vascular disease. The folate in oranges helps to lower homocysteine.

- ✔ **Oranges protect you from strokes.** Research published in *The Journal of the American Medical Association* in 1999 found that people who drank citrus juice such as orange juice every day had a lower risk of stroke.

- ✔ **Oranges prevent anemia.** Vitamin C makes it easier for your body to absorb iron from plant-based foods such as legumes, seeds, and vegetables and from dietary supplements.

Enjoying the ease of oranges

Select oranges that have smooth skin, but don't worry about a few blemishes. Ripe oranges feel a little heavier than those that are less ripe. You can find oranges in your local grocery store. Valencia oranges are best for juicing; navel oranges are easy to peel and eat. The more exotic mora orange, or blood orange, is just as good for you, with a slightly different flavor.

Navel oranges have a little "belly button" on one end. The larger the navel, the sweeter the orange will be.

Orange juice is available with or without pulp. Just be sure you're buying 100 percent orange juice and not orange-flavored beverages that have added sugar and less nutritional value. Freshly squeezed orange juice has more vitamin C than the orange juice you buy at the grocery store, but even one serving of store-bought orange juice has all the vitamin C you need for one day.

Oranges can be stored in the refrigerator or on your counter; it just depends on whether you like to eat them cold or at room temperature. Orange juice should always be refrigerated.

Preparing an orange is easy. First, wash the skin so that you remove any dirt or bugs that may contaminate the flesh. You can cut the orange in half and cut each half into two or three lengthwise slices, or you can peel the rind off and eat it section by section.

The Berry "Grenade": The Pomegranate

Pomegranates have gone from something rather exotic to a staple in many grocery stores. They're about the size and shape of a large orange, but have a smooth, reddish exterior. Rather plain looking on the outside, the real beauty of the pomegranate is found inside — each pomegranate contains dozens of red *arils* (berry-like seed casings) that resemble large garnet gemstones (see Figure 4-1).

Grenadine

Grenadine is a red syrup that colors and flavors many cocktails, from Shirley Temples to Tequila Sunrises. Real grenadine is made from pomegranate, sugar, and water. Unfortunately, most of the grenadine you see in the mixers section of your grocery store is composed of high fructose corn syrup and artificial flavors, with no pomegranate at all.

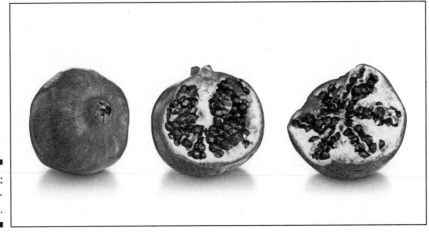

Figure 4-1: Pomegranates.

Pomegranate arils are deliciously sweet with different degrees of tartness, depending on the variety. The juice is rich in antioxidants and vitamins, while the seeds are a good source of fiber.

You can buy pomegranate juice at the grocery store. We recommend drinking 8 ounces of juice, three times a week.

Packing powerful polyphenols

Pomegranate juice is a good source of vitamin C, pantothenic acid (vitamin B5), potassium, and polyphenols that are similar to the *tannins* (another kind of plant polyphenols) found in wine and tea. Plus, you get a little bit of fiber if you eat the seeds inside the arils.

You don't need to eat the arils, however, because most of the health benefits are found in the juice. Most research studies focus on the juice, and pomegranate juice is quite a superfood.

- ✔ **It keeps your heart healthy.** The antioxidants lower your blood pressure and help keep your arteries clear and healthy. According to the journal *Clinical Nutrition* in 2004, drinking pomegranate juice also helps to keep so-called "bad" cholesterol low.

- ✔ **It protects against cancer.** According to research published in 2006 in the journal *Clinical Cancer Research,* pomegranate juice has a beneficial effect on *prostate specific antigen* (PSA), one of the lab markers for prostate cancer.

- ✔ **It may improve erectile dysfunction.** A preliminary study reported in 2007 in *The International Journal of Impotence Research* suggests that by promoting healthy arteries, pomegranate juice may improve blood-flow to the penis, thereby improving sexual function.

Fixing the fruit or buying the bottle

Pomegranates are easy to select because they are fully ripe when they arrive at the store. Look for fruits that aren't cracked or split, and choose the ones that feel heaviest for their size.

So what do you do with a pomegranate when you get it home? You can store it at room temperature, uncut, for about one week, or you can keep it up to a month in the refrigerator. After you remove the arils from the pomegranate, you can keep the arils in an airtight container in the refrigerator for a few days or in the freezer for up to one year.

Preparing a pomegranate to harvest the juicy arils inside may seem a little daunting, but it really isn't difficult if you follow these steps:

1. **Cut off the crown end of the pomegranate.**

2. **Score the rind of the pomegranate into several sections, but don't slice all the way through as you would an orange; you'll damage the arils.**

3. **Place the pomegranate into a large bowl of water and break it into sections along the score lines.**

4. **Hold the sections under water and use your fingers to separate the arils from the white connective membrane.**

   The arils will sink to the bottom of the bowl. The rind and membrane will float so you can easily scoop them off.

5. **Drain the arils in a colander.**

You can eat the arils as a snack or sprinkle them on top of oatmeal, pancakes, salads, and desserts.

If you prefer pomegranate juice, look for the words "100 percent pomegranate juice" on the label. Pure pomegranate juice is expensive. Beware of cheaper pomegranate juice drinks that contain lots of sugar or cheaper filler juices that dilute the actual amount of pomegranate juice.

If you find pomegranate to be a little too tart for your liking, mix it with sweeter juices such as blueberry, apple, or grape.

Savoring Sensational Strawberries

Strawberries land on the superfood list because of their terrific nutrition and powerful phytochemicals (plus a low calorie count). They're also a good source of fiber. These beautiful red berries are the most popular member of the berry family.

You may be familiar with strawberries on shortcakes, in pies, or on top of ice cream sundaes, but they really don't need the extra sugar. Strawberries are naturally sweet.

Because strawberries are so good for you and fairly inexpensive (compared to other fresh berries), we suggest you enjoy them three or four times a week.

Optimizing health with strawberries

Strawberries are a significant source of vitamin C and phytochemicals called phenols that help protect your health with their powerful antioxidant activity. The phenols in strawberries include anthocyanins and tannins, similar to the ones found in other berries.

Strawberries aren't far behind oranges when it comes to vitamin C. One cup of strawberry slices gives you more than 100 percent of the vitamin C you need each day for fewer than 50 calories, so strawberries are an excellent food for watching your weight.

Among the health benefits of eating strawberries are the following:

- **They keep your heart healthy.** Strawberries provide heart-healthy potassium while being low in sodium. Strawberries also contain natural anti-inflammatory agents that may help keep your arteries healthy. The folate found in strawberries reduces homocysteine levels (high levels are associated with heart disease). Folate is particularly important for pregnant women, as it helps to prevent spina bifida in babies. (See the "Keeping healthy with vitamin C, folate, and phytochemicals" section earlier in this chapter.)

- **They protect your vision.** Eating three or more servings of fruit every day may help reduce your risk of macular degeneration (the leading cause of blindness in the elderly). The antioxidant lutein (found in strawberries and blueberries) may be particularly potent.

- **They may help prevent cancer and rheumatoid arthritis.** The phenols in strawberries have powerful anti-cancer properties. According to *The Journal of Agricultural and Food Chemistry* in 2008, berries of all kinds may help to prevent several types of cancers. The phenols in strawberries may also prevent rheumatoid arthritis.

- **They're natural painkillers.** In 2008, *The Journal of Agricultural and Food Chemistry* explained that phytochemicals in strawberries are powerful anti-inflammatory agents that may work to reduce pain similar to the way ibuprofen and aspirin work — but without the side effects.

✔ **They keep your immune system strong.** Strawberries contain a lot of vitamin C, which strengthens your immune system. Vitamin C also keeps your connective tissue strong for younger-looking skin.

Selecting, storing, and savoring strawberries

These delicious, bright-red berries are available year-round in grocery stores. Look for fresh, plump strawberries in the produce section. Healthy berries should be a rich red in color and firm to the touch, with no sign of mold or spoilage.

Strawberries are also available in the frozen foods section. When you buy frozen strawberries, read the label to be sure the strawberries don't have any added sugar.

Strawberries are easy to grow in your garden, or you can go to a farm that lets you pick your own strawberries. This is a fun family activity and a nice way to spend a beautiful summer morning.

At home, keep the berries in the refrigerator just as they are; wait until you're ready to eat them before you wash them and cut off the stems. Strawberries are quite perishable, so only buy as many as you intend to eat over the course of about three days.

If you have more berries than you can eat in just a few days, you can freeze them by placing them in sturdy plastic containers just as they are. Freezing strawberries reduces the vitamin C content by about one-third. However, the phytochemicals remain intact, so frozen strawberries are still good for you.

When you're ready to use your strawberries, just rinse them under water and remove the stems. Strawberries taste delicious whole or sliced and served in a bowl with a little cream or mixed with whole-grain cereal. They also work well as an ingredient in fruit smoothies. You can make yogurt fruit parfaits by layering yogurt, strawberries, blueberries, and crunchy nuts or granola in tall dessert glasses. Higher-calorie treats include using strawberries as a topping on ice cream and strawberry shortcake.

Another way to use strawberries is to make a simple fruit salad by combining strawberry slices, blueberries, melon chunks, grapes, and pineapple pieces. Strawberries can also be added to a regular garden salad.

For a deliciously decadent (but healthy) superfood treat, try a large strawberry dipped in dark chocolate (see Chapter 9 for more on dark chocolate).

Watch out for strawberry toppings that are mostly sugar or syrup with very few strawberries. Use freshly sliced strawberries to top your desserts.

Chapter 5

Vegging Out in a Good Way

- -

In This Chapter

▶ Unlocking the health benefits of the superfood vegetables

▶ Choosing superfood vegetables

▶ Preparing superfood vegetables

- -

*W*hen you eat a superfoods diet rich in vegetables, you give your body what it needs to stay healthy. Eating lots of vegetables helps to prevent cancer, controls blood pressure, makes weight control much easier, and even keeps your brain healthy. The journal *Neurology* reported in 2006 that diets with lots of vegetables are associated with a slower rate of cognitive decline in the elderly. You should eat at least four servings of vegetables every day.

Are all vegetables good for your health? Absolutely. Some vegetables, such as potatoes and sweet corn, have gotten a bad reputation with the popularity of low-carbohydrate diets, but they really are healthful vegetables when you prepare them in healthful ways. A baked potato with the skin intact is good for you, for example, but French fries aren't. Other healthful vegetables include beans, peas, squash, cauliflower, radishes, and greens. These vegetables are all nutrient-dense, which means they have a lot of nutritional value without a lot of calories. So eating lots of vegetables helps keep you slim.

While all vegetables are good for you, some have added benefits from *phytochemicals* (natural compounds found in plants that can improve health and prevent disease) and high concentrations of vitamins, minerals, and fiber. The ones that have these additional benefits are our superfood vegetables.

Superfood vegetables are richly colored with red, orange, and green hues. The pigments contain phytochemicals called *flavonoids* (powerful antioxidants that fight cell damage in your body).

Choose vegetables of different colors every day to get a variety of phytochemicals that will affect different parts of your body. Dark green and brightly colored vegetables are your best choices.

As this chapter explains, superfood vegetables are easy to incorporate into your diet as snacks, side dishes, soups, and salads. Plus, they're easy to find in your local grocery stores; they store well; and, most important, they taste delicious.

Dipping into Holy Guacamole: The Avocado

Avocados, like tomatoes, are technically a fruit, but they're usually used in cooking as a vegetable. Avocados have a rough, thick, dark skin that has earned them the nickname "alligator pear." But don't let the tough skin fool you — the flesh inside is smooth, soft, and flavorful due to the avocado's fat content. Avocados are rich in monounsaturated fats that help keep your heart healthy.

Avocados are rich in healthy oils and fiber, so we suggest you eat at least one avocado each week.

Making the most of monounsaturated fats

One ounce of avocado (about 2 tablespoons) contains 50 calories and 2 grams of fiber, plus significant amounts of magnesium, potassium, folate, vitamin K, and lutein — quite a lot of nutrition for such a small amount of food.

Avocados have more calories than most vegetables, so you need to watch your serving sizes. One serving of avocado is only about 2 tablespoons.

Avocados help to keep your heart healthy, reduce the symptoms of an enlarged prostate, and increase your absorption of vitamins A, E, and K.

✔ **Protecting your heart:** Avocados contain *oleic acid,* a heart-healthy monounsaturated fat recommended by the American Heart Association. Oleic acid protects your cardiovascular system by reducing your total cholesterol (elevated levels of cholesterol are linked to an increased risk of heart disease) and increasing your HDL cholesterol (the good kind — higher levels of HDL help to protect your heart).

Avocados are also a good source of a plant sterol called *beta-sitosterol.* Sterols are a component of cell membranes in plants, and play a role similar to that of cholesterol in animal cells. Plant sterols are well-known for their ability to lower cholesterol in humans.

The combination of oleic acid, plant sterols, folate, and fiber makes for powerful protection from heart disease.

✔ **Reducing prostate symptoms:** Avocados are rich in beta-sitosterol. *The British Journal of Urology* reported in 2000 that men who were treated with beta-sitosterol had reduced urinary symptoms due to *benign prostatic hyperplasia,* or enlarged prostates. Follow-up studies found that beta-sitosterol therapy was still effective after 18 months.

✔ **Increasing absorption of fat-soluble vitamins:** Eating fat along with foods containing vitamins A, E, and K helps improve the absorption of those vitamins. Adding a little avocado to a garden salad is a great way to boost vitamin absorption while adding extra nutrition.

Adding avocado to your diet

Fresh avocados are found in the produce section of the grocery store. You can't tell much about an avocado by its tough exterior, but you can tell whether it's ripe by gently squeezing. A ripe avocado will yield just slightly to your touch. If it's too soft, you won't be able to slice it, but you can still mash it for use in guacamole or other recipes.

Avocados that are firm to the touch can be ripened at home. Place them in a brown paper bag and keep them at room temperature for up to five days.

Your avocados will ripen faster if you place an apple in the bag. Apples give off ethylene gas that ripens fruits and some vegetables.

Once your avocados are ripe, you can keep them in the refrigerator for two or three days. They don't keep well, so don't buy more avocados than you can use in a couple days.

When you're ready to use an avocado, wash it first to remove any dirt or bacteria. Cut the avocado lengthwise around the large seed. Twist the two halves in opposite directions to separate. Slide a spoon underneath the seed and lift it out. Place the halves cut side down, and peel away the skin. Slice or dice the flesh, and your avocado is ready to go.

You can enjoy avocados on sandwiches, in salads, or as guacamole — a delicious dip made with avocados (see Chapter 19). Add small chunks of avocado to burritos and tacos, too.

Feeling the Beet

Red beets are rich in nutrients and fiber and low in calories, with a deliciously sweet flavor. Beets also contain antioxidants and other healthy phytochemicals. Red beets are often passed over in favor of other, more popular vegetables. That's a real shame, because they're easy to prepare and so good for you. We suggest that you eat beets twice each week.

Beating heart disease, birth defects, and metabolic syndrome

The red pigments in beets contain antioxidants called *betalains* that may help to reduce risk of heart disease and other chronic disease. According to research reported in 2005 in *The Journal of Agricultural and Food Chemistry,* betalains protect your body from oxidative stress damage caused by *free radicals* (particles that occur as by-products from normal metabolism or from exposure to smoke, pollution, or too much sun).

Beets are also rich in a substance called *betaine* that reduces homocysteine levels (elevated homocysteine levels correlate with having a higher risk of cardiovascular disease). Betaine may also aid in digestion and improve your *metabolism,* the rate at which you burn calories.

Eating two cooked beets gives you 40 calories and 2 grams of fiber, plus magnesium, potassium, and folate. Beets are also rich in plant sterols. When you eat beets, you reap the following benefits:

- ✔ **They protect your heart.** The combination of folate, fiber, betaine, and sterols helps to protect your heart by reducing homocysteine levels and keeping cholesterol levels in check. And, according to an article published in 2006 in *The American Journal of Clinical Nutrition,* betalains prevent oxidative damage to blood cholesterol.

- ✔ **They may prevent a birth defect.** Beets are rich in folate. Mothers-to-be who are deficient in folate are more likely to give birth to babies born with *spina bifida,* a defect of the spinal cord and vertebrae.

- ✔ **They fight metabolic syndrome.** *Metabolic syndrome* is a combination of obesity, elevated cholesterol, elevated glucose (blood sugar), and high blood pressure. People with metabolic syndrome have a high risk of cardiovascular disease. According to an article published in 2008 in *The Journal of Nutrition,* research subjects with metabolic syndrome had lower concentrations of betaine in their blood. Beets are rich in betaine.

Choosing and enjoying beets

Look for fresh beets in the produce section of your grocery store. They should be a deep red color with smooth skins. Choose small- to medium-sized beets for the best flavor. Avoid beets that have damage to the skin, such as bruising or spots, and those that appear to be dry and shriveled. Store your beets in the refrigerator for up to two weeks.

You can cook red beets and serve them as a side dish, or you can grate raw beets over salads and soups. To cook beets, first wash the skin gently. Then cut off the greens (you can use them as salad greens), but leave an inch or two of the stem attached to the beets. Don't peel the beets until after they're cooked. Simply boil them until they're tender when you pierce them with a fork.

When you roast vegetables in your oven, add some beets for variety, flavor, and color. You can also purchase heat-and-serve beets in cans or pickled in vinegar.

Eating large quantities of beets may result in pink or reddish-colored urine. Don't be alarmed; this comes from the red pigments in beets and is harmless.

Betting on Broccoli: A Nutritional Powerhouse

Broccoli is a member of the *cruciferous family* (or mustard family) of vegetables that also includes cauliflower, Brussels sprouts, cabbage, bok choy, and kale (another superfood vegetable). Cruciferous vegetables contain several types of natural compounds called *glucosinolates,* phytochemicals that have a positive impact on your health by reducing your risk of cancer. Broccoli is a superfood vegetable because it contains both glucosinolates and large amounts of other nutrients that are crucial for good health.

The dark green pigment of broccoli contains antioxidant phytochemicals along with several vitamins, such as vitamins A, K, and C.

Broccoli is such a nutritional powerhouse that we suggest you eat broccoli (either raw or cooked) four times each week.

Providing a wealth of health benefits

One cup of chopped broccoli gives you a full day's supply of vitamin C, a water-soluble vitamin that your body can't store and therefore needs to replace frequently. Vitamin C keeps your immune system strong so you can fight colds, flu, and infections, plus it protects your skin by keeping the underlying connective tissue strong. Broccoli also contains lots of vitamins A and K, two fat-soluble vitamins that are important for normal vision, healthy cell growth, and normal blood clotting.

Eating broccoli also provides you with calcium, potassium, and magnesium. These minerals keep your bones strong and are necessary for your muscles and nerves to work normally.

Finally, broccoli is a great source of fiber (1 cup contains 3 grams), which is good for your digestive system and cholesterol levels. And because 1 cup contains a mere 30 calories, you can eat large portions of broccoli with no negative impact on your weight.

And as if all these benefits weren't enough, broccoli enhances your health in the following ways, too:

- ✔ **Preventing cancer:** Broccoli has been found to be effective in preventing several types of cancer, including prostate, bladder, colon, breast, and ovarian cancers. In fact, in 1994, *The American Journal of Clinical Nutrition* reported findings that broccoli was the best vegetable for preventing colon cancer.

  According to the American Cancer Society, this anti-cancer action may be attributable to the fact that the phytochemicals in broccoli boost detoxifying enzymes. Researchers also believe that two important glucosinolates found in broccoli — *sulphorophane* and *indole-3-carbonyl* — play a starring role. In particular, indole-3 carbonyl has been shown to prevent breast and ovarian cancers.

- ✔ **Promoting clear vision as you age:** Your eyes contain substantial amounts of lutein and zeaxanthin, two phytochemicals related to vitamin A that are also found in the dark green pigments of broccoli. *Archives of Ophthalmology* reported in 2007 that people who ate diets rich in lutein and zeaxanthin were less likely to suffer from macular degeneration.

- ✔ **Maintaining cardiovascular health:** The effect of lutein on the heart is similar to that of aspirin — without the side effects. The lutein in broccoli acts as an anti-inflammatory agent that reduces plaque in your blood vessels, including the arteries that feed your heart. Plaque build-up leads to *atherosclerosis* (a narrowing of the arteries), reduces blood flow to vital organs, and increases your risk for heart attacks and strokes.

  The folate found in broccoli helps to keep homocysteine levels low (high levels are associated with heart disease), and potassium helps to keep blood pressure normal. As an added benefit, broccoli is low in sodium, an important consideration if you're watching your blood pressure.

- ✔ **Preventing a birth defect:** The risk for spina bifida is higher when mothers-to-be don't get enough folate in their diets, especially during the initial stages of pregnancy. Broccoli, along with other dark green vegetables, is a good source of folate.

Buying, storing, and preparing broccoli

Fresh broccoli is available in the produce department of every grocery store. Look for dark green, tightly packed florets (the darker the green tint, the more phytonutrients it contains). The stem should not be woody and the leaves should not be wilted. You can also buy frozen broccoli, either alone or combined with other vegetables. You can even find broccoli sprouts in some stores.

Some frozen broccoli products include seasonings or sauces. Some sauces are light and healthy, while others are high in calories and sodium, so be sure to read Nutrition Facts labels before you buy.

Broccoli keeps well in the refrigerator. Store broccoli in the vegetable drawer and use it within a few days. Wash the broccoli just before you prepare it. Cut the florets off the stem and break into bite-sized pieces. Slice the stem into similar-sized chunks.

You can eat both the florets and the stem; however, the stems take longer to cook.

Broccoli can be steamed or boiled, but don't overcook it: Florets only need about five minutes. The stems need another minute or two. Broccoli also works well in stir-fry dishes. Add stem pieces to hot oil and stir for one minute before adding the florets, and cook everything for another minute or so. Broccoli is done when it is crisp-tender and very bright green.

Serve crunchy raw broccoli pieces with veggie dip or salad dressing, or add them to garden salads and side dishes. See Chapters 17 and 18 for delicious and healthy broccoli recipes. Use broccoli sprouts in salads or on sandwiches, just as you would use alfalfa sprouts.

Cutting Heart Disease with Carrots

Carrots are delicious any time of the year. Bright orange carrots contain lots of vitamin A, which helps keep your vision healthy, and antioxidants plus phytonutrients that may help to prevent cancer. Carrots are high in fiber and low in calories, so they're good for weight-loss diets. You don't need to be a rabbit to enjoy nibbling on fresh carrots.

Carrots are versatile and very nutritious whether you enjoy them as a raw crunchy snack or cooked as a side dish. We suggest you eat carrots two to three times each week.

Exploiting carotenes and phytochemicals

Carrots have lots of vitamin A, a substantial amount of vitamin C (about 10 percent of what you need for one day), and a lot of beta carotene. One cup of carrots contains 20,381 International Units of vitamin A, which is six times the amount you need for the day! Vitamin A has many health benefits:

- ✔ It sharpens your eyesight because a form of vitamin A called *retinal* is found in the retinas of your eyes.
- ✔ It triggers production of white blood cells that fight infection.
- ✔ It promotes normal cell growth and reproduction.

Vitamin C is important for strong immune system function and strong connective tissue under your skin, which helps to prevent wrinkles. Beta carotene is a powerful antioxidant that protects your cells and keeps you young. Carrots are also a good source of niacin (a B vitamin), potassium, and calcium.

Other benefits you can take advantage of by eating carrots include:

✔ **Preventing certain cancers:** A 2008 article in *Nutrition and Cancer* stated that diets rich in carotenoids (beta carotene, lutein, and zeaxanthin — all related to vitamin A) are associated with a lower risk of cervical cancer in women. Research published in 2005 in *The Journal of Agricultural and Food Chemistry* found that a phytochemical found in carrots called falcarinol prevented cancer in lab rats.

✔ **Preventing diabetes:** Research published in 2008 in the journal *Diabetes Care* confirms that high levels of carotenoids in the blood are associated with a lower risk of diabetes. Eating a healthy diet, watching your weight, and getting the carotenoids found in carrots can help prevent the onset of type II diabetes (which most often occurs in adults).

✔ **Helping you lose weight:** One cup of sliced carrots contains only 50 calories, plus lots of fiber, so eating carrots is a great way to feed your craving for crunchy foods while you're watching your weight.

Finding and preparing carrots

You can find carrots in the fresh produce section, the canned foods section, and the freezer section of the grocery store. You can also find carrots as ingredients in soups, salads, and slaws.

Canned carrots often lack the flavor of fresh or frozen carrots, but they're convenient. Be sure to read the label to avoid excess sodium. As for fresh carrots, choose ones that are bright orange and firm. Avoid fresh carrots that are soft or appear to be shriveled.

Baby carrots are really just grown-up carrots cut into small pieces. To save money, skip the baby carrots and buy full-sized carrots. Wash and slice them and place the pieces into snack-sized plastic bags for a less expensive, but still convenient, snack on the go or as lunch items for work or school. Add a little container of vegetable dip or your favorite salad dressing for extra flavor if you have a refrigerator handy.

Store carrots in the vegetable crisper in your refrigerator. Carrots keep well for about two weeks as long as they're not cut. After they're peeled and cut, they should be eaten within three or four days.

Carrots freeze well, either alone or with other vegetables. The freezer section in your grocery store offers mixed vegetables such as peas and carrots or more exotic blends that include seasonings and sauces (just look out for extra calories and sodium in the sauces).

Add extra chunks of carrots to soups and stews, or grate a carrot on top of a salad. Serve our ginger-glazed carrots (see Chapter 18) as a sweet side dish that even picky eaters will enjoy.

Kicking It Up a Notch with Kale

Kale is a sturdy, leafy green plant related to broccoli, Brussels sprouts, cauliflower, and cabbage. It's rich in vitamins and cancer-preventing phytochemicals called glucosinolates. And because kale is deep green in color, it also contains lutein and zeaxanthin, two more powerful antioxidants that are related to vitamin A.

We recommend that you eat kale two or three times per week, either raw (as a green in salads, for example) or cooked.

Meeting healthy objectives with kale

Kale is very rich in vitamin K and vitamin A (as the precursor of beta carotene, which is also an antioxidant). Vitamin K is important for strong bones and normal blood clotting, and vitamin A is necessary for vision, cell reproduction, and fighting infections. Kale is also a good source of potassium, folate, and magnesium, so kale is good for a healthy heart.

Eating kale plays a positive role in meeting the following objectives:

- **Managing your weight:** Kale is nutrient dense, which means it has lots of nutritional value and is low in calories. Kale has more fiber than other greens, so it keeps you full longer and you're comfortable eating less food.

- **Preventing cancer:** Cruciferous vegetables like kale contain the glucosinolates that help to prevent cancer. *The International Journal of Cancer* reported in 2007 that eating a diet rich in *kaempferol* (one of the glucosinolates found in kale) is associated with a decreased risk of ovarian cancer.

- **Building stronger bones:** The vitamin K in kale helps to regulate *osteocalcin,* a hormone involved in bone formation. Kale also contains magnesium and calcium, although the absorption of the calcium is inhibited by the presence of oxalic acid.

- **Feeling more energetic:** Kale is a good source of iron, which is needed for healthy blood cells that can carry plenty of oxygen and glucose (the fuel your body needs for energy) to all your cells.

- **Waging war against infections:** Kale contains a full day's worth of vitamin C and a lot of beta carotene. These nutrients help your immune system function properly by regulating the white blood cells that fight infections.

✔ **Protecting your eyesight:** Lutein and vitamin C were shown by the Age-Related Eye Disease Study in 2001 to slow down the effects of macular degeneration, the leading cause of blindness in the elderly.

Enjoying kale in the winter — and all year-round

Kale is available year-round in both the produce section and the canned vegetable aisle of your grocery store. Kale is also easy to grow in your own superfoods garden (see Chapter 14).

Look for fresh kale in the produce section near the lettuce and other greens. It should be dark green and fresh looking, with no wilted leaves. Choose kale with smaller leaves — they're tenderer than larger, overgrown leaves. Kale is also available in cans and can be used just like cooked spinach.

Kale is in season during the winter, so it's a good buy during a time when other vegetables are at their highest prices. It's also available just in time for the cold and flu season. Eat lots of this superfood to help keep your immune system healthy and reduce your risk of getting sick.

Store kale in your refrigerator; it doesn't do well in warmer temperatures.

Prepare kale by removing and discarding the tough stems. Just use the tender leaves, tearing them into bite-sized pieces. Kale can be used raw as a salad green, served warm in soups and side dish recipes, or roasted with a little bit of olive oil and a bit of salt for a nutritious, crispy snack. Canned kale can be used just like cooked spinach (see the later section "Selecting and savoring spinach" for more ideas).

Getting Strong with Spinach

Spinach is a leafy green vegetable rich in nutrients, including many important vitamins and minerals, plus fiber. Spinach can be eaten raw or cooked. Either way it's low in calories — 1 cup of raw spinach has just 7 calories, while a cup of cooked spinach has about 32 calories (cooked spinach leaves are denser than raw ones).

The dark green pigments of spinach contain the antioxidants lutein and zeaxanthin, which are good for your heart and your eyes, plus flavonoids called *luteolin* — phytochemicals that have anti-cancer properties, according to research published in 2008 in the journal *Nutrition and Cancer*.

The source of Popeye's strength

E.C. Segar created the comic strip character Popeye in 1929 as a part of Thimble Theatre. Popeye was a sailor who had to regularly depend on his strength to fight the bad guys, especially his arch nemesis, Bluto. What was the source of Popeye's muscular power? Spinach! Before each fight, Popeye gulped down spinach — straight from the can.

Because spinach is so nutritious, we suggest you eat it four times per week.

Bursting with antioxidant protection

Spinach is a good source of vitamins A, E, and K. All the cells in your body need vitamin A to promote reproduction through cell division. Vitamin E may help to prevent some cancers and cardiovascular disease, and vitamin K helps your blood to clot properly. Spinach also provides large amounts of beta carotene. Besides being a raw material for vitamin A production, beta carotene functions as an antioxidant that protects your body's cells.

Spinach is rich in folate, potassium, and magnesium, which are important for your cardiovascular system and for healthy nerves and muscles. Spinach is also an excellent source of vitamin A (as good as carrots) and is a good plant source of iron (perfect for vegetarians).

When you eat spinach, you reap a host of health benefits, including the following:

- ✔ **Keeping cancer at bay:** The journal *Nutrition and Cancer* reported in 2003 that several antioxidant compounds in spinach have anti-inflammatory and anti-cancer properties. A 2004 article in *The Journal of the National Cancer Institute* stated that folate may reduce the risk of ovarian cancer.

- ✔ **Maintaining heart health:** The folate in spinach reduces homocysteine levels that are associated with an elevated risk of cardiovascular disease. The antioxidant lutein has been shown to reduce inflammation and plaque build-up in the arteries. Spinach also improves heart health with an ample amount of potassium while being naturally low in sodium.

  If you have high blood pressure, be sure to choose fresh or frozen spinach to avoid sodium. If you want canned spinach, look for a brand that's low in sodium.

- ✔ **Strengthening bones:** Vitamin K activates the protein osteocalcin that's involved in bone formation. A vitamin K deficiency may lead to weaker bones. Spinach also contains magnesium and calcium, which are also helpful for strong bones. However, the calcium in spinach is not absorbed as easily as calcium in dairy products, due to a substance called *oxalic acid* that's also in spinach.

✔ **Seeing clearly:** Your eyes need vitamin A to function properly because one form of vitamin A, retinal, is an important component of your retina. Lutein, vitamin E, and beta carotene have all been studied for their ability to impair the development of macular degeneration, the leading cause of blindness in the elderly.

✔ **Staying sharp:** The antioxidants found in spinach help to keep your mind sharp. *The Annals of the New York Academy of Sciences* reported in 2007 that diets rich in fruits and vegetables, especially berries and spinach, help to maximize cognitive function long into old age. According to the journal *Clinical Nutrition* in 2008, decreased blood levels of B vitamins, including folate, correlate with a decline in cognitive function.

While folate appears to be important for healthy brain function, folic acid supplements may not do the trick. A 2008 study in *The Journal of the American Medical Association* reported that B vitamin supplementation had no positive effect on slowing the progression of Alzheimer's disease. For optimal brain function, rely on fruits and vegetables rather than folic acid supplements.

✔ **Boosting energy:** Spinach contains iron and folate, both of which are important for preventing anemia. This can be especially important for women who regularly have heavy menstrual periods.

✔ **Preventing spinal cord malformation:** Women who are deficient in folate are much more likely to give birth to babies with spina bifida, which affects the spinal cord and bones.

✔ **Fighting infections:** Vitamin A acts as an immune system regulator by making white blood cells that kill viruses and bacteria. Vitamin E, which is found in spinach, also impacts immune function. *The Journal of the American Medical Association* published a study in 2004 showing that extra vitamin E improved the immune systems of the elderly.

Selecting and savoring spinach

Fresh spinach is available year-round in just about every grocery store, usually right next to the salad greens. In fact, spinach can be substituted for lettuce in many salads to make them healthier and, oftentimes, less expensive, because spinach usually costs less than the upscale greens. Choose fresh spinach that is dark green in color and looks fresh — not wilted.

Frozen and canned spinach are also available. Canned spinach usually contains added sodium, so if you're on a sodium-restricted diet, be sure to read the labels to find brands with little or no sodium added.

Irradiation of spinach and other greens

Several breakouts of food-borne illness from spinach contaminated with E. coli bacteria have resulted in a decision by the United States Food and Drug Administration to allow irradiation of spinach leaves and other greens before they are shipped to grocery stores. The irradiation does not harm the spinach, but it kills bacteria and other organisms responsible for the outbreaks of food-borne illness.

Store unwashed spinach in your refrigerator until you want to use it — washing the leaves beforehand causes them to deteriorate. Rinse the leaves with cold water thoroughly to remove dirt and bugs. For convenience, you can purchase pre-washed spinach in bags; however, you may still want to give these spinach leaves a good rinse before eating them.

Serve fresh spinach salad with a little bit of olive oil to improve the absorption of vitamin A and lutein. Fresh spinach leaves can also replace lettuce on sandwiches for an easy nutritional boost.

Both frozen and canned spinach are good in recipes that call for cooked spinach (see Chapters 16 and 18 for spinach recipes), or you can just heat and serve for a simple side dish.

You can add spinach to pasta sauce or use it as a pizza topping. Spinach can also be incorporated into mashed potato recipes (delicious when you also add some parmesan cheese and garlic) or added to stuffing. Make breakfast healthier by using spinach in your omelets and quiches.

The Fruit that Eats Like a Vegetable: The Tomato

Tomatoes contain several vitamins, and the beautiful red coloring holds phytochemicals that support your heart, immune system, and vision and may prevent cancer. You may have expected to see tomatoes included in Chapter 4 on superfood fruits. Technically, tomatoes are fruits, but in most culinary circles, tomatoes are treated as vegetables, so we include them with the superfood vegetables. But there's no controversy about the health benefits of tomatoes; in fact, we think you should eat one serving of tomatoes four or five days each week.

From poison to superfood

North Americans generally believed that tomatoes were poisonous until 1820. Colonel Robert Gibbon Johnson ate a tomato on the courthouse steps in Salem, New Jersey, and proved to onlookers that tomatoes were safe to eat.

Today, according to California Tomato Growers, every American eats about 80 pounds of tomatoes per year, and it is one of the most common vegetables grown in home gardens.

Loving the perks of lycopene and more

Tomatoes offer vitamins A and C, plus lutein, zeaxanthin, and lots of lycopene (a carotene that's closely related to vitamin A and beta carotene), while being very low in calories. According to an article published in 2000 in *The Canadian Medical Association Journal,* lycopene is linked to having a lower risk of cardiovascular disease and a variety of cancers.

Lycopene is activated by heat and processing, so when you eat tomato juice, spaghetti sauce, or even ketchup, you actually get more lycopene than you would from a fresh tomato.

Tomatoes are also rich in potassium and very low in sodium, so they can be part of a healthy diet to reduce high blood pressure (just watch out for high-sodium sauces and tomato soups).

We suggest that you eat tomatoes (or tomato products) five times each week to cash in on the following benefits:

- ✔ **Keeping your eyes healthy:** Vitamin A, lutein, and zeaxanthin are important for healthy vision. Research published in *The British Journal of Nutrition* in 2009 reported that those antioxidants, plus lycopene, may help to reduce the risk of retinopathy (disease of the retina inside the eye) in diabetics.

- ✔ **Protecting your heart:** In *The Canadian Medical Association Journal* in 2008, researchers stated that diets rich in tomato and tomato products reduce the risk of cardiovascular diseases, with the credit again going to lycopene. The other antioxidants in tomatoes help combat inflammation and plaque build-up in your arteries.

- ✔ **Reducing your risk of cancer:** According to the same article, eating tomatoes is associated with a reduced risk of several cancers, including prostate, breast, and digestive tract cancers. The researchers believe lycopene prevents cancer by protecting the DNA in cells.

✔ **Boosting your immune system (and feeling better when you have a cold):** Vitamins A and C boost your immune system, and in 2008, *The Journal of Nutritional Biochemistry* reported that lycopene helps to reduce inflammation in your airways caused by cold viruses. Eating tomatoes may help to reduce some of your suffering when you catch a cold.

Tempting your taste buds with tomatoes: Selecting, storing, and serving tips

Fresh tomatoes come in a variety of shapes and sizes and are available year-round in the produce section of your grocery store, but there is a definite difference in flavor. The vine-ripened tomatoes of summer are much more flavorful than tomatoes that are harvested while immature and artificially ripened.

Take advantage of farmers' markets during the summer months, where you'll find juicy, vine-ripened tomatoes (along with other fresh vegetables).

Choose fresh tomatoes that are a deep red in color, firm, and heavy. Avoid tomatoes with bruised skins and those that feel too squishy.

Store your fresh tomatoes, just as they are, at room temperature. Refrigerated tomatoes lose their flavor.

When you're ready to enjoy a tomato, simply rinse the skin, remove the stem, and slice or chop the tomato. Some people prefer to remove the seedy part and serve just the flesh.

For soups and sauces, you need to remove the skin first. Simply slice a small X through the skin in the bottom of your tomato, and then place it in simmering water for a minute or two until the skin starts to break away from the tomato. Remove the tomato from the hot water, chill in cold water, and slide the skin right off.

Tomatoes are also sold in cans as tomato sauce, tomato pieces, or stewed whole tomatoes. Canned tomatoes are great for soups, stews, and sauces because they're ready to use — you don't have to remove the skins. If you're watching your sodium intake, look for low-sodium varieties of canned tomatoes, soups, and sauces.

Getting tomatoes into your diet is easy. Sliced tomatoes are perfect for sandwiches. Smaller pieces of tomatoes are perfect for a salad, or you can pop a few cherry tomatoes in your mouth as a quick snack.

Make an aromatic and simple salad by alternating tomato slices with thinly sliced mozzarella cheese on a plate. Garnish with fresh basil leaves — whole or roughly chopped. Drizzle olive oil over the top, and add salt and pepper.

Other ideas for tomatoes include topping a baked potato with salsa, and adding slices of sun-dried tomatoes to your favorite vegetables. Broil thick tomato slices with a little bit of parmesan cheese, garlic, and bread crumbs. See Chapters 17 and 18 for some great recipe ideas for tomatoes.

Chapter 6

Gathering Nuts and Seeds

. . . .

. . . .

During the autumn months, you may notice that squirrels are busy gathering nuts and seeds to store for the long winter ahead. That's because nuts are both nutritious and packed with energy. Nuts and seeds are rich in healthful fats and phytochemicals, plus lots of vitamins and minerals. It makes a lot of sense if you think about it. Nuts and seeds (actually, nuts are really seeds, too) contain enough energy and nutrients to feed a sprouting tree.

Nuts and seeds are very healthful, but they're often high in calories, so if you're watching your weight, you'll want to watch your serving sizes. Luckily, you can get a lot of nutrition from eating even a small amount of nuts. If you're trying to gain weight, eating nuts and seeds is a healthful way to add extra calories. They're quite delicious and can be added to any meal or eaten alone as a healthful snack.

In this chapter, we discuss our super nuts and seeds, how they work to keep you healthy, how many you should eat, and how often you should eat them.

The fats in nuts and seeds are sensitive to oxygen and go rancid if they aren't stored properly. Nuts in the shell can be stored in a cool area and don't need any care beyond that (the thick shells provide a natural oxygen barrier that protects the fats from going rancid). Nuts and seeds that have been shelled and packaged in cans, jars, or bags can be stored in your pantry, but after you open the package, the nuts and seeds need to be stored in airtight containers in your refrigerator. Nuts that need to be stored for more than a few months can be frozen.

Steer clear of shelled nuts that are sold in bulk bins; they're exposed to air and may not be as fresh as packaged nuts or nuts still in the shells. Unless you know when they were added to the bulk bin, you have no way of knowing how fresh bulk nuts really are.

Adding Almonds to Your Diet

Almonds are crunchy, delicious, and very good for you. They're rich in fiber, monounsaturated fats, and phytochemicals that fight free radicals to keep the cells in your body healthy.

Almonds also contain *polyphenols* (phytonutrients that provide health benefits) — especially in the thin brown skin that covers the nut. According to an article published in 2008 in *The Journal of Food Science,* roasting almonds with the skin intact actually concentrates the amount of polyphenols.

The almonds you buy in the grocery store are sometimes called sweet almonds. Bitter almonds are processed and used to make pure almond extracts and liqueurs. Raw bitter almonds are actually toxic, but fortunately, the sale of raw bitter almonds is prohibited in the United States.

We suggest you eat 1 ounce of our superfood nuts every day, such as one serving of almonds (up to 23 nuts).

Filling up on fiber, healthful fats, and antioxidants

Almonds weigh in at 165 calories per ounce. They contain vitamin E and substantial amounts of magnesium, manganese, and copper. Magnesium is involved in many of the biochemical reactions that take place in your body. Manganese is an antioxidant and is necessary for healing wounds and keeping bones strong. Copper is essential for the formation of healthy blood cells. In addition to all this, almonds offer the following health benefits:

- **Lowering cholesterol:** Almonds are rich in *phytosterols* (a plant version of cholesterol that's good for you) that help regulate cholesterol levels in your body. Phytosterols and monounsaturated fats are particularly beneficial when they replace saturated fat, which increases cholesterol. Vitamin E, magnesium, and polyphenols also may increase the heart-healthy effects of eating almonds.

- **Preventing anemia:** Almonds supply copper, which is necessary for normal red blood cell production. Copper and manganese also work as enzymes in some of the chemical reactions in your body that produce energy.

- **Easing weight loss:** Although almonds have a lot of calories, according to *The British Journal of Nutrition* in 2006, substituting monounsaturated fats for saturated fats (found in red meats) may help to increase weight loss, even if you don't cut many calories. Almonds also help keep you full between meals because they're rich in proteins and fiber.

✔ **Protecting your prostate:** According to research published in 2000 in the journal *BJU International, beta-sitosterol,* a phytosterol found in almonds, is effective for decreasing the symptoms of benign prostatic hyperplasia (BPH) in men. BPH is a common condition where the prostate gland enlarges, resulting in difficulty in urination and sexual performance.

✔ **Preventing diabetes:** Research published in 2006 in *The Journal of Nutrition* states that almonds slow down the rises in blood sugar that occur after eating carbohydrate-rich meals. The polyphenols and vitamin E in almonds also help to protect you from damaging free radicals.

Buying and enjoying almonds

Almonds are easy to find in any grocery store. The best almonds are still in the shells, which protect the delicate fats inside the nuts. Look for almonds with shells that are unbroken and free of mold. Use a nutcracker to open them — you may make a little mess with the broken shells, but freshly shelled almonds are quite a treat (and the added effort of cracking the shell makes for automatic portion control, because you can't eat them by the handful).

While fresh almonds are best, they aren't very convenient for cooking. For this purpose, you can find sealed packages of shelled, blanched almonds in the baking section of your grocery store.

You can buy whole blanched almonds and chop them up in a coffee grinder to retain the polyphenol-rich skin. Alternatively, you can buy sliced or slivered almonds (they lose the skins, but they still retain the good fats).

You can find roasted almonds in bags or cans in the snack section of the grocery store. Be careful with these almonds, because they're usually roasted in unhealthy oils and contain extra salt and artificial flavorings (as is the case with smoked almonds) that may not be good for you.

Store shelled almonds in a covered container in the refrigerator to protect the healthful fats. If you have a large amount (more than you can eat in a week), keep some in the freezer.

You can enjoy a handful of almonds as a protein- and fiber-rich afternoon snack (both protein and fiber will keep you feeling full until dinnertime). Or you can add them to many of your favorite dishes for extra crunch. Almonds have a delicious flavor that works well with savory foods as well as sweet foods.

Here are some delicious ideas for eating almonds:

✔ Enjoy almond butter in place of peanut butter on your sandwiches.

✔ Eat a handful of almonds with an apple for a superfoods snack.

> ✔ Sprinkle sliced almonds on a salad or on vegetables.
>
> ✔ Make a yogurt and berry parfait and top it with chopped almonds.
>
> ✔ Sprinkle slivered almonds over trout.

You can use raw almonds or toast them briefly before adding them to recipes. Toasting (or roasting) almonds is best done just before eating. Toasting almonds is easy and augments the flavor. Place a nonstick skillet over medium heat and add sliced or slivered almonds. Stir frequently until they're golden brown, about three to five minutes. You can also toast almonds by baking them in an oven heated to 350 degrees Fahrenheit for about 15 minutes.

Getting Antioxidants with Brazil Nuts

Brazil nuts are rich in antioxidants and minerals that serve a wide variety of functions, such as the formation of thyroid hormones and immune system function, plus they give you protein and fiber. As with most nuts, eating Brazil nuts adds a balance of energy and nutrients to your superfoods diet. We suggest you eat six Brazil nuts twice a week.

Souping up your diet with selenium

Brazil nuts are rich in minerals, especially selenium, which works as an antioxidant to protect the cells in your body and is needed for normal thyroid function (your thyroid works like a thermostat in your body to regulate energy use). Brazil nuts contain other minerals along with the selenium. They're rich in magnesium, which is used in many chemical reactions in your body and is needed (along with calcium) for normal muscle and nerve function. Brazil nuts also contain calcium, potassium, zinc, and copper. As an added bonus, Brazil nuts are a good source of vitamin E, a natural antioxidant that protects your heart.

Nut butters

Everyone's familiar with peanut butter (who doesn't love a PB and J sandwich?), but there are several nut and seed butters that can be fun to try for a little variety. Popular nut butters include almond butter, cashew butter, sunflower seed butter, and pumpkin seed butter. They aren't always easy to find at the local grocery store, but you can find them in online stores (see Chapter 13 for tips on online shopping). They're usually minimally processed and quite delicious.

Look to Brazil nuts to provide the following benefits:

- **Immune system support:** Selenium and zinc are important for fighting bacterial and viral infections. Selenium also protects cells, which may slow down diseases such as HIV/AIDs, according to a 2007 article in the journal *Medical Hypotheses*.

- **Cancer prevention:** Research published in 2007 in the journal *BioFactors* explains how selenium may prevent cancer by protecting normal, healthy cells and by slowing down the growth of cancerous cells.

- **Heart protection:** Brazil nuts contain lots of the monounsaturated fats that are also found in olive oil. The combination of these healthful fats and antioxidants helps to protect your heart and blood vessels, especially when you substitute Brazil nuts for foods high in saturated fats, such as red meat.

Breaking Brazil nuts

Brazil nuts are protected by a hard, thick shell. You can buy Brazil nuts with these shells intact in the produce section of your local grocery store. They're also available already shelled and chopped in the baking goods section. They can be eaten as a snack or used in recipes.

Make the shells easier to crack by plunging whole Brazil nuts into boiling water for three minutes. Remove and let cool before cracking.

Brazil nuts are commonly found in packages of mixed nuts, along with cashews, almonds, and peanuts; however, they're usually heavily salted and roasted in oil that adds extra calories from unhealthy fats. As an alternative, you can make your own mixed nuts by roasting coarsely chopped Brazil nuts, almonds, and walnuts at home.

Toast Brazil nuts in a sauté pan over medium heat for three to five minutes. They're quite big, so you may want to chop them into ¼-inch-long pieces first.

Brazil nuts can be used in many interesting ways. Here are some ideas:

- Replace the meat in stir-fry recipes with chopped Brazil nuts.

- Add some variety to pesto recipes by using Brazil nuts in place of pine nuts or walnuts (see Chapter 17).

- Sprinkle chopped Brazil nuts on a green salad or on top of your favorite green vegetable.

- Stir chopped Brazil nuts into wild rice or rice pilaf.

- Mix chopped Brazil nuts into stuffing and dressing.

Loading Up on Lignins and More with Flax Seeds

These small seeds are powerful because they're rich in omega-3 fatty acids and phytochemicals called *lignins* (a type of polyphenol). Lignins are antioxidants that protect the cells in your body. Flax seeds also pack a powerful punch of fiber.

Flax seeds also add fiber, B vitamins, magnesium, and manganese, all of which are important for many different chemical reactions that occur in your body, to your daily superfoods diet.

We suggest you eat milled flax seeds every day. Start with 1 tablespoon and work your way up to 2 tablespoons, which you can eat all at once or throughout the day.

Reaping the rewards of fiber and (good) fats

One tablespoon of ground flax seeds contains 2 grams of fiber and 37 calories. Whole flax seeds contain soluble and insoluble fiber. Soluble fiber dissolves in water (similar to the fiber in fruits) and helps regulate blood sugar and eliminates extra cholesterol. Insoluble fiber does not dissolve in water, but it adds bulk to the intestinal contents and helps to keep your digestive system regular.

The oil in flax contains large amounts of alpha-linolenic acid (ALA), which is converted to eicosapentaenoic acid (EPA) and docosahexaenoic acid (DHA), just like the fats in fish. Omega-3 fatty acids are good for your cardiovascular system and your bones, and eating them helps you lose weight. Flax seeds' many other health benefits include the following:

✓ **Protecting your heart:** The fiber and healthful fats in flax seeds reduce cholesterol levels and inflammation in your blood vessels, both of which are risk factors for cardiovascular disease. Research published in 2008 in *The Journal of American College of Nutrition* found that flax seeds also lower the levels of lipoproteins (complexes of fats and proteins — increased levels of certain lipoproteins correlate with an increased risk of cardiovascular disease).

✓ **Reducing inflammation:** The fats and the phytochemicals in flax seeds work together to reduce inflammation in the body. According to the journal *Nutrition, Metabolism, and Cardiovascular Disease*, research in

2008 in Denmark found that eating muffins made with the addition of flax seed lignins called *secoisolariciresinol diglucoside* lowered C-Reactive Protein (CRP) levels in the study subjects. CRP is a blood test that measures inflammation in the body that may be caused by rheumatoid arthritis or other disorders such as cardiovascular disease, diabetes, and some cancers.

✔ **Improving digestive function:** The fiber in flax helps to keep your bowel movements regular.

✔ **Maintaining strong bones:** Omega-3 fatty acids help to maintain strong bones by reducing the amount of calcium that is lost from the bones, according to 2001 research published in The Journal of Nutrition.

✔ **Preventing cancer:** According to *The International Journal of Cancer* in 2005, the lignans in flax inhibit the growth of cancer cells in the lab. A study published in the journal *Urology* found that men who ate diets rich in flax seed tended to have a lower risk of prostate cancer.

✔ **Easing symptoms of BPH:** The hormonal effect of the lignins helps to reduce urinary symptoms of benign prostatic hyperplasia (BPH), according to research published in *The Journal of Medicinal Foods.*

✔ **Eliminating the discomfort of dry eyes:** *The American Journal of Clinical Nutrition* reports that increasing dietary levels of omega-3 fatty acids reduced the incidence of dry eyes in participants of the Women's Health Study (a large study involving more than 3,500 female health professionals).

✔ **Keeping blood sugar levels normal:** Chinese-American research found taking flax lignins daily helped improve blood sugar levels in patients with type 2 diabetes. The soluble fiber also helps to regulate blood sugar.

Grinding for good health

You can buy flax seeds or flaxseed oil (or both, if you'd like). You'll get the most health benefits from whole flax seeds that you grind in your kitchen (just a few seconds in a coffee grinder will do) just before you eat them. If you eat the seeds whole, you won't get as much of the fatty acids as grinding them provides. You can also buy milled flax seeds that have already been ground — just be sure they're in airtight packaging.

Flaxseed oil contains the omega-3 fatty acids, but it doesn't contain the lignins or the fiber. Only buy flaxseed oil that's sold in opaque bottles that have been kept in the refrigerator case to keep the delicate oils from spoiling.

While it's okay to add milled flax seeds to recipes for baked goods, don't use flaxseed oil as cooking oil. It doesn't handle heat well at all and is best added to foods that have already been cooked.

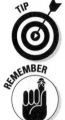

If you want more omega-3 fatty acids in your cooking oil, use canola oil instead of vegetable oil. Canola oil is rich in monounsaturated fats (like those found in olive oil), so it is much better suited for cooking than flaxseed oil.

Milled flax seeds and flaxseed oil lose their healthful properties more quickly than whole flax seeds, so if you buy oil or milled seeds, buy them in small amounts and keep them refrigerated.

Flax seeds have a nice nutty flavor, so you can sprinkle them on other foods or just take a spoonful or two every day like a dietary supplement. This works just fine; however, taking large amounts (more than 2 tablespoons) at one time may lead to some temporary digestive discomfort. Some tips for getting your daily flax:

- Sprinkle ground flax seeds on your morning oatmeal for a healthful superfoods breakfast.
- Add ground flax seeds to muffin, waffle, or pancake recipes (see Chapter 16 for our superfood versions of these recipes).
- Top your salad or soup with ground flax seeds, or add them to your favorite vegetable side dishes.
- Stir ground flax seeds into some plain yogurt sweetened with a little honey.
- Add some fiber to your smoothies with ground flax seeds.

You can also use flaxseed oil to increase your intake of omega-3 fatty acids every day. Take it by the spoonful (1 or 2 teaspoons per day) or add the oil to foods:

- Drizzle flaxseed oil on pancakes, waffles, or toast at breakfast.
- Pour a teaspoon of the oil on cooked vegetables.
- Make a salad dressing by blending 1 cup flaxseed oil, $1/2$ cup balsamic vinegar, and 1 teaspoon mustard.
- Add flaxseed oil to pasta, potatoes, or rice dishes.

Discovering the Perks of Pecans

Pecans are another nut rich in monounsaturated fats, which lower LDL cholesterol (the bad cholesterol). They contain other nutrients and phytochemicals that improve your health as well.

We suggest you eat 1 ounce of pecans (about 19 nuts) at least once a week as one of your daily servings of nuts.

Helping the heart and more

With a calorie count of 196, 1 ounce of pecans (about 19 halves) offers 2.7 grams of fiber, plus a healthy dose of minerals and vitamins. Pecans contain magnesium and manganese, two important minerals in many bodily chemical reactions. Pecans are a good source of potassium, which helps keep your heart healthy and your blood pressure in check. You get a good dose of zinc from pecans too, which your body needs to have a strong immune system. Zinc is also an important component of male health.

There are plenty of vitamins in pecans, like vitamin E, an antioxidant that protects the cells in your body, and B vitamins: niacin, pantothenic acid, and thiamin. B vitamins are necessary for your body to produce energy from the foods you eat.

Adding pecans to your superfoods diet gives you a lot of bang for the buck, including

- ✔ **Keeping your heart healthy:** Pecans are rich in oleic acid, the monounsaturated fat found in olive oil (see Chapter 9). Monounsaturated fats help to reduce cholesterol and improve heart health, especially when they're eaten in place of saturated fats.

  Research published in 2001 in *The Journal of Nutrition* showed that eating pecans in place of other foods effectively lowered total cholesterol, LDL cholesterol (the bad stuff), and triglycerides (another type of blood fat that, when elevated, raises your risk for heart disease), without adding any additional weight.

- ✔ **Improving prostate health:** Pecans are rich in beta-sitosterol, a phytosterol that has been studied for prostate health. Beta-sitosterol effectively decreases the symptoms of benign prostatic hyperplasia (BPH) in men, as reported in the journal *BJU International* in 2000. BPH is a common condition that results in difficulties in urination and sexual performance.

- ✔ **Losing extra fat:** According to *The Asia-Pacific Journal of Public Health* in 2003, diets rich in monounsaturated fats resulted in weight loss even though study participants weren't required to count any calories. Although pecans are high in calories, they also contain a lot of fiber and protein that help you feel full much longer than many other foods.

- ✔ **Fighting cancer:** Oleic acid, the monounsaturated fat found in pecans, has been shown to inhibit breast cancer cells in the lab, according to 2005 research in the journal *Annals of Oncology*. The journal *Nutrition and Cancer* published research in 1999 that showed diets rich in nuts, such as pecans, were associated with a reduced risk of prostate cancer.

Preparing pecans

Pecans that are still in the shell are available in the produce section of your local grocery store. The shells should be smooth and light brown in color, with no evidence of holes, cracks or breaks, or mold growth.

Shelled pecans are sold in the baked goods section of the grocery store or in the bulk foods area. They look a little like walnuts but have a brown skin similar to almonds. Shelled pecans are more convenient than unshelled pecans for cooking. You can choose from whole pecans, pecan halves, or chopped pieces.

Pecans make great snacks when you crack them open with a nutcracker, or you can just munch on a handful of shelled pecan halves.

Pecans are often included in commercial packages of mixed nuts. Unfortunately, mixed nuts contain lots of salt and the nuts are roasted in unhealthy oils that add extra calories.

Toasting pecans enhances their flavor. Simply place one layer of pecans in a skillet or sauté pan over medium heat. Stir frequently and toast for about three to five minutes. Serve as a warm snack or add to your favorite recipes.

Pecans work well as an ingredient in sweet or savory dishes. You'll frequently find pecans in delicious and healthy recipes (sorry, pecan pie doesn't count). Check out our Spinach Quiche with Pecans in Chapter 16. Pecans make a great addition to many foods:

- ✔ Sauté broccoli, green beans, or asparagus with pecans in a little olive oil for a deliciously healthful side dish.

- ✔ Add chopped pecans to muffin recipes.

- ✔ Combine chopped pecans and bread crumbs to coat fish or skinless chicken breasts. Sauté until fish or chicken is cooked thoroughly.

- ✔ Add pecans to chicken or tuna salads.

- ✔ Mix chopped pecans into your morning oatmeal (see Chapter 16 for our Banana Cream Oatmeal recipe).

- ✔ Toast pecans and add them to your own granola mix (see our recipe in Chapter 16).

Getting Seeds from the Great Pumpkin

If you've ever carved a jack-o-lantern, you've seen raw pumpkin seeds covered in pumpkin pulp. They don't look so great covered in all those "pumpkin guts," but those seeds are actually very good for your health. They contain lots of nutrients and healthful fats. We suggest you eat pumpkin seeds two or three times each week.

Relieving anxiety while promoting good health

Pumpkin seeds contain the healthful omega-3 fatty acid, alpha-linolenic acid, which works as an anti-inflammatory agent. The seeds are also very rich in phytosterols, the plant version of cholesterol.

Pumpkin seeds contain a large amount of magnesium, which you need for normal nerve and muscle function and many chemical reactions in your body. Pumpkin seeds are a good source of iron and B vitamins, which your body needs for energy, and potassium, which helps protect your heart and regulates blood pressure.

One ounce of pumpkin seeds contains 148 calories. The payback comes in the following forms:

✔ **Lowering cholesterol:** According to *The Journal of Agricultural and Food Chemistry* in 2005, pumpkin seeds are rich in phytosterols that help to reduce cholesterol. The omega-3 fatty acids in pumpkin seeds also help to reduce inflammation and decrease the risk of cardiovascular disease.

✔ **Avoiding bladder stones:** Research from Thailand found that eating pumpkin seeds reduced the risk of bladder stones (small masses of minerals that form in the urinary bladder). This benefit was attributed to the high levels of phosphorus in the seeds.

✔ **Treating anxiety:** Pumpkin seeds are rich in tryptophan, an amino acid that's important for the production of brain chemicals that affect your mood. *The Canadian Journal of Physiology and Pharmacology* reported on a small study in 2007 that discovered that tryptophan in seeds helped to relieve symptoms of social anxiety disorder. Tryptophan is also used as a sleep aid.

✔ **Protecting your prostate:** Eating pumpkin seeds may help to reduce the risk of benign prostatic hyperplasia. According to research published in 2006 in *The Journal of Medicinal Foods,* pumpkin seed oil reduces prostate hyperplasia in rats by inhibiting testosterone.

Picking pumpkin seeds

Pumpkin seeds are available in the snack section of the grocery store; however, most are roasted in oils that add extra fat and calories. Look instead for pumpkin seeds in the baking area of your grocery store. Or, for a fun project, toast your own pumpkin seeds at home — a great thing to do after carving those Halloween pumpkins.

Cut open a pumpkin and remove the pulp and seeds. Clean the pulp from the seeds and soak them in water overnight. Some people, especially those who have a hard time digesting raw nuts and seeds, find they can enjoy these foods more often if they're soaked and roasted or dehydrated. But if you don't have any digestive issues with seeds, or if you don't have the time or inclination to soak the seeds overnight, you can skip that step. Spread the seeds on a paper towel to dry, then spread them on a cookie sheet, drizzle with olive oil, and add a few sprinkles of salt. Roast in an oven heated to 325 degrees Fahrenheit for 20 to 25 minutes, stirring occasionally, until the seeds are golden brown.

Pumpkin seeds can also be roasted in your microwave. Spread the seeds on a glass tray, place it in the microwave, and cook on high for seven minutes or until seeds are light golden brown.

For variety, sprinkle curry powder or any other seasoned powder on the pumpkin seeds before roasting.

Keep the pumpkin seeds in an airtight container. Munch on the seeds as a healthful snack or add them to vegetables, salads, or your own granola (see Chapter 16 for a granola recipe). You can also buy dark red pumpkin seed oil, which is delicious drizzled over salads or vegetables.

Cracking Wonderful Walnuts

Humans have been eating walnuts for thousands of years. And for good reason — walnuts help keep your heart healthy. They're rich in vitamins, minerals, fiber, and ALA — the plant version of omega-3 fatty acids.

Almost all walnuts found in grocery stores are English walnuts (although they probably originated in Persia). They're delicious as a snack or as an addition to main dishes, sides, and salads.

Black walnuts are native to North America and are edible; however, they have a very thick, tough shell. In fact, a typical nutcracker won't break them open. You can find shelled black walnuts online or in some specialty stores.

We suggest you eat 1 ounce of walnuts every day; that's about 14 halves.

Providing marvelous melatonin and more

Walnuts are one of the few foods rich in melatonin, a hormone that protects the cells in your body. As you age, your body makes less melatonin and you lose some of that protection. Melatonin also helps you have normal sleep cycles, which are often disturbed as the body's natural levels of melatonin fall with age.

Along with melatonin, walnuts have several antioxidants like vitamin E and polyphenols. A Norwegian study published in 2006 in *The American Journal of Clinical Nutrition* ranked walnuts very high on a list of foods with the highest amounts of antioxidants per servings; they came in second only to blackberries.

Walnuts contain healthful monounsaturated fats and omega-3 fatty acids, which are necessary for normal nervous system and brain function, plus they function as anti-inflammatory agents. While the omega-3 fatty acids aren't exactly the same as those found in fish and seafood, your body can convert a lot of the ALA to the two forms found in fish: EPA and DHA.

You also get plenty of protein and fiber from walnuts. One ounce of walnuts (about 14 halves) contains 4 grams of protein and 2 grams of fiber. Walnuts also have magnesium, potassium, and plant sterols like beta-sitosterol. Magnesium is needed for many chemical reactions in your body, plus normal muscle and nerve function. Potassium helps keep your blood pressure normal. Plant sterols reduce cholesterol and promote prostate health.

And if all that's not enough, you can count on walnuts to provide the following benefits, too:

- **Keeping arteries healthy:** The journal *Circulation* published studies in 2004 that found that people who ate walnuts showed improved blood vessel function. That same study showed that eating walnuts also reduces total cholesterol and LDL cholesterol (the bad kind). Lowering cholesterol helps to protect your heart.

- **Strengthening bones:** *The Nutrition Journal* reported in 2007 that diets rich in plant-based omega-3 fatty acids reduce bone loss. The magnesium in walnuts also helps to keep bones strong.

- **Making weight loss easier:** Although they're energy-dense and contain about 185 calories per ounce, research published in *The British Journal of Nutrition* indicated in 2005 that adding walnuts to diets did not contribute to weight gain. The protein and fiber in walnuts make for a very satisfying superfood that can help keep you going until the next meal.

- **Helping diabetics:** Research published in *Diabetes Care* showed in 2004 that eating walnuts helped improve the cholesterol levels of patients with type 2 diabetes. This is important because people with type 2 diabetes are at a higher risk for cardiovascular disease.

- **Staying youthful:** The melatonin and other antioxidants in walnuts have strong anti-aging properties because they protect your cells from damage.

Selecting and enjoying walnuts

You may find walnuts in the shell in the produce section of your local grocery store. Walnuts in the shell are easy to find in the fall, but you may have a tougher time finding them the rest of the year. Look for walnuts that feel heavy and aren't cracked or broken, and be sure they show no signs of mold growth.

Shelled walnuts are sold in bags containing walnut halves or chopped walnut pieces. Walnuts don't have a skin like almonds, so you can go with either halves or pieces without sacrificing nutrition. They're usually located in the baking goods section of the grocery store, but you may also find them near the fresh produce.

Walnuts make a great snack with a piece of fresh fruit. Use a nutcracker to crack open the shells of fresh walnuts. Here are some other ideas for enjoying walnuts as part of a superfoods diet:

✔ Add walnuts to a bowl of fresh berries.

✔ Top a green salad with $1/4$ cup of walnut pieces.

✔ Make your own granola with walnuts, whole-grain cereals, and dried fruits.

✔ Sauté chopped walnuts in a little olive oil and substitute them for meats in pasta dishes or on pizzas.

To bring out the flavor in walnuts, toast halves or pieces in a dry, nonstick skillet over medium heat for 4 to 5 minutes, stirring constantly.

Getting the goodness every day

We recommend you eat 1 ounce of nuts every day and either a spoonful or two of flax seeds or 1 ounce of pumpkin seeds every day. Here's a sample of how to get the proper amount of nuts and seeds each week:

✔ **Sunday:** Add 1 tablespoon of flax seeds to your morning smoothie, and top your lunchtime salad with 1 ounce of walnuts.

✔ **Monday:** Munch on 1 ounce of pumpkin seeds for a midmorning snack, and have six Brazil nuts after dinner.

✔ **Tuesday:** Stir 1 tablespoon of flax seeds into a serving of yogurt, and serve your green beans with 1 ounce roasted almonds per serving at dinnertime.

✔ **Wednesday:** Spread 1 tablespoon of flaxseed oil on your toast in the morning, and enjoy 19 toasted pecans with fresh apple slices, whole-grain crackers, and your favorite cheese for a light evening meal.

✔ **Thursday:** Chop 1 ounce of walnuts and add to a bowl of oatmeal in the morning, and top a bowl of fresh berries with light whipped topping, 1 tablespoon flax seeds, and six chopped Brazil nuts for a snack or dessert.

✔ **Friday:** Enjoy 23 almonds as a midmorning snack, and drizzle 1 tablespoon of flaxseed oil over your vegetables at dinner.

✔ **Saturday:** Chop 19 pecans into small pieces and add them to a lunchtime pizza topped with spinach and tomatoes, and make a simple salad dressing with flaxseed oil and balsamic vinegar.

Chapter 7

Angling for Super Seafood

. . . .

In This Chapter

▶ Understanding why fish is so good for you

▶ Deciphering worries about mercury

▶ Exploring the wonders of salmon, tuna, sardines, and trout

. . . .

*S*eafood makes a delicious and healthy addition to a superfoods diet, and our four superfood fish — salmon, tuna, sardines, and trout — make the best choices. So, what qualifies these fish as superfoods? Although fish don't contain phytochemicals or fiber like plant-based foods, they do contain several vital nutrients.

An even bigger benefit is their fat content, particularly a type of fat called *omega-3 fatty acids*, which are lacking in many people's diets. The fish that live in cold water have the highest amounts of omega-3 fats per serving.

Many experts suggest that eating fish every week (or taking omega-3 fatty acid supplements daily) is a great idea to keep your heart healthy. But eating fish does a lot more than that. In this chapter, we tell you what makes fish so good for you, outline the health benefits of omega-3 fatty acids in fish, and help you figure out how to choose fish at the grocery store or on a restaurant menu.

Catching On to the Benefits of Superfood Fish

When you replace high-fat red meats with baked, grilled, or broiled fish at least twice a week, you do your heart — and the rest of your body — a healthy favor. There are so many reasons to enjoy fish in your superfoods diet that we encourage you to eat at least 12 ounces of low-mercury superfood fish each week. If fish isn't your thing, or if you're worried about being exposed to mercury, never fear: Taking omega-3 fatty acids as dietary supplements (2,500 milligrams of fish oil) is also acceptable, as we explain in the following sections.

Keep fish healthy by preparing it right. Baked, broiled, grilled, or pan-fried fish are best. Stay away from heavy, creamy sauces that add extra calories and unhealthy fats. And stay away from deep-fried fish, too. Fish is healthy; fish sticks are not.

Enjoying the mega-boost of omega-3 fatty acids

Superfood fish offer many advantages, including high levels of omega-3 fatty acids. *Omega-3 fatty acids* (also known as *linolenic acid*) are one type of *polyunsaturated fatty acid* (polyunsaturated refers to the chemical structure — it means there is more than one double bond in the fatty acid molecule). Fish and seafood are rich in a form of linolenic acid that's made up of two different fatty acids called *eicosapentaenoic acid* (EPA) and *docosahexaenoic acid* (DHA).

There's another type of polyunsaturated fatty acid called *omega-6 fatty acid,* found mainly in vegetable oils (like corn oil and safflower oil). Both omega-3 and omega-6 are considered essential because you have to get them from your diet; your body can't manufacture them.

Even though most people know that both of these fats are important, many experts agree that few people eat these two fats in the proper balance. Generally, most people eat too many omega-6 fatty acids and not enough omega-3 fatty acids. This imbalance of fatty acids leads to your body being in a *pro-inflammatory state,* whereby your body is more prone to develop inflammation that can lead to chronic disease and pain.

The average person's diet has a 15 to 1 ratio of omega-6 to omega-3 — or worse. No one knows what the optimal ratio should be, but many experts think it should be closer to 4 to 1 — that is, no more than 4 times as many omega-6 fatty acids as omega-3s. Omega-3 fatty acids are found in some plant foods such as flax seeds, chia seeds, pumpkin seeds, soy, canola oil, and walnuts, but the best source of these fats is fish and seafood.

Omega-3 fatty acids fight inflammation, but they do so much more. They're particularly important for brain development and cognitive function, plus they may be important for eye health. Omega-3 fats also protect your heart by keeping your blood vessels healthy, lowering your cholesterol, and, in some cases, regulating the rhythm of your heartbeats.

Pumping up your brain

Omega-3 fatty acids, especially DHA, are crucial for the formation of the brain during the last trimester of pregnancy and the first three months of infancy.

Studies published in 1994 in the *European Journal of Clinical Nutrition* showed that premature infants who were fed DHA-enriched formulas had better cognitive function. Many more studies have confirmed the importance of DHA for brain development. A study published in 2008 in the *Journal of Child Development* showed that children born from mothers with higher levels of DHA had better cognitive function. Although the exact amount needed for pregnant women has not been established, a common recommendation is 250 mg of DHA daily.

Of course, infants can't eat fish, but pregnant and breast-feeding mothers can get ample amounts of DHA in their diets eating safe fish and dietary supplements. The FDA states that salmon and light pink canned tuna are safe, along with shrimp and Pollack. (Unfortunately, pregnant women also have to be concerned with potential mercury toxicity in fish. See the section "A few words on mercury," later in this chapter.)

Omega-3 fatty acids are also important for keeping your brain healthy as you age. *The Journal of Clinical Nutrition* reported in 2007 that elderly men who ate diets high in fish had better brain function than those who did not.

Helping your heart

Eating fish high in omega-3 fatty acids helps keep your heart healthy in several ways. The omega-3 fatty acids help normalize cholesterol levels and lower triglycerides. Both cholesterol and triglycerides are fats found in the blood; high levels of either fat are related to a higher risk of cardiovascular disease.

Omega-3 fatty acids are valuable for the rhythm of heartbeats. *The American Journal of Clinical Nutrition* reported in 2000 that omega-3 fatty acids may help to prevent *arrhythmias* (irregular heartbeats) and that fish should be included in the diet in order to help prevent deaths from heart disease.

Opting for plant-based omega-3 fatty acids

If you don't want to eat fish or seafood, you can get omega-3 fatty acids from some plant foods, such as walnuts, pumpkin seeds, and flax seeds in a form called alpha linolenic acid (ALA). Your body can use EPA and DHA just as they are; however, your body needs to make some changes in the ALA to convert it to the EPA or DHA forms. Most of the time, that works just fine. However, if you need larger amounts (if you want to reduce cholesterol or inflammation, for example, or if you're a breast-feeding mother), your body may not be able to make enough EPA and DHA from the ALA. In this case, your best choice is to take mercury-free fish oil or algal oil (from ocean algae) capsules.

An article in *Cardiovascular Research* in 2003 explained how fish oil improved the health of blood vessels. The authors contend that adding two or three servings of fish to your diet each week may be beneficial for having strong blood vessels. When your blood vessels are healthy, you're less likely to have heart disease or suffer a stroke.

The American Heart Association suggests that everyone eat fish (preferably oily fish) at least twice a week to help prevent heart disease. The AHA also suggests that people who already have heart disease or elevated triglycerides take extra fish oil in the form of dietary supplementation.

Easing pain and inflammation

The omega-3 fatty acids found in fish act as natural anti-inflammatory agents. The journal *Rheumatology* reported in 2008 that omega-3 fatty acids from cod liver oil work as an effective pain reliever in patients with rheumatoid arthritis. Patients who took cod liver oil were able to use fewer non-steroidal anti-inflammatory drugs.

Omega-3 fatty acids may also help to reduce the suffering of dry eye syndrome. A study reported in 2007 in the journal *BMC Ophthalmology* found that omega-3 supplements improved the visual acuity in patients who have *macular degeneration* (a common complication of diabetes and the leading cause of blindness in the elderly).

Discovering what else fish has to offer

In general, fish is a good source of several nutrients, including the following:

- **Magnesium** is crucial for many chemical reactions in your body and helping your muscles and nervous system to function properly.

- **Selenium** is an antioxidant mineral that helps protect the cells in your body from damaging free radicals. It's also important for healthy sperm counts in men.

- **Many of the B vitamins** have a variety of roles in your body, including the breakdown of carbohydrates into glucose (the fuel your body needs), the breakdown of fats and proteins (for more energy and for building body tissues), the production of red blood cells, and normal nervous system function.

- **Potassium** helps control your blood pressure.

- **Calcium** is important for strong bones and teeth, as well as normal muscle and nerve function.

- **Iron** is needed for healthy blood.

- **Zinc** is involved in thousands of processes in your body, such as wound healing, immune function, and protein synthesis.

Fish is also a terrific source of protein. It's a complete source of protein, containing all the essential amino acids. A 3-ounce serving of fish has between 15 and 20 grams of protein, depending on the type of fish you're eating. Fish can be especially beneficial for those watching their weight, because it's not only high in protein but also low in fat.

Fish provides your body with so-called "good" fats while being very low in artery-clogging saturated fats. That makes fish an excellent main course for a heart-healthy meal.

A few words on mercury

Methyl mercury is a toxic metal that has polluted our waters across the globe. The fish and seafood that live in the water are exposed to that mercury, and when you eat mercury-contaminated fish, your body, in turn, is exposed to this metal.

While your body can detoxify and eliminate a small amount of mercury, if you get too much, you can become quite sick with central nervous system disorders. Mercury may have an even stronger negative effect on the cognitive development of babies.

So, this could pose a problem. Fish is a very healthy food with all the nutrients and omega-3 fatty acids it has to offer, but methyl mercury contamination is bad. What to do?

You have a few options:

- ✔ You can skip the fish and eat plants that have omega-3 fatty acids, like flax or chia seeds.
- ✔ You can take omega-3 fatty acid supplements that are mercury-free.
- ✔ You can eat fish that's considered to be low in mercury, such as salmon, sardines, trout, and tuna (our superfood fish).

Which fish should you avoid? Older, larger fish like shark, swordfish, and king mackerel tend to have the highest levels of mercury, according to the U.S. Food and Drug Administration.

If you want more omega-3s for therapeutic reasons, you can take omega-3 supplements, but be sure to speak to your doctor before you start gulping down mega-doses (more than 2,500 milligrams a day) of fish oil. This is especially important if you're taking certain medications such as blood-thinners: The combination of blood thinners and high doses of omega-3 fatty acids may increase your risk of bleeding.

Choosing wild or farmed fish

The fresh or frozen fish you buy in the grocery store or at a restaurant may be wild or farm-raised. Are there any differences? Some experts believe the fat content of farmed fish isn't as healthy as the fat content in wild-caught fish.

The American Dietetic Association sponsored a study on the omega-3 levels in several farm-raised fish and found that farm-raised salmon and trout had healthy levels of omega-3 fatty acids, but that farm-raised tilapia and catfish had less omega-3 fats in contrast to higher levels of omega-6 fats. This ratio of higher omega-6 fats is considered by many experts to be pro-inflammatory.

This study suggests that at least two of our superfood selections — salmon and trout — are good for you whether they're farm-raised or wild-caught. Typically, farm-raised fish are less expensive, and it isn't clear that higher-priced wild-caught fish are worth the extra cost — at least as far as the fat content is concerned.

Seeing What Salmon Has to Offer

Salmon is a very richly flavored fish found in cold ocean waters. It has the highest levels of omega-3 fatty acids of commercially available fish. The fat content makes it pretty easy to cook because, unlike some other types of fish, salmon is less likely to become dry if you overcook it.

Getting the lowdown on nutrition

Salmon is a good source of healthful protein, vitamins, and minerals. A 6-ounce salmon fillet has 240 calories and favorable amounts of these important nutrients:

- **Magnesium** helps regulate muscle contractions and can also help relax the muscles within artery walls. This makes magnesium important in reducing migraines and blood pressure. Magnesium is also necessary for the absorption of calcium.

- **Potassium** is important for regulating the electrolytes in your body and the movement of water inside the cells. It helps the heart beat regularly and it supports the nervous system.

- **Selenium** is a trace mineral needed only in small amounts to produce healthy benefits. Selenium binds with protein to become an antioxidant and can help reduce the risk of diseases such as cancer.

✔ **B vitamins** consist of eight individual vitamins that are important for many functions of the body, including your immune system, metabolism, and cognition.

✔ **Omega-3 fats** help reduce inflammation in muscles, which is good for athletes, and they also help reduce inflammation associated with heart disease. Omega-3 fats reduce the levels of bad cholesterol and can help lower blood pressure.

Serving up salmon

Buying and preparing salmon is a cinch. Fresh salmon may be available at your local grocery store, or you may find frozen salmon fillets, smoked salmon, or canned salmon chunks — they're all good for you. Salmon is also commonly found on the menus of many restaurants if you'd rather order it ready-made. In fact, salmon could easily be the healthiest choice on the menu because it's usually baked, grilled, or broiled and served with vegetables and salad. Compare that to a typical plate of white fish (like cod or haddock) that's often deep-fried and served with French fries. With so many great salmon options, you may have to sample each one to see which is your salmon of choice.

About 90 percent of North American salmon comes from Alaska. Varieties of salmon found in the Pacific Ocean include the Chinook or King salmon, the Coho or Silver salmon, and the Sockeye or Red salmon. The one variety of salmon found in the Atlantic Ocean is the Atlantic salmon, which is mostly farm-raised rather than wild-caught. Any variety is a good addition to your superfoods diet, so choose the one with the taste and texture you like best.

When you decide to buy fresh salmon, first check out the food safety practices of the store. The seafood area should be clean and have the aroma of fresh fish. The fish should be on ice, preferably under a cover.

If you're looking at a fillet, it should be pinkish in color with no milky fluids. The skin should be fresh and shiny and the fillet should smell fresh, without a strong fishy odor. The flesh should be firm, not mushy.

Fresh salmon lasts in the refrigerator for 48 hours, so it must be eaten or stored securely in a freezer-safe bag or container within that time period. Salmon fillets can be frozen; however, they should be cooked and eaten within three months.

If you're shopping for the whole fish, the eyes should be clear, the skin should be shiny, and the gills should be bright red. Older fish have cloudy eyes and brownish-red gills. As with fillets, don't buy a fish that has a strong fishy odor.

Salmon fillets can be grilled, broiled, poached, seared in a pan, or baked in the oven. Whole salmon can be grilled or baked in the oven. Many recipes are available for salmon: We offer two recipes for baked salmon in Chapter 17.

Salmon cooks quickly. Broil it about 10 minutes per each inch of thickness, or bake fillets at 350 degrees Fahrenheit for about 20 minutes.

Canned salmon is convenient and ready to use for sandwiches, salads, and recipes for dishes like salmon cakes (see our recipe in Chapter 19). Canned salmon may also include skin and soft bones that you eat right along with the flesh.

Salmon is often smoked and served with crackers as an appetizer, on bagels with cream cheese, or combined with cream cheese and lemon juice.

Making the Most of Super Sardines

The word *sardine* refers to any of a variety of species of small oily fish, including herring, pilchard, and sprats. These small fish are found in both the Atlantic and Pacific oceans and in both northern and southern hemispheres.

Sardines have edible bones that you may often find packed into flat cans. If you're fortunate enough to have a fish market close by, you may be able to find fresh sardines. Either way, sardines are very rich in omega-3 fatty acids and other nutrients, which make them a superfood fish.

Packing a big nutritional punch

For being small fish, sardines really pack a nutritional punch. Three ounces of sardines contain about 175 calories and are a rich source of

- **Calcium:** The most abundant mineral in the body, calcium is mostly stored in the bones and teeth. About 1 percent of calcium circulates around the body and is very important for muscle and blood vessel contractions. Calcium is important for bones because if there isn't enough calcium in the blood, the body takes it from the bones, making them weak and susceptible to a disease called *osteoporosis*.

- **Iron:** The most important function of iron is the transportation of oxygen throughout the body. Iron is a component of *hemoglobin*, which is the oxygen-carrying protein in the red blood cell.

> ✔ **Zinc:** Most commonly associated with strengthening the immune system, zinc is also important for many other functions, such as wound healing and the development of taste and smell.

> ✔ **Omega-3 fatty acids:** These good fats can help reduce inflammation and improve cholesterol levels in the body.

Enjoying sardines — really

Fresh sardines may be difficult to find, but if you have a local fish market, you may want to buy some. Don't buy more than what you need for a meal, though, because fresh sardines don't last long, and they don't freeze well, either.

Canned sardines are much more convenient and widely available. When you open the tin, you'll find that the heads, gills, and internal organs have been removed. They're usually packed in olive oil or water.

A popular way to serve sardines is to grill them and serve them on toast. Sardines can also be served cold with your favorite seasonings, a drizzle of olive oil, and a sprinkle of lemon juice.

Need more calcium and you don't drink milk? Sardines are packed with calcium as well as other minerals that help keep your bones strong and healthy.

Paying Tribute to Trout

Trout are related to salmon, so they have lots of omega-3 fats, but they have a much milder flavor. Trout is the perfect choice for people who don't like the strong flavor of oily fish like salmon and sardines.

Trout can be found in both fresh water and salt water. There are several varieties, with the rainbow trout being the best known. Other varieties include spotted trout, brown trout, and silver trout. Like other fish, trout varieties vary in terms of the taste, texture, and color of the meat, so you should give them all a try.

Tapping into the benefits of trout

This is one fish that definitely deserves to be called super. One 6-ounce trout fillet has 200 calories and serves as a good source of the following:

- **Omega-3 fatty acids** keep the heart healthy by reducing the amount of triglycerides and bad cholesterol (LDL) in the blood. They can also help reduce the amount of inflammation in the body, which is good for preventing many diseases.

- **Calcium** helps reduce the risk of thinning of the bones called *osteoporosis*. Calcium is also important for the contraction of muscles, including the heart.

- **Magnesium** can help regulate muscle contractions and is very valuable in reducing blood pressure and helping people who suffer from migraines.

- **B vitamins** are used for several functions of the body, such as regulating hormones and stabilizing blood sugar.

- **Selenium** is a great antioxidant, helping to prevent the inflammation that can lead to cancer and other diseases.

Buying and preparing trout

When you buy whole trout, look for fish that are clean and have bright eyes, bright red gills, and no fishy odor. Trout fillets should have a firm texture that springs back when pressed lightly with your finger, and the fish should have a fresh aroma.

Fresh raw trout can be refrigerated for a day or two or frozen for up to one month; however, it's best to cook your fish right away.

Trout may be cooked as the whole fish, or in fillets with the skin intact — you don't need to remove scales. Trout is typically prepared by pan-frying, poaching, grilling, steaming, or baking in an oven, usually with a little butter and lemon. Turn to Chapter 17 to see our recipe for Trout Almandine.

Trout is best cooked at high temperatures, and it cooks very quickly — often in as little as 3 minutes on each side when grilled or fried. It's done when the flesh flakes easily. Take care not to overcook it.

Trout has a delicate flavor that can be altered by the fat used for cooking. If you pan-fry your trout, use a lightly flavored fat such as butter or peanut oil.

Opening a Can of Tempting Tuna

Tuna is an oily ocean fish that offers omega-3 fatty acids. It has a milder flavor than salmon, and it has been the most popular canned fish in the United States for many years.

Not only is tuna tasty and convenient, it's also good for your health because it contains those omega-3 fats. Plus, tuna is a healthy source of protein and several vitamins and minerals.

Varieties of tuna include two dark red-fleshed tuna: bluefin, which is highly prized in Japan for sashimi, and yellowfin, which is less expensive but almost as tasty as bluefin. Skipjack tuna is the variety that you usually find in cans. It has the strongest flavor and the highest fat content. Albacore tuna has the mildest flavor — perfect for people who don't care for the heavier taste of many oily fish — but albacore also has been found to have higher mercury levels than the other tunas.

Combining vitamins, minerals, and healthy fats

A typical can of light tuna chunks packed in water has about 200 calories and contains valuable amounts of the following nutrients:

- ✔ **Magnesium** can regulate muscle contractions, help relax muscles of the heart and blood vessels, and improve heart disease.

- ✔ **Selenium** is a powerful antioxidant that helps heal damaged cells, thereby preventing the development of many chronic diseases.

- ✔ **Vitamin B3 (niacin)** is very effective at increasing the levels of HDLs, or good cholesterol, in the blood. It also supports the conversion of carbohydrates into sugar, which is then used for energy.

- ✔ **Vitamin B12** is important for maintaining the cells of the nervous system. It has been found to be helpful for treating and preventing nerve-related diseases such as Alzheimer's and Parkinson's.

- ✔ **Omega-3 fats** increase good cholesterol and are a great natural anti-inflammatory for the body.

Tuna, like other fish, is also a healthy source of protein, which your body needs for building muscles and organs. The minerals and B vitamins help various bodily systems function properly.

Choose low-sodium varieties of canned tuna if you need to watch your sodium intake. Fresh tuna steaks are not a significant source of sodium.

Bringing tuna to your table

Canned tuna is easy to find at your grocery store, where you'll probably have a choice between light tuna or white tuna (albacore). Albacore is firmer and has a deliciously mild flavor compared to regular tuna.

Tuna displaces sardines as favorite fish

Sardines were the canned fish of choice until 1903, when Albert Halfill packed his empty sardine cans with albacore, which was thought of as a nuisance fish. Today, Americans enjoy more than one billion pounds of canned or pouched tuna every year.

Check your cans of tuna to see whether they wear the "dolphin-free" label. This voluntary label means that observers on the fishing vessels have ensured that no dolphins were killed or seriously injured during the tuna fishing season.

You can choose tuna packed in water or oil. We prefer tuna packed in water because the oil adds extra calories with no particular benefit. Low-sodium varieties are also available, and at least one brand offers flavorful yellowfin tuna in a can. Some brands offer tuna in pouches that are more convenient (and less messy) than canned tuna. (They also tend to be significantly more expensive, however.)

Fresh or frozen tuna steaks are available in many grocery stores, too. When you choose fresh tuna steaks, look for flesh that's deep red in color, with a fresh aroma and firm texture. Fresh tuna steaks will keep in the refrigerator for a day or two, but they're best when cooked the same day that they're purchased.

Canned tuna is commonly used in sandwiches, salads, and casseroles. It's delightful for use in sandwich wraps with dark greens, tomatoes, sprouts, and a little light dressing. In a salad, tuna adds healthy fats and protein and turns a simple salad into a meal. Check out our recipe for tuna wraps in Chapter 17 and a salad recipe incorporating beans and soy in Chapter 18.

Raw tuna is popular in sushi and sashimi. Sushi-grade tuna is frozen almost as soon as it's caught, so it retains its firm texture and fresh flavor.

The best methods for cooking tuna steaks are grilling or broiling, usually to a medium rare to medium temperature of 125 to 140 degrees Fahrenheit.

However you choose to enjoy tuna, just remember that the healthiest recipes don't drench the tuna in mayonnaise or heavy sauces. Keep it light.

Don't care for salmon? Tuna can be substituted for salmon in most recipes.

Chapter 8

Going with the Grains and Legumes

*H*umans have been eating grains for thousands of years. They're easy to cultivate, transport, and store, plus they're rich in nutrients and fiber that nourish the human body. It's no coincidence that civilization began to flourish when humans learned how to grow grains. The most common grain is wheat, which is ground into flour and used in everything from bread and pasta to cookies and cakes.

Legumes include peas, peanuts, lentils, and dry beans. They're high in protein, fiber, and phytochemicals, so they make a terrific substitute for red meats, which are high in saturated fats that can raise your cholesterol and increase inflammation.

While grains (especially whole grains) and legumes are good for you, a few in particular are super. In this chapter, we tell you about the superfood grains and legumes you need for your superfoods diet.

Packing in the Protein: Dry Beans

Dry beans are a staple food that has been traced back through different civilizations. So what exactly are dry beans? They're the group of legumes like pinto beans, black beans, and navy beans that come in a variety of colors and flavors, and they're all superfoods. They have an amazing amount of fiber and protein, which is linked to improved health and reduced risk of several diseases.

The most popular dried beans are kidney, black, navy, pinto, and lima beans. According to the Unites States Department of Agriculture, red kidney beans are rated the highest in antioxidant function, even above blueberries. Pound for pound, dried beans give you filling, healthy meal options for an unbelievably low price. The fact that dried beans as a group makes our superfood list is a major statement about how nutritious this food group really is. We suggest you eat dry beans three times each week.

Getting super healthy with super beans

The health benefits of dry beans are about the same across the board. In addition to about 14 to 16 grams of protein and 10 to 15 grams of fiber, 1 cup of cooked beans contains substantial amounts of magnesium, potassium, iron, folate, and vitamin K, and about 200 to 250 calories.

When you add dry beans to your superfoods diet, you improve your health by

- **Keeping your heart healthy.** Dry beans are a great source of soluble fiber that helps to lower cholesterol and the associated risk of cholesterol plaque in your arteries.

- **Stabilizing blood sugar.** The fiber in dry beans helps keep your blood sugar from rising after a meal, which makes beans a great option for diabetics. Beans stabilize blood sugar by slowing the absorption and digestion of carbohydrates.

- **Reducing the risk of cancer.** Studies have shown that women who eat more beans have a reduced risk of breast cancer. A study by researchers with the National Cancer Institute found that eating significant amounts of dry beans reduced recurrence of colon polyps and the overall risk of colon cancer.

- **Healing your digestive system.** Dry beans are a great source of insoluble fiber. The insoluble fiber reduces the risk of bowel disease and acts as a bulking agent to help prevent constipation and regulate bowel movements.

  While you can't digest the fiber in dry beans, the friendly bacteria that live in your intestinal tract can. As a by-product, the bacteria produce short chain fatty acids that help to heal the walls of your digestive system, and, according to the *Journal of Nutrition* in 2001, reduce the risk of colon cancer.

Selecting and preparing dry beans

Look for dry beans in the grocery store near the rice or canned vegetables. Dehydrated dry beans are available in bags or in the bulk area. Hydrated dry beans are also available near the canned vegetables and the "pork and beans."

If you're getting your beans in bulk, check out the bins and make sure there's no moisture in the containers and there aren't any obvious foreign objects or broken beans mixed in.

When you get the beans home, package them in bags or airtight containers and store them in a dry area at room temperature. You don't want to keep them in the refrigerator or any damp area that might allow the beans to absorb water. If the beans get moist, they'll spoil quickly.

When you're ready to prepare the beans, place them in a colander and look for any debris. After going through the beans and getting rid of any abnormal-looking ones or other non-edible substances, rinse them well to remove any dust.

Many people soak dry beans in water to reduce cooking time, but it isn't an essential step. Soaking the beans causes them to expand to two to three times their original dry size. You can soak beans overnight (or at least six to eight hours) by keeping them in room-temperature water. You can also quick-soak beans by boiling them in water for two to three minutes. Remove the beans from the heat and keep them covered for about one hour.

Cooking beans is easy. Add your dry beans (soaked or not) to a large pot and cover them with at least 2 to 3 inches of water. Cook the beans for one to three hours until tender. (Soaked beans take less than two hours to fully cook.) After cooking, they're ready to serve as a side dish, or you can place them in the refrigerator to use later as an ingredient in another dish or to top a salad.

Canned beans are easy to use. Simply rinse the beans thoroughly in a colander and heat them or add them to recipes.

Children occasionally sing about the connection between eating legumes and suffering from *flatulence* (intestinal gas). That's because dry beans contain fiber that your body can't digest, but the friendly bacteria that live in your colon can. The bacteria produce gas as a by-product. You don't want to avoid legumes, though, because the advantages definitely outweigh the disadvantages.

Loving Life with Luscious Lentils

Lentils are legumes that come in an assortment of colors, like red, yellow, and black. Lentils are easier to prepare than other legumes, and they're very inexpensive. They're a staple food in many countries, especially India. Fat-free, filling, and affordable, lentils make a great superfood option for everyone.

We suggest you add them to your regular rotation of superfoods by eating them twice each week.

Looking at what lentils have to offer

All colors of lentils provide you with fiber, protein, and folate, with almost no fat. Lentils are about 25 percent protein, and are second only to soybeans for the highest protein count in the legume family. One cup of cooked lentils packs 18 grams of protein.

A cup of cooked lentils contains 226 calories and a whopping 16 grams of fiber to keep you feeling full and satisfied between meals. A serving of lentils also gives you 90 percent of the daily recommended amount of the B vitamin folate and is a good source of iron, which you need to get oxygen to all the cells in your body.

When you eat lentils, you improve your health by

- **Taking care of your heart.** Lentils have a lot of fiber. Fiber binds to cholesterol and removes it from the body in the stool. This not only reduces cholesterol levels but also decreases the risk of cholesterol plaques in your arteries.

  Lentils are also an excellent source of folate, which has been shown to reduce homocysteine levels (elevated homocysteine levels are associated with an increased risk of cardiovascular disease).

- **Preventing a birth defect.** Pregnant women who are deficient in the B vitamin folate are more likely to have babies with a birth defect of the spine and spinal cord called *spina bifida*. Lentils contain a large amount of folate.

- **Weighing less.** Lentils are a good source of complex carbohydrates, fiber, and protein that are digested slowly and keep you feeling full between meals. The combination of protein and fiber also helps to keep your blood sugar at a healthy level. This makes lentils a great carbohydrate option for diabetics or those with signs of insulin resistance (which often leads to diabetes).

- **Reducing the risk of cancer.** According to studies based on the 1989 Nurses' Health Study II (which included more than 90,000 women), women who ate more legumes such as lentils had a 24 percent reduced risk of breast cancer.

✔ **Keeping your digestive system regular.** Lentils contain a large amount of both insoluble and soluble fiber. Insoluble fiber allows the stool to absorb water. The insoluble fiber reduces the risk of bowel disease and acts as a bulking agent to help prevent constipation.

Selecting and preparing lentils

You'll find lentils in your grocery store. They come in several colors:

✔ **Black** lentils may also be called "Beluga Lentils." They have a shiny black appearance when they're cooked.

✔ **White** lentils are simply black lentils that have been cooked and had the skins removed, revealing the white legume with a firm texture.

✔ **Brown** lentils are also known as "Egyptian Lentils." They're the most popular variety and have the shortest cooking time.

✔ **Green** lentils are named "French Lentils" or "Continental Lentils." They're the largest and most expensive lentils, and are often used to top salads because they stay firmer when cooked.

✔ **Yellow** lentils are gold before cooking and turning a lighter yellow. They have a short cooking time.

✔ **Red** lentils have a sweeter flavor than other lentils and also take longer to cook.

Lentils are usually packaged in a dry form that stores very well — up to 12 months. You can also buy canned lentils, but rinse them to remove some of the excess salt, which isn't good for your blood pressure and your heart.

Unlike dry beans, lentils don't have to be soaked before you cook them. Add 1 cup of lentils to 3 cups of boiling water and cook, covered, for 20 to 30 minutes. The longer you cook them, the softer they become. Firmer lentils can be added to salads; softer lentils work best as a side dish.

Lentils can be served on salads, as a side dish, or as an ingredient in soups and stews. Try our Tomato and Lentil Stew in Chapter 17.

Starting the Day with Wholesome Oatmeal

Whole-grain oatmeal has warmed many bellies at breakfast, which may be the most important meal of the day. Whole grains (with the bran and husk intact) are high in fiber, so they're digested more slowly than foods made up of mostly simple carbohydrates (sugars). Whole-grain fiber helps stabilize blood sugar and gives you sustained energy.

Oatmeal may be one of the oldest — and smartest — choices for a breakfast food. In fact, a Tufts University study found that children who ate oatmeal for breakfast scored higher on cognitive tests than kids who ate other breakfast cereals.

Oats have some super benefits to get you ready for the day. They're packed with fiber and other nutrients that are important for your health. We suggest you eat oats at least two times per week.

Good carbs versus bad carbs

Grains and legumes are both rich in carbohydrates, which have gotten a bad rap over the last decade or so with the popularity of low-carb diets. That's unfortunate, because your body needs carbohydrates for energy — you just need to pick the good carbs and avoid the bad ones. So what's the difference?

All carbohydrates are made up of chains of sugar molecules known as *glucose, fructose*, and *galactose.* Simple carbohydrates like table sugar, high fructose corn syrup, and honey contain small chains of sugar — just two molecules long. Each one is a combination of fructose and glucose. It's very easy for your digestive system to break these molecules apart, so you absorb them rapidly, which raises your blood sugar levels after you eat meals high in these ingredients. Your body deals with the excess sugar by making insulin, which helps to remove the extra sugar from your blood and converts it to fat that's stored somewhere on your body — usually your belly, butt, and thighs. Sugars like this are considered "bad" carbs because they add calories, but no other nutritional value. Plus, higher insulin levels in the blood are associated with obesity and an increased risk of cardiovascular disease.

This doesn't mean simple carbohydrates are always bad, though. Fruit is very healthful even though it contains fructose, because it's also high in vitamins, minerals, phytochemicals, and fiber. The fiber in fruit helps to slow down the digestion and absorption of the sugars it contains. Fruit and fruit juices are good carbs.

Complex carbohydrates are made up of longer chains of sugar molecules. Starch and cellulose are two types of complex carbohydrates found in the plant foods you eat. Your body digests starch a little more slowly than simple sugars, but it doesn't digest cellulose at all. Cellulose is a main component of dietary fiber, so when starch and fiber are found in the same food, it takes longer for your body to digest and absorb the starch. This is good because now your body has a more sustained source of energy rather than the flood of sugar that rushes into the blood when you eat simple carbs. Complex carbohydrates combined with fiber are good carbs. Good carb sources include vegetables, whole grains, and legumes.

The difference between good carbs and bad carbs is big enough that the World Health Organization recognizes overconsumption of refined sugars as the leading factor driving the obesity epidemic around the world. So, although carbohydrates are important, try to get most of your daily consumption of carbohydrates from healthful food sources.

Exploring the proven benefits of oats

One cup of cooked oats contains 6 grams of protein, 4 grams of fiber, and 166 calories. The type of fiber oatmeal contains, *beta-glucan,* seems to be more effective than other types of fiber for lowering cholesterol.

Oats also contain polyphenols called *avenanthramides*, which, according to an article published in 2004 in the *Journal of Nutrition*, help reduce your risk of cardiovascular disease. These polyphenols fight inflammation and work with vitamin C to keep your blood fats at healthy levels.

Last but not least, oats are a good source of minerals like magnesium, manganese, zinc, and selenium. These minerals are important for several chemical reactions that take place in your body, plus selenium is a powerful antioxidant. Oats also contain lutein, a phytochemical related to vitamin A that's important for normal vision.

When you eat oats, you improve your health by

- **Lowering cholesterol.** The beta-glucan helps lower levels of LDL, the bad cholesterol. Normally, your body excretes cholesterol into your digestive system and reabsorbs it to be used again. When you eat oatmeal, the beta-glucan fiber binds with cholesterol in the intestinal tract and prevents it from being reabsorbed, thus lowering the cholesterol levels in your body. The bound cholesterol is simply eliminated through the stool.

  A large study published in 1993 in the *Archives of Internal Medicine* found that people who ate the most fiber every day had the greatest reductions in cholesterol, which also lowered their risk for cardiovascular problems.

- **Decreasing cardiovascular disease.** A study published in 2004 in the *Archives of Internal Medicine* showed that men who ate one bowl of oatmeal a day reduced their risk of heart failure by 29 percent. Other studies have also indicated the reduction of high blood pressure with regular intake of oats.

- **Strengthening your immune system.** According to research published in 2004 in the journal *Surgery,* beta-glucan helps your white blood cells recognize and fight bacterial infection quickly.

- **Stabilizing blood sugar.** The fiber in oats slows down the absorption and metabolism of sugar, which reduces the need for insulin. Eating oatmeal may help diabetics reduce their blood sugar. The American Diabetes Association recommends you eat 20 to 35 grams of fiber every day. If you have diabetes, be sure to speak with your doctor about incorporating oatmeal into your diet.

To make your oatmeal even healthier, add a tablespoon of chia seeds or flax seeds to increase your fiber and add some healthy omega-3 fatty acids. This combination is even more effective in lowering cholesterol and improving heart health than oatmeal alone.

Buying and eating oatmeal

Oatmeal is made by removing the outer husk of oat grains while leaving the bran and germ intact, so the oats are still whole grains. The husked oats are known as groats and are minimally processed into the forms you see in the grocery store. You can choose from the following varieties:

- ✔ **Steel-cut oats or Irish oats** are chopped into small pieces by sharp steel blades. Steel-cut oats have a chewy texture and require a longer cooking time compared to rolled, quick, or instant oats.

- ✔ **Rolled oats or old-fashioned oats** are steamed and rolled into flattened flakes. They have a creamy texture and require less cooking time than steel-cut oats.

- ✔ **Quick oats** are processed in the same manner as rolled oats, but are rolled until they're even thinner, so they require even less cooking time.

- ✔ **Instant oats** are precooked and rolled very thin so that they only need to be mixed with a hot liquid. They're very convenient and are usually flavored with berries, syrup, brown sugar, and spices.

Read the labels if you buy instant oatmeal. Many brands of instant oatmeal contain excess sugar that you don't need. Look for plain instant oatmeal from reputable brands such as Quaker, and add just a little honey, sweetener, or fresh fruit.

Uncooked oatmeal is best stored in an airtight container in a dry area of your kitchen. Oatmeal will keep well for about two months.

See Chapter 16 for our recipe for Banana Cream Oatmeal.

A Grain Out of the Ordinary: Quinoa

If you haven't heard of quinoa before, you're not alone. Quinoa (pronounced kee-*noh*-uh or *keen*-wah) is native to South America and, like the superfood chia (see Chapter 10), was used by Native Americans as an energizing food that could help their warriors stay strong in battles. The Incas considered quinoa a sacred food, and it was a staple of their diets for many years.

Quinoa has a mild nutty flavor and crunchy texture. Quinoa is really a seed, but in cooking it's treated like a grain. It's related to spinach, which is a superfood as well (see Chapter 5). Quinoa may not be as popular as oats, wheat, or other well-known grains, but it's a great superfood with many health benefits. We suggest your enjoy quinoa at least once each week.

Understanding quinoa's superfood powers

Quinoa is a complete source of protein, which means it contains all the essential amino acids (which is important for vegetarians and vegans). One cup of cooked quinoa has 8 grams of protein — about twice as much protein as other cereal grains — plus a good amount of fiber (5 grams), all for just 222 calories.

Quinoa is a good source of minerals, including magnesium, manganese, iron, and copper, plus B vitamins. All these nutrients are involved in chemical reactions that your body uses to make energy out of the foods you eat. Quinoa also has some healthful fats and potassium that are good for your heart and blood pressure.

By adding quinoa to your superfoods diet, you reap the following health benefits:

- ✓ **Keeping your digestive system healthy:** The large amount of insoluble fiber (fiber that doesn't dissolve in water) in quinoa helps you have regular bowel movements. Insoluble fiber passes through the intestinal tract and helps move stool through the colon by adding bulk. Keeping the bowels regular reduces the risk of bloating, pain, and gas associated with irregular movements. It also reduces the risk of *diverticulosis* (small pouches that arise from weak spots in the intestine that can get inflamed or infected) and hemorrhoids.

- ✓ **Reducing your risk of gallstones:** Fiber has been found to reduce the secretion of bile acids, which are associated with gallstone formation. A large study published in 2004 in the *American Journal of Gastroenterology* indicated a 17 percent reduction in gallstones in the group of people who consumed the most insoluble fiber.

- ✓ **Getting antioxidants and more energy:** The minerals manganese and copper both help in the production of *superoxide dismutase,* an enzyme that helps the body fight off cellular damage throughout the body. This antioxidant activity helps prevent cardiovascular disease, cancer, and other inflammatory conditions. Quinoa is also rich in riboflavin (vitamin B2), which is necessary for energy production.

- ✓ **Easing migraine headaches:** The strong concentration of magnesium makes daily consumption of quinoa a good option for those with migraines. Magnesium helps prevent migraines by relaxing blood vessels, which is the hallmark treatment for these vascular headaches.

✔ **Making weight loss easier:** The combination of protein and fiber in quinoa makes for a very filling food. A scientific study published in 2005 in the *British Journal of Nutrition* found that quinoa had a high satisfaction index compared to grains like wheat, so eating quinoa may help keep hunger pangs at bay.

Finding, keeping, and using quinoa

Although quinoa is relatively unknown, it really isn't difficult to find. Some major grocery chains carry prepackaged quinoa in the same area where they sell oatmeal and other breakfast cereals; others carry it near the rice and couscous. Most natural foods stores carry quinoa in packages or in bulk. Food items that use quinoa, such as pasta, tortillas, crackers, cookies, and other baked items, also may be available.

Once you've opened a package of quinoa, keep it in an airtight container in a cool, dry place, where it will stay fresh for several weeks. Refrigerated quinoa will keep up to six months.

Just before cooking, rinse quinoa seeds thoroughly in a colander to remove any saponin residues that may impart a bitter taste. *Saponin* is a bitter covering that naturally repels insects. It's removed during the processing of the seeds, but you should rinse your quinoa to remove any residues.

Add the quinoa to a pot of boiling water and simmer, covered, until the quinoa looks transparent — usually about 10 to 15 minutes. Use one part quinoa to two parts water — the seeds will expand. You can also cook quinoa in a rice cooker.

As the quinoa cooks, the germ that surrounds the grain pulls off and creates a small tail. A unique characteristic of quinoa is that when it's cooked, the grain softens but the tail remains crunchy.

Serve hot quinoa just like oatmeal, with fresh berries, nuts, flax, or chia, and a little milk or cream (see Chapter 16 for a recipe). You can also serve quinoa as a side dish, similar to rice.

For a different flavor, cook quinoa in chicken broth. Add chopped cooked onions, mushrooms, or any other cooked vegetables to make a delicious and healthful pilaf.

You can grow quinoa sprouts at home in a container garden. Sprouted quinoa is quite tasty and can be used to season soups and salads. See Chapter 14 for more information on growing your own superfoods.

Staying Healthy with Soy

Soy makes our superfoods list rather effortlessly. Soy has been consumed in Asian diets for thousands of years and is still a very popular food choice — in fact, it's considered to be the most popular legume in the world. Soy is a complete protein source, containing all of the essential amino acids, and it has more protein per volume than meat.

Soy tastes delicious and has great nutritional value, and research has found numerous health benefits. It has plenty of vitamins and is full of antioxidants that reduce the risk of disease and fight inflammation.

Exploring the proven perks of soy

The health benefits of soy have been so well established that the Food and Drug Administration (FDA) has approved this claim to be placed on labels of foods that contain soy as an ingredient: "Diets low in saturated fat and cholesterol that include 25 grams of soy protein a day may reduce the risk of heart disease."

One cup of cooked soybeans delivers 29 grams of protein and 10 grams of fiber for 298 calories. The beans are nearly half protein, and soy flour has an even higher protein count.

Soybeans are not just protein packages; they're also a good source of vitamin E and the B vitamins: B1 (thiamin), B2 (riboflavin), B6 (pyridoxine), and folate. Soy contains large amounts of calcium and iron, too.

Soybeans contain healthy omega-3 fatty acids with no cholesterol. Compared to other legumes, soybeans are a better source of essential fatty acids. Soybeans contain *lecithin* (a fat molecule that has high concentrations of the amino acids *inositil* and *choline*) and *isoflavones* (health-promoting compounds found in plants). Two isoflavones, *daidzein* and *genisten* are considered *phytoestrogens* (plant chemicals with estrogen-like activity).

If you go online, you can find many detractors of soy and soy foods. The main argument against the use of soy is that soy (like all legumes) contains phytates that reduce absorption of minerals like calcium, and trypsin inhibitors that reduce the availability of an important enzyme. While these so-called "anti-nutrients" are present in raw soybeans and legumes, cooking and processing removes the phytates and trypsin inhibitors, rendering a very healthful and beneficial superfood.

When you eat soy, you improve your health by

- ✔ **Lowering cholesterol.** The fiber in soy helps to keep cholesterol in check. A study at Tufts University found that soy not only reduced LDL (bad cholesterol) but also increased the size of the LDL particles and raised HDL (good cholesterol) levels. Increasing the size of the LDL may be beneficial because smaller particles may cause more damage to blood vessel walls. The American Heart Association reports that isoflavones in soybeans exert cholesterol-lowering effects and also reduce blood vessel wall inflammation that may lead to heart disease.

✔ **Preventing osteoporosis.** Isoflavones have very weak estrogenic activity when compared to human estrogen (a major female hormone that's present in both men and women), but researchers still feel that these phytochemicals help prevent bone destruction and may also help bone formation. This may explain why there's a lower incidence of osteoporosis in Asian countries.

✔ **Reducing the risk of cancer.** The estrogenic activity of the isoflavones may be of value in treating hormone-sensitive cancers such as breast, prostate, and endometrial cancer. The estrogenic activity is found to work similarly to some anti-cancer drugs. Studies have shown women who have the highest soy consumption have a lower incidence of endometrial cancer. Research published in 2003 in the *Journal of Nutrition* suggests that the isoflavones in soy may work synergistically with indole-3-carbonyl (found in broccoli; see Chapter 5) to reduce the risk of estrogen-sensitive cancers. More studies are underway that will tell us more about how soy reduces the risk of cancer.

Although there is promising research supporting soy's role in cancer treatment and reduction, discuss using soy with your doctor first if you have had or are currently being treated for breast cancer.

✔ **Protecting your prostate.** Isoflavones in soy not only may help reduce the risk of prostate cancer, but evidence also shows that it may help fight enlargement of the prostate, *benign prostatic hyperplasia (BPH)*, which is a common problem for men. Regular consumption of soy may reduce the symptoms of urinary frequency and erectile dysfunction associated with an enlarged prostate.

✔ **Improving nerve function.** Soy contains large amounts of a fatty substance called lecithin, which is a major component of cell membranes. This may open doors to aid in the treatment of some neurological disorders, such as Parkinson's, Alzheimer's, and other conditions that affect the nervous system.

Selecting and serving soy

You may be able to find soybeans at your local grocery store near the canned vegetables or rice and dry beans. If you choose dehydrated soybeans, be sure there's no sign of moisture or broken packaging. Look for soy beverages in the dairy case or near other beverages. You'll find tempeh and tofu in refrigerated cases.

Health foods stores usually have a much larger selection of soy, including soy flour and soy cheese. You may even find hot dogs and burgers made from soy, along with other vegetarian ingredients.

Dried soybeans can be stored in a dry, cool place for up to one year. To cook them, place 3 cups of water or broth in a pot for every 1 cup of dried soybeans. Soybeans take about 1½ hours to cook.

Eating cooked soybeans is the best way to get all of the nutritional goodness of soy; however, there are other ways to add soy to your superfoods diet. Soy can be found in beverages, snack bars, vegetarian foods, and protein powders.

Of the many options for soy consumption, the following are some of the most popular:

- ✔ **Whole soybeans** can be roasted and eaten plain or added to salads, soups, or other recipes. *Edamame,* a popular food and common appetizer in certain restaurants, consists of soybeans that are boiled while still in the pods and then sprinkled with salt or a seasoning of choice.

- ✔ **Soy beverages** are a common choice for vegans and as a milk replacement for people who are lactose intolerant. Soy beverages are made from crushed, cooked soybeans. Not only do you get a higher amount of protein than from cow's milk, you also gain the benefits of soy's isoflavones.

- ✔ **Tofu** is one of the most popular meat substitutes and is especially popular among vegetarians and vegans. It has a cheese-like consistency with a very bland taste that takes up the flavors of sauces and vegetables that are combined with it. Tofu comes in a few different consistencies (soft to firm) that allow you to use it in a variety of ways, from smoothies to stir-fries.

- ✔ **Tempeh** is another soy product that's easily incorporated into meals as a meat substitute. *Tempeh* is a fermented form of soy sold in flat, rectangular pieces. It has more of a nutty flavor than tofu. Tempeh can be kept in the refrigerator for a week to ten days.

About 1 in every 200 people has an allergy to soy. Soy allergies are more common in children, but if you're not sure whether you have an allergy, you should start taking soy slowly and pay attention to any changes or symptoms that may develop. Call your doctor or go to the emergency room if you feel that you're having a reaction to soy.

Chapter 9

Spicing It Up with Flavor (and Flavonoids)

. . . .

In This Chapter

▶ Indulging in dark chocolate and red wine

▶ Pouring on the phenols in olive oil and green tea

▶ Adding some super spices

. . . .

*E*very successful diet allows room for some zesty flavors (and even a little indulgence now and then), so we flavor our superfoods diet with a few extra *flavonoids* (phytochemicals found in the pigments of plants that have health benefits). Of course, they're all superfoods, too.

In this chapter, we show how dark chocolate and a little red wine can be good for you (really!), and how replacing a little of that coffee with some luscious green tea can help your health. We include olive oil, which is good for your heart, and garlic, which has been used for many years in folk remedies. We also show you how to spice things up a bit with two sensational spices — turmeric and zesty cayenne pepper.

The key to enjoying most of the superfoods in this chapter is keeping your serving sizes small. One little piece of chocolate each day is good for you, but a lot of chocolate adds too much fat and too many calories, which is not only bad for your waistline, but also negates a lot of the benefits you get from the flavonoids.

Bringing the Heat with Cayenne Peppers

Cayenne peppers are red hot and spicy and will add a bit of zing to your superfoods diet. Cayenne peppers are related to bell peppers, jalapenos, and many other varieties of red and green peppers.

The amount of cayenne you use is a matter of taste. You may want to use up to a teaspoon of cayenne, depending on how spicy you like your foods. We suggest you add a little spice to your meals three or four times per week.

Fighting with fire

Capsaicin is the main compound in cayenne pepper that gives it its heat. Capsaicin heats up your body, too, because it's a *vasodilator*, which means it increases blood flow by opening up your blood vessels. Cayenne peppers are rich in beta-carotene, the precursor to vitamin A, which is necessary for a healthy immune system, normal vision, and regular cell reproduction. Cayenne peppers also contain lutein and zeaxanthin, powerful antioxidants that help protect your vision and your cardiovascular system.

Cayenne pepper acts as all of the following when added to foods:

- ✔ **A pain fighter:** Capsaicin helps to relieve pain when you eat it or when you rub it into the skin over a painful part of your body. Capsaicin reduces the amount of *substance P*, a neurochemical associated with inflammation. When substance P is diminished, so is pain. Reducing inflammation is also good for your heart and cardiovascular system.

- ✔ **A congestion reliever:** Capsaicin stimulates drainage of the mucous membranes in your nasal passages, providing an effect similar to that of some cold medications.

- ✔ **A weight controller:** According to research published in 2006 in the *American Journal of Clinical Nutrition,* cayenne pepper revs up your metabolism and increases your body's ability to burn calories. Cayenne peppers also help control insulin levels, which may help to control diabetes.

Selecting, handling, and serving cayenne peppers

You can buy whole, fresh, or dried cayenne peppers in the produce aisle of your local grocery store, or you can choose powdered cayenne pepper, which you'll find in the herb and spice aisle. You're also likely to see a few varieties of cayenne pepper sauce, which is a combination of red pepper and vinegar.

Fresh cayenne peppers are sometimes used in recipes. To prepare a pepper, just remove the stem, slice it open, and remove the seeds inside.

When you handle fresh peppers, be sure to wear gloves and don't touch your eyes — the capsaicin will sting and irritate them. When you're finished, wash your hands and cooking utensils thoroughly. Rinsing your hands with milk also helps to reduce the burning sensation.

Remember that cayenne is hot, so a little bit is all you need for recipes and for seasoning.

Try a dash of red pepper sauce on our vegetable omelets (see Chapter 16) or our salmon cakes (see Chapter 19).

Indulging in Decadent Dark Chocolate

We spend a lot of time telling people to avoid candy, so it's a lot of fun to be able to recommend chocolate as a superfood. There is one stipulation — it has to be dark chocolate, because it contains more cocoa than the typical milk chocolate candy bar. Cocoa is rich in natural compounds that are powerful enough to make dark chocolate a superfood.

Cocoa is made from seeds harvested from the pods of cacao trees. The seeds are processed into cocoa powder, which finds its way into a wide range of sweet treats ranging from candy bars to cakes, cookies, truffles, and ice cream sundaes. Most of these foods are high in fat, sugar, and calories, but, if you're careful, you can enjoy chocolate treats and improve your health.

We recommend that you eat 1 to 2 ounces of dark chocolate every day, but not more. Too much chocolate adds fats and sugar that may contribute to unwanted weight gain.

Getting a boost from cocoa

Cocoa is rich in flavonoids, especially one called *epicatechin*. In general, flavonoids reduce inflammation and protect the cells in your body from damage.

One ounce of dark chocolate (about 60 to 70 percent cocoa) has about 160 calories; is rich in magnesium, a mineral that your body needs for normal nerve and muscle function; and provides 5 percent of your daily need of selenium, a mineral that works as an antioxidant. An article published in the *Journal of American Dietetic Association* in 1999 states that magnesium deficiency may have a connection to chocolate cravings. (One ounce of dark chocolate has 55 milligrams of magnesium — more than two slices of whole-grain bread and about 10 percent of what you need each day.) Chocolate cravings may also involve some neurotransmitters (brain chemicals) like serotonin that lead to a feeling of well-being. Dark chocolate contains tryptophan, an amino acid that your body uses to produce serotonin. Chocolate also contains the stimulants caffeine and theobromine, as well as phenolethylamine, a biochemical that mimics the feeling of being in love.

When you eat small amounts of dark chocolate every day, you partake of cocoa's health attributes:

✔ **Improving vascular health:** Several studies point out the vascular benefits of the flavonoids in dark chocolate. Research published in 2004 in the *Journal of the American College of Nutrition* found that eating about 1½ ounces of Dove dark chocolate every day improved blood vessel function. A 2007 German study published in *The Journal of the American Medical Association* discovered eating one dark Hershey's Kiss a day was effective for lowering blood pressure.

You need healthy blood vessels to let blood flow to your brain, your heart, and, of course, the rest of your body. Eating a small amount of dark chocolate daily reduces your risk of *atherosclerosis* (thickening of the arteries), a big risk factor for heart disease and stroke, and helps keep your blood pressure at a healthy level.

✔ **Curbing insulin resistance:** The *American Journal of Clinical Nutrition* reported in 2005 that flavonoids in dark chocolate help to improve *insulin resistance,* an inability of the body to respond properly to insulin, thereby leading to diabetes. The flavonoids' effect on blood vessels may be very helpful for diabetic patients, because vascular problems are a common complication with diabetes.

✔ **Having a healthier pregnancy.** A 2008 study from Yale University found that pregnant women who ate more chocolate and had higher levels of theobromine (a chemical in chocolate that's similar to caffeine) in their systems were less likely to suffer from *pre-eclampsia,* a condition that effects pregnant women who have high blood pressure.

Choosing the best dark chocolate

You can buy dark chocolate almost anywhere, from local convenience stores and vending machines to exclusive gourmet chocolate shops. Quality and price vary widely. Look for dark chocolate that contains more than 65 percent cocoa: The flavonoids are in the cocoa, not the sugar or fat that accompanies them, so the higher the cocoa content, the better. Avoid Dutch-processed cocoa, however (see the nearby sidebar to find out why).

The easiest way to enjoy dark chocolate is to buy dark chocolate bars. They vary in size, ranging from 1 ounce to 3 ounces. Just eat one smaller bar, or break the larger bars into smaller pieces. Chocolate should be stored in a dark, dry place at about 60 to 70 degrees Fahrenheit. Chocolate that is still wrapped will last up to a year at this temperature. If you live in a warm climate, keep your chocolate in the refrigerator. Be sure to wrap the chocolate in foil or plastic to protect it from food odors. Let it warm up to room temperature before eating it. Note that some chocolate candies, such as truffles, may only last up to a month at room temperature.

Any dark chocolate bar that is not Dutch-processed (read the label) offers plenty of flavonoids; however, you also can buy CocoaVia bars, which contain soy products (see Chapter 8) that are good for heart health.

The pitfalls of Dutch-processed cocoa

Dutch-processed cocoa is treated with an alkaline substance to reduce the natural acidity and bitterness of cocoa. Unfortunately, this process also destroys cocoa's healthful flavonoids. Many people prefer the taste of Dutch-processed cocoa, which has a smoother, milder flavor that works well for many recipes.

It's important to note, however, that Dutch-processed cocoa has a neutral pH (rather than acidic), which can throw off the chemical balance of some baked good recipes: They may not rise properly, unless the recipe also calls for baking soda.

Some research has found that sugar-free dark chocolate may be more effective than sugar-sweetened dark chocolate. Unsweetened chocolate is very bitter, but you may find dark chocolate sweetened with artificial sweeteners, such as sucralose.

Livening Up Foods with a Clove of Garlic

Pungent, cream-colored cloves of garlic add more than flavor to your foods; they also bring good health to you and your family. Garlic has been used as medicine for a very long time to fight infections and to ward off evil spirits (not to mention vampires). Today, garlic is used to reduce cholesterol and prevent cancer and as an anti-microbial agent.

Garlic has a distinctive aroma and flavor due to a compound called *allicin,* which is released when the clove is sliced or crushed. Garlic is used in many recipes, and although the heat from cooking reduces some of the active compounds in garlic, the garlic retains most of its health benefits.

We suggest you eat one clove of garlic every day, or take garlic supplements two or three times each week.

Gauging garlic's health benefits

The main active compounds in garlic are allicin and other sulfur-containing compounds. Garlic also contains some B complex vitamins and selenium, which are important for many chemical reactions in your body. Selenium is a mineral that works like an antioxidant. Garlic is also very low in calories — one clove has only 4 calories.

You can rely on garlic to assist with the following:

- ✔ **Lowering blood pressure:** A study published in 2008 in the *Annals of Pharmacotherapy* determined that garlic reduces high blood pressure, which is a risk factor for heart disease and strokes.

- ✔ **Preventing cancer:** Eating garlic appears to increase antioxidant activity, according to research published in 2008 in the journal *Gerontology*. Boosting antioxidants may help to prevent cancer and help you live longer.

- ✔ **Fighting microbes:** Garlic inhibits a variety of fungi, viruses, and bacteria and has been used as an anti-microbial for thousands of years. The *Journal of Antimicrobial Chemotherapy* reported in 2003 that garlic inhibits the growth of the bacteria that cause *methicillin-resistant Staphylococcus aureus* (MRSA), a type of antibiotic-resistant infection, in mice. Garlic also inhibits *candida albicans,* a common cause of yeast infections.

- ✔ **Promoting digestive health:** Garlic contains the prebiotic compound *fructose oligosaccharide* (FOS). Prebiotics support the growth of friendly bacteria that reside in the intestinal tract. These bacteria are necessary for making vitamin K and for normal, healthy digestion.

Selecting, keeping, and using garlic

Fresh garlic is available in the produce section of your grocery store. Garlic is also often available pre-chopped, in jars or bottles.

To roast garlic, just remove the outermost layer of papery covering and place the bulb in a baking dish. Drizzle some olive oil on top of the bulb, cover the baking dish with aluminum foil, and bake in an oven heated to 375 degrees Fahrenheit for about one hour. Serve the roasted garlic with whole-grain bread.

To prepare garlic for cooking, simply break the cloves you need off the bulb. To make peeling the papery covering off the cloves easier, heat the cloves in your microwave on high for about ten seconds or so. This loosens the covering. Then chop the peeled cloves with a knife or a garlic press, a device that squeezes the clove through several small holes.

You get the most health benefits from fresh garlic cloves that you chop or crush just before you add them to your recipes. According to research published in 2008 in the *Journal of Agricultural and Food Chemistry,* the amount of allicin decreases rapidly. In fact, garlic preserved in oil lost half of its allicin content in just six hours. Garlic stored in water fared better, but half of the allicin disappeared within six days.

Pre-chopped garlic is not as powerful as fresh garlic; however, it retains much of its health benefit and many people like the convenience. If you choose pre-chopped garlic, buy it in small jars and store the garlic in the refrigerator after it has been opened.

Garlic supplements, such as Garlique, are available. Many people prefer taking supplements to avoid the after-effect of "garlic breath." The garlic odor can be diminished by using an enteric coating on the capsules, which ensures the garlic is released in the small intestine instead of the stomach.

Brewing Up a Cup of Green Tea

Humans have been brewing tea for a very long time — perhaps as many as 500,000 years, according to archeological evidence. One tea in particular — green tea — makes our superfoods list. You may be more familiar with the many popular varieties of black tea that are available in nearly every restaurant or grocery store, such as orange pekoe and Earl Grey. These black teas are very popular in the United States, but in Asian countries, green tea is actually preferred. Green tea contains more polyphenols, which are the antioxidants that protect your body and promote good health.

We suggest you drink 2 or 3 cups of green tea four or five days each week, perhaps in place of your regular cup of coffee.

Catching some catechins

Green teas contain several types of *catechins* (flavonoids) that appear to protect your body from a variety of cancers. They also keep your blood vessels healthy. Green tea also contains caffeine, along with theobromine and theophylline, which act as stimulants, although coffee contains much more caffeine. If you prefer to avoid caffeine, green tea is available in decaffeinated form.

Green, black, white, or oolong tea?

All four of these types of tea are made from the leaves of the same plant, Camellia sinensis. The difference is in how they're processed. The leaves are harvested at the same time for green, black, and oolong teas; however, green tea leaves are dried immediately, whereas the leaves for black and oolong teas are fermented before drying. Fermentation reduces the amount of polyphenols found in the tea, so that's why green tea is considered the healthiest of the teas. Oolong tea isn't fermented as long as black tea, so oolong has more antioxidants than black tea, which has the least. A fourth version, called white tea, is harvested while the leaves are immature. Like green tea, white tea is processed immediately without fermentation, and, in fact, white tea may have more antioxidants than green tea. However, it's more expensive and more difficult to find in stores.

Epigallocatechin gallate (EGCG) is a catechin that has received the most attention in research studies because it appears to have several biological actions, including anti-cancer activity and blood pressure reduction. It also may help you burn calories.

Green tea is beneficial in a host of health endeavors:

- **Preventing breast cancer:** Research involving the dietary patterns of large groups of people showed lower rates of cancer in people who drank green tea every day. An article in *Breast Cancer Research and Treatment* reported in 2008 that green tea stops cancer cells by blocking *angiogenesis*, which is the growth of new blood vessels that feed a cancerous tumor.

- **Reducing the risk of ovarian cancer:** The *Archives of Internal Medicine* published research in 2005 showing the more tea (both green and black) women drank every day, the lower their risk of ovarian cancer. EGCG is thought to be the main catechin responsible for preventing this type of cancer.

- **Decreasing prostate cancer:** Catechins stopped the growth of prostate cancer cells in lab research. Australian studies of large groups of people showed that drinking green tea appears to protect men against prostate cancer.

- **Protecting your cardiovascular system:** The journal *Nutrition* confirmed in 2005 that green tea extracts reduce inflammation, blood pressure, and LDL cholesterol (the bad cholesterol) in about three weeks. Green tea also keeps blood vessels healthy.

- **Preventing diabetes:** Catechins improve blood sugar control. The journal *Obesity* published research in 2008 that found diabetics who drank green tea had lower hemoglobin A1C levels (a blood test that measures blood sugar). Drinking green tea also keeps blood vessels healthy, which is very important for diabetics.

- **Aiding weight loss:** *The American Journal of Clinical Nutrition* explained in 2008 that the catechins in green tea help burn more fat calories during moderate exercise. Drinking green tea (or taking green tea extract) before working out may improve your odds of losing weight and keeping it off.

Buying and brewing green tea

You can find green tea online and in most grocery stores. Some tea and coffee shops sell loose green tea, or you can purchase it in regular tea bags.

The easiest way to brew green tea is to buy tea bags that already contain the perfect amount of tea leaves to make 1 cup of tea. To maximize the amounts of polyphenols, let the tea bag steep in very hot water for two to five minutes.

Some people prefer loose tea over bags. To brew loose-leaf tea, you need a device for straining the leaves. You can use a tea ball, a mesh metal ball that you fill with tea leaves and place into a cup of hot water. Tea infusers that look like small baskets can also hold your tea in the water until it's brewed to your liking.

Green tea extract is available as a dietary supplement if you'd prefer not to drink tea. Be sure to follow the directions on the product label.

According to the University of Maryland Medical Center, green tea may possibly interact with some types of chemotherapy. If you're undergoing any form of treatment for cancer, speak with your doctor before drinking green tea or taking supplemental green tea extracts.

Pouring It On! Olive Oil

Olive oil is one of the main features of the Mediterranean diet, which appears to be one of the best diets for reduction of heart disease risk and for living longer. Olive oil contains *oleic acid* (an omega-9 monounsaturated fat that's good for your health), and virgin and extra-virgin olive oils also contain phytochemical antioxidants.

Olives are harvested and taken immediately to mills, where they're cleaned and ground into paste. The oil is separated from the solids (the pomace) and bottled. Oil pressed in this manner is called *virgin* or *extra virgin* olive oil (depending on the oleic acid content). Virgin and extra virgin olive oils are rich in polyphenols. Olive oil that is *refined* has fewer polyphenols than virgin or extra virgin olive oils.

Because olive oil is so good for you and so easy to use, we suggest you consume 2 tablespoons of olive oil every day, preferably in place of saturated animal fats. Two tablespoons may not seem like much, but oils are high in calories, so a little bit goes a long way.

Reaping the benefits of olive oil

Two tablespoons of olive oil supply 239 calories plus vitamins E and K, mono-unsaturated fats, and polyphenols, such as *tyrosol* and *hydroxytyrosol*. These polyphenols, in addition to oleic acid, elevate olive oil from just another healthy food to superfood status.

Olive oil has a positive impact on cholesterol and can help prevent heart disease when you use it to replace unhealthy saturated fats (from fatty red meats and high-fat dairy products, for example). Other sources of oleic acid include canola oil and avocados.

Adding a little olive oil to your diet imparts several important benefits.

- **Protecting your heart:** The monounsaturated fats and polyphenols in olive oil help to lower your total cholesterol while raising the good HDL cholesterol. Olive oil also helps to lower blood pressure and keeps your arteries healthy by decreasing inflammation.

- **Preventing cancer:** The polyphenols in olive oil may help to reduce the risk of breast cancer by inhibiting the growth of cancer cells, according to research published in 2008 in the *International Journal of Molecular Medicine*. Research published in the *Journal of Agricultural and Food Chemistry* in 2007 discovered that those same polyphenols kill H. pylori in the lab. H. pylori is the bacteria that's been linked to peptic ulcers and stomach cancer.

- **Longevity:** According to a study published in 2000 in the *British Journal of Nutrition*, people who follow a Mediterranean type of diet rich in olive oil, poultry, and vegetables tend to live longer compared to people who eat more pasta and red meat.

A super diet — The Mediterranean Diet

The Mediterranean Diet was introduced in 1993 by the Oldways Preservation & Exchange Trust, Harvard School of Public Health, and the World Health Organization. It's based on the traditional foods eaten by people living in the Mediterranean region, especially Greece and Italy. The Mediterranean diet features olive oil, lots of fish and seafood, fresh fruits and vegetables, legumes, nuts, and seeds. The diet also includes moderate consumption of whole grains, red wine, and dairy, but is very low in the consumption of red meat.

Although the inhabitants of this region of the Mediterranean eat diets high in fat, they have much lower rates of cardiovascular disease and cancer than people who eat high-fat diets in other parts of the world. This is unusual, because most high-fat diets are correlated with a higher incidence of disease and death. The difference could be due in part to the use of omega-9-rich olive oil and the large amounts of omega-3 fatty acids from fish and seafood.

You can re-create a Mediterranean diet by using olive oil in place of other fats and oils, increasing your intake of fruits and vegetables (like our superfoods in Chapters 4 and 5), and eating more fish (see Chapter 7). You should reduce your consumption of red meat and highly processed foods and sweets; however, it's okay to enjoy a glass of wine with dinner.

Selecting, storing, and pouring olive oil

Olive oil is available in every market and grocery store. Olive oils vary in price, from refined olive oil, which is the least expensive, to delicately flavored (but not delicately priced) olive oils found in exclusive gourmet shops. Extra virgin olive oils are more expensive than virgin or refined olive oils, but they're worth the cost. In fact, they have a dedicated following with aficionados, just like wines do.

If you're fortunate enough to have a gourmet food shop in your area, such as a Dean & Deluca, check to see whether they hold olive oil tastings. You'll be able to discover more about the subtle differences among the different varieties and find out which oils pair best with your favorite foods.

Store olive oil in a dark glass bottle or stainless steel container in a cool area, away from heat sources. You can also store your olive oil in the refrigerator; however, it may alter the flavor of extra virgin olive oil.

You can use olive oil for salad dressings, sauces, and cooking a variety of savory dishes. Here are some ideas:

- ✔ Extra virgin olive oil loses flavor when cooked, so it's better for making dressings or for using on top of cooked foods.

- ✔ Replace butter with olive oil, or blend the two into a spread that has less saturated fat than butter alone.

- ✔ Dip whole-grain bread in olive oil mixed with a little parmesan cheese and red pepper.

- ✔ Dress your salads with extra-virgin olive oil and a bit of balsamic vinegar.

- ✔ Top your cooked vegetables with a drizzle of olive oil and lemon juice.

- ✔ Make pesto (see Chapter 17) and serve with pasta.

Some people even choose to bake their cookies and cakes with olive oil, although others may not associate the flavor of olive oil with sweets.

Sipping a Small Glass of Red Wine

Enjoying a glass of red wine with your dinner may be good for your heart. Red wine contains flavonoids called catechins, a substance called *resveratrol*, and *gallic acid,* which are all antioxidants. Drinking red wine (in moderation) may be one of the reasons for the "French paradox," which is the observation of good heart health among the French despite their rich, high-fat diet.

Don't start drinking wine if you normally don't drink alcohol or if you have problems with alcohol dependency, are under age, or are pregnant or nursing. You can find other superfood beverages such as fruit juices (see Chapter 4) or green tea (see the section "Brewing Up a Cup of Green Tea" earlier in this chapter). If you do drink wine, remember that *more is not better*. One serving of wine is 5 ounces, or little more than $1/2$ cup. While several health benefits are associated with enjoying small amounts of alcohol, there are no health benefits (and some risks) in having more than one or two drinks each day.

If you drink alcohol already, we suggest that you enjoy one 5-ounce glass of wine daily. The American Heart Association recommends one glass a day for women and up to two glasses a day for men. You may also choose to drink nonalcoholic red wine.

More than truth in red wine

One 5-ounce serving of red wine has 125 calories. Red wine also contains potassium, which is good for your heart and your muscles, plus fluoride for your teeth. You can enjoy a glass of red wine with the knowledge that you are

- ✔ **Improving cardiovascular health.** The flavonoids and resveratrol in wine keep your blood vessels healthy and prevent platelets from sticking together to form blood clots. According to the Mayo Clinic, drinking red wine may prevent heart attacks and strokes. Red wine also helps to increase your HDL cholesterol (the good kind).

- ✔ **Preventing cancer.** According to the National Cancer Institute, the antioxidants in red wine may help to prevent cellular damage that results in cancer. In addition, resveratrol appears to inhibit the growth of cancerous cells in the lab.

- ✔ **Living longer.** The antioxidants that prevent cancer and heart disease may lead to living a longer life. A study published in 2008 in the *Journal of Agricultural and Food Chemistry* states that drinking red wine with red meat actually reduces the harmful effects of eating red meat. Other studies have found a correlation between drinking one or two alcoholic drinks each day and living longer.

Selecting and serving red wines

There are several types of red wine. The most common types include cabernet sauvignon, pinot noir, merlot, syrah (or shiraz), chianti, malbec, and zinfandel. Red wine is available at liquor stores and wine shops, some grocery stores, and many restaurants.

Antioxidants are found in the skins of red grapes, and the alcohol produced during fermentation draws the antioxidants out of the skins. Deeper red wines have a much higher concentration than the lighter rose wines because the grape skins are removed during the process of making lighter wines.

If you don't know which wine you like best, check out a local wine shop to see when they have wine tastings or ask for advice on choosing wine. You can also refer to *Wine for Dummies,* 4th Edition, by Ed McCarthy and Mary Ewing-Mulligan (Wiley) for more information.

All red wines are good sources of flavonoids and resveratrol, even wines that have had the alcohol removed. Resveratrol is also found in other foods, such as peanuts, and you can get some resveratrol when you eat grapes or drink grape juice.

You can enjoy a glass of wine with dinner, or you can use red wine as an ingredient in many dishes (the alcohol will usually be cooked away by heat, but the heat won't damage the resveratrol). Our tomato and lentil stew (see Chapter 17) contains red wine as one of the ingredients.

Relieving Pain with Turmeric

Turmeric is a golden yellow powder that's used in curry dishes from India and sometimes as a yellow food coloring. The powder is ground from *rhizomes* (a portion of plant stem that grows underground) of the *Curcuma longa*, which is in the same family as ginger.

Besides adding flavor to food, turmeric helps to reduce pain and may slow down the progress of Alzheimer's disease. It has been used in India as an Aruvedic medicine, which is a form of traditional medicine. One serving of turmeric is about $1/4$ teaspoon. We suggest you use this seasoning twice a week.

Taking advantage of turmeric

Turmeric contains *curcumin*, which is a polyphenol, antioxidant, and anti-inflammatory agent. Using turmeric or curcumin capsules may help to improve your health by providing the following benefits:

- ✔ **Battling autoimmune diseases:** Curcumin affects the immune system and inhibits some diseases, such as multiple sclerosis and rheumatoid arthritis, by regulating signaling mechanisms called *cytokines*. According to the *Journal of Clinical Immunology* in 2007, these regulating mechanisms are the reason curcumin is beneficial for people with diabetes, arthritis, asthma, allergies, and cancer.

- **Providing pain relief:** Curcumin functions as a COX-2 inhibitor, just like some prescription pain medications, but with fewer side effects. Research in Israel suggests that curcumin makes prescription COX-2 inhibitors more effective at lower doses, thus also reducing side effects.

  Curcumin reduces pain by fighting inflammation. Curcumin has been studied for pain relief in the treatment of autoimmune diseases such as rheumatoid arthritis and multiple sclerosis.

- **Fighting cancer:** The polyphenols in turmeric have anti-cancer properties due to their ability to regulate cytokine. *Biochemical Pharmacology* reported in 2007 that curcumin also slows the growth of breast cancer cells in a laboratory setting.

- **Aiding memory:** Turmeric may help fight Alzheimer's disease due to the antioxidant and anti-inflammatory properties of curcumin. A study in the *American Journal of Epidemiology* reported in 2006 that elderly Asians who ate curry regularly were less likely to suffer from Alzheimer's disease than Asians who rarely or never ate curry.

While eating turmeric as a seasoning is perfectly safe, please speak with your doctor if you want to take curcumin as a dietary supplement, because it may have an impact on blood clotting and blood sugar control.

Using turmeric

You can buy turmeric alone or in curry powder in the baking section of your grocery store. Curry powders are popular in Asian and Indian cooking. Different curries vary in ingredients. All curries are well-seasoned, and some are downright hot. Store curry powder in an air-tight container at room temperature for up to two months.

Try sprinkling some curry powder instead of salt and pepper on your poultry, rice, and vegetable dishes.

Turmeric is the ingredient in mustard that gives it its yellow color, and it's a component of Worcestershire sauce. Turmeric goes well with chicken, turkey, and vegetable dishes.

Chapter 10

Exploring Exotic Superfoods

In This Chapter

▶ Introducing the exotic superfoods

▶ Getting the exotic superfoods into your diet

▶ Knowing where to find them

*T*he word *exotic* refers to something that's different, unusual, or foreign. Our exotic superfoods are well-known in other parts of the world and include fruits, grains, grasses, and marine life that all pack a powerful punch when it comes to helping your body. These exotic superfoods are all great examples of why we call certain foods super.

In the world of superfoods, being exotic also means being a little harder to find. Some of our exotic foods may not be available on the shelves of your favorite grocery store — yet. However, with time, these exotic superfoods will become better known, and, most likely, more readily available.

In this chapter, we introduce you to some superfoods that you may never have seen in the grocery store, or even heard of. We show you what makes them superfoods, where to find them, and how to add them to your superfoods diet.

The foods in this chapter tend to be harder to find and often are fairly expensive. So, although we offer recommendations for regular consumption, you can always treat these foods as extras — something you indulge in occasionally as part of your overall superfoods regimen.

South America's Açaí

Açaí berries (pronounced ah-*sigh*-ee) are grown on palm trees in the Amazon rainforest of northern Brazil. The trunks of these palm trees grow in groups and can reach up to 80 feet tall. The Açaí berries hang down in clusters from the branches, and each tree can produce a large amount of berries.

An açaí berry is dark purple to almost black in color and is about the size of a blueberry (see Figure 10-1). Brazilians use the berries not only as fruit, but also for juice, wine, and as an ingredient in desserts. The berries are usually used soon after picking.

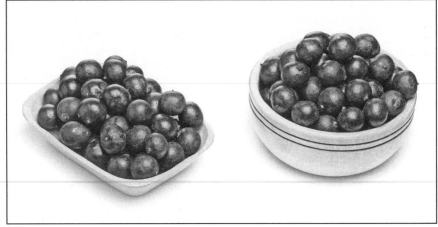

Figure 10-1:
Açaí
berries.

©Lew Robertson/Getty Images

Fighting cancer and inflammation

Like all of our other superfood berries, açaí berries are rich in nutrients and antioxidants that can help fight the inflammation that's associated with many chronic diseases. A few recent studies have shown that extracts from açaí berries may destroy cancer cells, particularly those associated with leukemia. The beautiful dark pigments that color the açaí berries contain flavonoids called *anthocyanins*. One serving of açaí juice contains large amounts of anthocyanins and plant sterols, as well as calcium, vitamin A, amino acids, and oleic acid.

One ounce of açaí pulp has 15 calories per ounce and the powder has 19 calories per 3-gram scoop. Açaí juice is often blended with other juices, so 1 cup of juice usually has from 100 to 150 calories.

Adding açaí berries to your diet can aid you in the following endeavors:

✔ **Fighting leukemia.** A study done by the University of Florida and published in the January 2008 *Journal of Agriculture and Food Chemistry* found that extracts of the açaí berry destroyed human cancer cells grown in a lab.

Studies on humans will have to follow to give more concrete evidence, but this is a positive start.

✔ **Reducing inflammation.** A study published in the 2006 *Journal of Agricultural and Food Chemicals* found açaí juice contained several anthocyanins that have powerful antioxidant properties, which, along with oleic acids, may reduce inflammation associated with chronic diseases.

Açaí berries also inhibit COX enzymes, which means drinking açaí juice may have an effect similar to that of aspirin in relieving chronic pain.

✔ **Taking care of your heart.** Açaí pulp contains lots of fiber that helps keep your digestive system healthy and reduces cholesterol. The oleic acid and beta-sitosterol found in açaí pulp are also good for healthy cholesterol levels. Add in the anti-inflammatory effects mentioned in the preceding bullet, and this berry is great for cardiovascular health.

Finding açaí berries

Açaí berries are most often sold as juice or in a pulp or purée because the berries are too delicate to ship fresh. Shopping for açaí berries is easiest to do online; however, you may find açaí juice, pulp, and supplements at some retail stores like Whole Foods, Trader Joe's, and other health food stores.

Açaí juice is very expensive, especially 100 percent açaí juice. You can find less expensive juice blends that contain açaí. That's fine as long as the other juices are also high in antioxidants, such as blueberry juice. Just be sure to read the label, and avoid juices with added sugar that you don't need.

V-8 now has an açaí version of its V-8 Fusion juice — an easily found alternative to açaí berries or supplements.

Açaí berry supplements are made from freeze-dried berries (freeze-drying helps preserve their nutritional value) or extracts. Supplements vary in cost, but they have a longer shelf-life than the juice or pulp. You can keep the pulp in the refrigerator for a few days, or two to three months in the freezer.

Açaí juice or pulp can be added to fruit smoothies or blended with other juices. A traditional Rio Bowl is made by blending açaí pulp with a banana and apple juice, and serving it with granola on top.

Algae and Kelp from Lakes and the Sea

These two exotic superfoods come from the ocean and from freshwater lakes. Blue-green algae are one-celled organisms called *cyanobacteria* and aren't really true algae. Kelp, which is commonly considered a seaweed, actually is an algae. But don't let these technical details confuse you — both of our superfoods from the sea are very good for you.

There are two popular strains of blue-green algae: *spirulina* and *aphanizom-enon flos aquae* (AFA). Kelp (technically known as *Ascophyllum nodosum sea-weed*) is a marine plant.

We suggest you eat a little raw or dried kelp once a week and 3 to 5 grams of algae daily. Manufacturers may have different amounts of each in their products, so make sure you compare different brands and check their recommended daily intake.

Taking advantage of kelp and algae

Algae and kelp both pack a powerful punch, nutritionally speaking. They're among the lowest-calorie superfoods available and have been considered the most complete food sources you can find. They're the best superfoods for trace minerals and have been a major part of Asian diets for decades.

With so many vitamins, minerals, essential fatty acids, and other food chemicals with antioxidant properties, these superfoods provide many different health benefits. They can reduce inflammation, aid in weight loss, boost your immune system, and help reduce the risk of heart disease and other chronic diseases.

Seeing what algae can do

Blue-green algae are good sources of omega-3 fatty acids, B complex vitamins, vitamin C, beta carotene, and several minerals, including iron. Blue-green algae also contain lots of complete protein (proteins that contain all of the essential amino acids). In fact, algae have one of the highest protein contents per serving of all the superfoods. Algae are very rich in beta-carotene and chlorophyll, too, making them powerful antioxidants. One tablespoon of powdered blue-green algae contains 4 grams of protein and about 20 calories.

According to information published by the National Institutes of Health, blue-green algae may help to reduce symptoms of nasal allergies, lower cholesterol, and help to remove toxic arsenic from the body.

If you take a blue-green algae supplement, you may benefit from

- **Anti-viral activity.** Research at Harvard showed that an extract of spirulina actually inhibited the replication of the HIV virus. There has also been speculation that this could have benefits for the common cold.

- **Cancer prevention.** One component of spirulina extract, called *polysaccharides,* has been shown to repair damaged DNA in a laboratory setting. This could help fight cancers, which are a result of this type of damage.

- **Treating anemia.** A substance called *phycocyanin* found in blue-green algae may stimulate the body to make red blood cells, which in turn may help to treat some forms of anemia.

✔ **Weight loss.** The high protein content of algae helps control appetite because it keeps you feeling fuller longer. Powdered algae has been used in various diets and weight loss supplements.

✔ **Treatment of degenerative nerve diseases.** Researchers in Switzerland found that a compound derived from blue-green algae may counter the effects of Alzheimer's disease and other degenerative nerve disorders by reducing inflammation.

Staying healthy with kelp

Kelp is rich in nutrients and can be an interesting way to add flavor and good health to your diet. Kelp is rich in potassium, iron, calcium, and omega-3 fatty acids. It's also a good source of iodine, a mineral that's important for optimal thyroid function. One-quarter cup constitutes one serving of raw kelp, and contains 8 calories.

If you're pregnant or have a history or family history of thyroid disease, consult your doctor before using kelp or iodine supplements. Some people are sensitive to iodine and may develop thyroid dysfunction. In any case, be sure to follow the label directions and consult with your doctor if you have any questions about the consumption of kelp.

When you eat kelp, you may improve your

✔ **Thyroid function.** Your thyroid gland acts like a thermostat that regulates many bodily processes. Normal thyroid function requires iodine. If you don't get enough iodine, you may suffer from an underactive thyroid, but if you get too much, you may overstimulate the thyroid. If your underactive thyroid isn't related to iodine deficiency, taking iodine can make it worse. If you have a history of thyroid dysfunction, discuss the pros and cons of taking kelp with your doctor. If you have no history of thyroid disease, supplementing with kelp can have great benefits, but you should limit yourself to the quantity recommended on the product label.

✔ **Weight control.** Proper thyroid function helps control your weight.

✔ **Cardiovascular health.** Kelp is a good source of folate, which reduces your levels of the protein *homeocysteine* (high levels are associated with inflammation and damage to blood vessels).

✔ **Odds of preventing breast cancer.** This theory is still in the research stages, but kelp might have anti-estrogen effects that could help prevent and treat breast cancer.

✔ **Odds of passing on birth defects.** The folate in kelp helps to prevent a birth defect of the spine called *spina bifida*. Women who may become pregnant must get enough folate from their diet or in supplemental form as folic acid.

Why is there iodine in salt?

A disease called *goiter* used to be a little too common in the United States. A goiter is a swollen, underactive thyroid gland that makes the person who has it appear to have a large, thick neck. Goiters occur when a person's diet is deficient in iodine for a long time. The widespread iodine deficiency that caused so many goiters was almost wiped out when iodine was added to table salt. There are still some iodine deficiencies in the United States, but the real problem lies in underdeveloped countries. Children who have iodine deficiency suffer from stunted growth and mental delay.

Getting the superfoods of the sea

It's important to purchase blue-green algae from sources that you can trust. The organisms in blue-green algae are harvested and then freeze-dried so they can be used in powders for supplementation, but the government doesn't regulate the conditions for harvesting algae. Unscrupulous companies could possibly harvest toxic types of algae. Thus, make sure the company you purchase your supplements from harvests the algae, usually spirulina, from controlled, fresh-water ponds that are checked regularly for toxins.

Kelp can be purchased in Asian markets or retail stores that carry Asian food items. One variety of kelp is kombu, which is used in soups and stews or as a garnish.

You may also use *nori,* which is dried seaweed paper that can be found in many grocery stores. Nori is dark green and papery with a slight flavor of oily ocean fish. It's used as a wrapper in a variety of sushi dishes.

Alginate is a carbohydrate extracted from kelp that's used as a thickener for processed foods and snacks. You may see it on the list of ingredients when you buy ice cream, jams, jellies, soups, and other products.

Peruvian Camu-Camu

The camu-camu bush grows in the rainforests of Peru and Brazil and bears a fruit that resembles a large purplish grape with yellow flesh — one of the richest sources of vitamin C of any food (see Figure 10-2). That alone might make camu-camu a superfood, but the juice also contains anthocyanins (from the pigments), which means it's an antioxidant with anti-inflammatory properties.

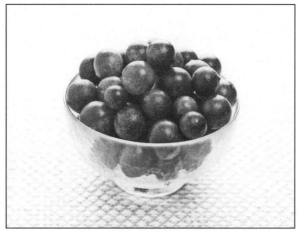

Figure 10-2:
Camu-camu.

Camu-camu isn't well-known as a superfood yet, but the health claims for camu-camu are impressive.

Providing copious amounts of vitamin C

A Brazilian study determined that camu-camu has so much vitamin C that pulp that has been stored for one month still contains more of the water-soluble vitamin than most other well-known fresh sources. One-half teaspoon of dried camu-camu powder contains up to 380 milligrams of vitamin C. You would have to eat about five whole oranges or 4 cups of sliced strawberries to get that much vitamin C (and they'd have to be fresh).

Furthermore, the November 2005 *Journal of Agricultural and Food Chemistry* published research investigating the anthocyanin content of camu-camu. Anthocyanins are natural antioxidants, and further research will determine what additional health benefits may come from camu-camu.

The scientific world is just learning about camu-camu. However, anecdotal evidence supports the use of camu-camu for

- ✔ **Fighting depression.** The *Clinician's Handbook of Natural Healing* lists camu-camu as one of the top plants for balancing mood and treating depression. Vitamin C is also important for the production of *serotonin,* a brain chemical that affects your mood.

- ✔ **Improving attention.** Camu-camu may improve attention by improving neurotransmitter function. More research is required to determine exactly how — and how much — camu-camu improves attention.

✔ **Supporting your immune system.** Vitamin C is crucial for a healthy immune system, and anthocyanins work as antihistamines and anti-inflammatory agents. Camu-camu is loaded with both.

✔ **Hurting the herpes virus.** The *Clinician's Handbook of Natural Healing* points to camu-camu as being effective in battling the herpes family of viruses, which cause cold sores and shingles (the same virus that causes chicken pox), among other ailments.

Finding and using camu-camu

Camu-camu powder is available online at Sunfood.com and other Web sites. You may also purchase health drinks that contain camu-camu juice along with other healthful fruit juices. Camu-camu is sold in some health food stores as a powder, but you may not be able to find much camu-camu in local retail stores just yet.

Coca-Cola sells a beverage called Camu-Camu and Vitamins that's very popular in Japan, but it hasn't made its way to the United States yet. Most camu-camu is harvested in the wild and therefore is expensive. Full commercial production of camu-camu could take quite a few years, but when it does happen, the cost should drop considerably.

Although it's expensive, a little powder goes a long way. One serving of camu-camu is only ½ teaspoon, which you can mix with water or fruit juice. You can also stir your camu-camu into applesauce or add the powder to your favorite smoothie recipe. Drink powder and capsules can be stored at room temperature for several months.

Mexico's Chia Seeds

Chia is a member of the mint family and is native to Mexico, where it has been used for thousands of years in cooking. The ancient Aztecs and Mayans ate chia seeds before entering into battle or making long treks to sustain their energy, give them endurance, and control their appetites when food would be difficult to find. Even a small amount of seeds (as little as ¼ cup) was said to keep them satiated for a whole day. Chia seeds were once a major crop in Mexico; however, production was reduced after the Spanish Conquest.

Chia seeds are relatively unknown outside of Central America, but they're increasingly gaining recognition as a superfood and, no doubt, demand will grow as the word spreads.

Cashing in on the health benefits of chia

Chia is making a name for itself in nutrition due to its neutral flavor and the fact that it contains large amounts of an omega-3 fatty acid called *alpha-lino-lenic acid* (ALA), similar to the fats found in our superfood fish (see Chapter 7) and flax (see Chapter 6). In fact, chia seeds contain more omega-3 fats than flax seeds — and you don't have to grind them up first. This fatty acid helps your heart and makes it easier to watch your weight.

Chia seeds are rich in calcium, manganese, and fiber, which are important for strong bones and good digestion. Chia contains two antioxidants, *chlorogenic acid* and *caffeic acid,* which are also found in coffee beans. Chia has a high percentage of protein, and it has all the essential amino acids (the building blocks of protein), so it's a terrific source of protein for vegans.

There are two types of chia: black and white. Although the white seeds are harder to find and therefore more costly, there isn't much difference nutritionally. Both black and white chia seeds offer lots of nutrition in a small package. One serving of chia seeds is about 1 ounce and contains 10 grams of fiber and 139 calories.

When you eat chia seeds, you can feel good knowing that you are

- ✔ **Preventing cardiovascular disease.** A study in the 2007 *Journal of Diabetes Care* showed that regular chia consumption can lower blood pressure and reduce inflammation. The omega-3 fatty acids are great for lowering cholesterol, which also helps reduce your risk of cardiovascular disease.

- ✔ **Keeping your gut in check.** The fiber in chia is great for bowel regulation and overall gastrointestinal health. You can also use chia to reduce the pain of heartburn.

- ✔ **Watching your weight.** Chia helps you feel full longer because it's absorbed and metabolized slowly, which helps regulate *insulin* (a hormone that controls blood sugar) so that you won't feel a blood sugar drop that causes hunger. ALA may also make weight loss easier.

- ✔ **Controlling blood sugar.** Preventing and treating diabetes is all about blood sugar control and insulin regulation. Because chia is beneficial in both of these areas, it may aid in treatment of diabetes.

- ✔ **Getting an energy boost.** Chia seeds can absorb seven to ten times their weight in water, forming a gel that's digested slowly, which helps to keep energy levels high.

Incorporating chia in your diet

Chia seeds are easy to find online, and you may also find them in health food stores and other retail stores. Storing them is easy, too. Keep them at room temperature out of direct sunlight, and they'll keep for up to two years — that's one durable superfood.

There are several ways to get your daily dose of chia. Chia seeds have a neutral flavor, so they can be added to almost any type of food. You can sprinkle chia seeds on a salad or stir them into a soup. You can also add them to recipes for bread and muffins.

Alternatively, you can take 1 or 2 tablespoons of chia seeds or chia gel every day as a supplement. Make chia gel by adding 9 ounces of water to 1 ounce of chia seeds, and then mix until a gel forms. Let the gel stand at room temperature for 15 minutes, then store it in the refrigerator. Add the gel to fruit juice or a glass of water, or mix it into your morning bowl of oatmeal. The gel will keep in your refrigerator for up to two weeks.

 If you have one of those grassy little Chia Pets — the clay pots, often in the shape of cartoon characters, that come with a seed-laden paste and sprout a green mini-forest after a couple weeks — don't eat your pet's seeds, even though they're the same. Make sure the chia seeds you buy are packaged as a food product. You can eat the sprouts from your Chia Pet, but we don't recommend it because Chia Pet sprouts aren't approved as a food product by the U.S. Food and Drug Administration (FDA). Get your chia from a local health store. You can grow your own in a container garden, too; just make sure the seeds you use are labeled as a food product. See Chapter 14 for more information on container gardens.

Asia's Goji Berries

Goji (pronounced *go*-gee) berries, which is the commercial name for wolfberries, have been used in traditional Chinese medicine for thousands of years. True goji berries originate in Mongolia, but goji and wolfberries are very similar and hence are both considered goji berries. They're rich in antioxidants that help to protect the cells in your body. In fact, some experts believe they're even more powerful than blueberries, which are at the top of the superfood chart for antioxidant properties.

The goji berry plant is a member of the nightshade family, which includes another superfood, the tomato, as well as peppers, eggplants, and potatoes. Goji berries are very delicate and cannot withstand shipment as fresh fruits, so they're sold as juice or tea or in dried form (they resemble raisins, but with a lighter red color, see Figure 10-3). They have a slightly sour flavor, similar to cranberries or cherries (although some people think they taste more like plums).

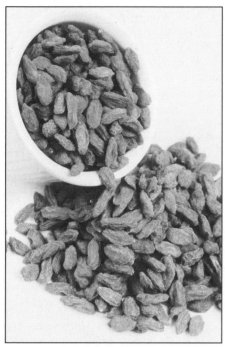

Figure 10-3:
Goji berries.

©Rosemary Calvert/Getty Images

The goji berry from Tibet has a sweeter flavor than the more bitter tasting wolfberries of China. Both are the same nutritionally. Most goji berries you'll find in the stores and online are wolfberries, and they will most commonly be cheaper than true goji berries.

Goji berries fall into the recommended five-to-nine daily servings of fruits and vegetables, but they're most often taken as a drink. We recommend 4 ounces of goji juice or one serving of berries daily.

Getting the goods on goji berries

Goji berries contain large amounts of phytochemical antioxidants like beta carotene and zeathanxin (which are related to vitamin A) and vitamin C. Goji berries are also rich in iron and fiber. Goji berry juice is packed with the same nutrients, but without the fiber. One ounce or 28 grams of goji berries has about 110 calories and 24 grams of carbohydrates.

Goji berries also contain the phytochemical *betaine* and a plant sterol called *beta-sitosterol*. Plant sterols are similar to the cholesterol found in animals, but sterols actually lower your cholesterol when you eat them. According to the March 2007 journal *Cellular and Molecular Neurobiology,* these compounds may also have powerful anti-aging effects by protecting your nerve cells and the retinas of your eyes.

Antioxidant effects on cancer

One of the most exciting health benefits of superfoods is their positive effects on cancer prevention and treatment. Many of the superfoods contain high levels of antioxidants, which are important for protecting cells from the damage created by free radicals. Free radicals are unstable molecules that travel through the body and can cause inflammation and cellular destruction. Antioxidants fight the free radicals and stabilize them to keep them from doing any more damage to the cells. Studies have supported that antioxidants can protect cells and reduce inflammation that can cause disease, including cancer. Large studies currently underway are looking specifically into the effects of antioxidants on cancer.

When you eat dried goji berries or drink goji berry juice, you may be

- ✔ **Preventing age-related macular degeneration.** The goji berry has high levels of the carotenoids beta-carotene and zeaxanthin, which are important for normal vision. Zeaxanthin helps protects the retina and may reduce the risk of age-related macular degeneration (AMD).

- ✔ **Fighting cancer.** The phytochemicals in goji berries may have powerful anti-cancer effects. One study published in the *Chinese Journal of Oncology* in 1994 found that goji berries had a positive effect on treatments when used along with other medical cancer regimens.

- ✔ **Helping with weight loss.** Your body needs betaine to make *choline* and *methionine* (natural compounds found in your body). Both these compounds are *lipotropic;* that is, they help to carry fat away from the liver and burn excess calories. Goji berries have an abundant amount of betaine.

- ✔ **Protecting your heart.** Beta-sitosterol helps lower cholesterol by blocking absorption of cholesterol in the gastrointestinal tract. The goji berry has also been found to increase the amount of a powerful antioxidant called *superoxide dismutase* (SOD), which your cells make as a natural defender against free radical damage. Betaine can help reduce high levels of *homocysteine,* a protein associated with a higher risk of heart disease and inflammation.

- ✔ **Boosting your libido.** Goji is thought to help raise testosterone levels in both men and women, thereby increasing your sex drive. Beta-sitosterol may also help to prevent or reduce swelling of the prostate in men.

The goji berry has blood-thinning properties, so talk to your doctor *before* you add goji berries to your diet. This is especially important if you take any heart medications or blood thinners.

Getting your goji berries

You may not find these berries at your local grocery store, but you can find them online, at some health food stores, and at herbalists' shops. (See Chapter 13 for tips on shopping for superfoods.) If you want to try goji juice, be prepared for some sticker-shock; it's very expensive.

Dried goji berries make a delicious snack just as they are, or you can use them to make your own granola, similar to our superfood granola in Chapter 16. Just add a few dried goji berries with the dried cranberries. You can also use goji berries in any recipe that calls for raisins. Add them to your morning oatmeal, or mix them into your next batch of muffins.

Dried goji berries keep for several months when stored at room temperature in a dry, dark place. If you soak the berries for eating, use them the same day you soak them; they spoil quickly after being exposed to water. Many goji juices will keep for 30 days when refrigerated, but check for brand differences after opening.

You can also get your goji as an extract or supplement, which is a convenient way to boost your daily antioxidant intake.

Thailand's Mangosteen

Mangosteen, known as the "queen of fruits" because Queen Victoria supposedly offered handsome rewards to those who brought her the fresh fruit, comes from a tree that grows in the southeast Asian countries of Indonesia, Sri Lanka, Malaysia, Philippines, and Thailand. The tree grows to be about 50 to 80 feet tall, and the fruit is about the size of a tangerine.

The white *aril* (the fleshy pulp) of the mangosteen is sweet and tangy and is very popular for its taste. The aril resembles a peeled citrus fruit with four to eight wedged segments. A thick maroon rind surrounds the white aril. See Figure 10-4.

The mango isn't a mangosteen

Although the word "mango" is in the name, there's no relationship between mangoes and the mangosteen fruit. Mangoes, which are also popular in southeast Asia, are red to yellowish fruits with a sweet golden flesh — and they're quite healthful as well. While mangoes used to be considered rare and exotic fruits, they're now commonly available in grocery stores.

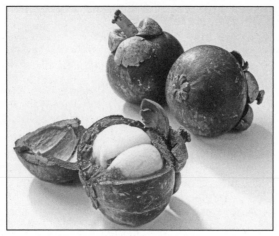

Figure 10-4:
Mango-
steens.

©Teubner/Getty Images

When the mangosteen is ripe, both the rind and pulp are used for medicinal purposes. Mangosteens have been used in traditional Asian medicine to treat digestive disorders, infections, wounds, and ulcers. The thick maroon rind contains most of the antioxidants that make mangosteen so super.

Zeroing in on xanthones

This exotic superfood contains a high concentration of *polyphenols* (compounds found in some plants that have health benefits) called *xanthones.* There are 40 different xanthones in the mangosteen that may exert some antioxidant effects. These powerful compounds go throughout your body, destroying free radicals that can cause inflammation and disease. The main xanthones are beta-, gamma-, and alpha-mangostin, and garcinone.

And that's not all. According to a review in the October 2008 issue of the journal *Food and Chemical Toxicology,* the xanthones found in mangosteen also exhibit anti-cancer, anti-allergy, antibacterial, and antiviral properties — at least in the lab. Adding mangosteen to your superfoods diet may prove to be very beneficial to your health. One cup (196 grams) of mangosteen contains 140 calories and about 35 grams of carbohydrates.

In order to reap the benefits of the xanthones, you need to find mangosteen juice or purée that includes the whole fruit. The white aril is delicious and does contain some vitamins and minerals, but the powerful polyphenols are in the maroon rind.

When you drink mangosteen juice or purée, you may improve your health by

- **Keeping your digestive system healthy.** The rind may be dried and ground into a powder to help with diarrheal illnesses and may be beneficial for other gastrointestinal disorders as well.

- **Fighting microbes.** Several of the xanthones have antibacterial properties. Some of the extracts have been found to stop the growth of fungi and viruses as well. According to research performed in Thailand, mangosteen may also inhibit the organisms that cause tuberculosis.

- **Lowering cholesterol.** The xanthones keep the bad cholesterol (LDL, or low density lipoproteins) from sticking to your blood vessels, which reduces your risk for *atherosclerosis* (clogged arteries). Atherosclerosis can lead to cardiovascular disease.

- **Fighting cancer?** A Dutch study found that the rind was able to reduce cancer growth in rats, but no human studies have been performed. There is plenty of evidence to support further studies on the potential for treating cancer.

- **Caring for your skin.** Well . . . not by eating it, but by using mangosteen topically. The rind contains *tannins* (polyphenols that tighten mucous membranes and skin — also found in tea and red wine). When the rind is ground into a powder, the tannins can be used as an astringent for wound care. The extracts have also been used to treat eczema and other skin diseases. In some countries, mangosteen is mixed with a few other substances for use after circumcision.

- **Alleviating allergies.** The xanthones, especially gamma-mangostin, have been found to have antihistamine properties, which, along with the anti-inflammatory effects, make drinking mangosteen a good option for relieving some symptoms of airborne allergies.

Some allergies are life-threatening. Don't expect mangosteen to protect you from exposure to peanuts or other similar, dangerous allergies.

Getting your hands on mangosteen

Fresh mangosteen fruits are available at Asian markets. Look for mangosteens that are a rich purple or maroon with healthy green stems. Mangosteen also is sold as a juice, purée, or supplement online and in some health food stores and retail stores such as Costco. Pure mangosteen juice is expensive, so it's usually mixed with other fruit juices. One of the first mangosteen drinks was a beverage called XanGo.

Because the beneficial antioxidants come from the not-so-tasty rind, many people prefer to get their mangosteen in supplement form. If you choose supplements, be sure to follow the instructions on the label.

You can prepare fresh mangosteens by cutting through the rind around the middle of the fruit. Pry open the rind to find the beautiful white arils inside. If stored in a dry, dark area at room temperature, the fruit can keep for about three weeks; a ripe fruit can last a month in the refrigerator. Mangosteen juices typically stay fresh for several days, but refer to directions on individual bottles.

North America's Wheat Grass

Wheat grass is a homegrown superfood that has been quietly used as a superfood juice and supplement since the 1930s. Wheat grass is simply the green, grassy portion of wheat that's harvested while the plants are young, within two weeks of sprouting. Wheat grass is an excellent source of vitamins, amino acids, and enzymes. There's anecdotal evidence that wheat grass helps to detoxify your body, helps heal your digestive system, and gives you a boost of energy.

Harnessing the power of wheat grass

Wheat grass is rich in nutrients and chlorophyll, the substance that gives wheat grass its green color. Wheat grass is also rich in enzymes called *glutathione peroxidase* and *catalase*, which may increase your levels of SOD — an enzyme in the body that acts as a natural antioxidant and targets a specific free radical that can damage cells. This is important because you can't take SOD as a dietary supplement; you need to get the enzymes to make SOD from your diet.

A typical dose of wheat grass is 3.5 grams of powder or a 1-ounce shot of wheat-grass juice. Wheat grass contains vitamin A, B complex vitamins, vitamin C, vitamin K, iron, and potassium. When you drink a shot of wheat-grass juice, you not only boost your energy, you boost your nutrient intake too. And all for only five calories per ounce.

Getting a 1-ounce serving of wheat-grass juice may improve your health by

✔ **Healing your digestive tract.** An article published in 2002 in the *Scandinavian Journal of Gastroenterology* found that wheat grass was beneficial for the treatment of individuals with *ulcerative colitis* — an inflammatory disease of the colon — as well as other diseases of the gastrointestinal tract.

✔ **Caring for wounds.** Chlorophyll has antibacterial properties that stimulate the healing of wounds.

✔ **Making you more energetic.** More than 60 years of research has been performed that compares chlorophyll and the oxygen carrier in the blood called *hemoglobin*. Drinking wheat-grass juice may improve the oxygen-carrying capacity of blood and help increase your red blood cell count.

✔ **Preventing cancer.** Because SOD is a powerful antioxidant that protects your cells from damage due to free radicals, it may help to reduce your risk of some forms of cancer.

Buying or growing wheat grass

Wheat grass has a natural fiber content that isn't digestible in humans, so it has to be juiced to get the benefits of its phytochemicals and nutrients. Wheat grass can also be dried and used as a supplement.

You can buy wheat grass as a juice, powder, or in tablets or capsules that may be taken as dietary supplements. It's available in many retail stores, health food stores, and online.

You can grow wheat grass at home with kits available in stores and online. Wheat grass makes a nice addition to any indoor superfoods garden. See Chapter 14 for more information on growing your own superfoods.

You can drink wheat-grass juice alone or mix it with fruit or vegetable juices and other healthful beverages. You can make your own superfood smoothie by blending one banana with some frozen blueberries and cranberries, plus a little applesauce and a shot of wheat grass.

You can also find "wheat-grass boosters" at juice bars and places that sell fruit smoothies, where supplemental wheat grass is added in order to boost your energy.

Part III

Launching Your Superfoods Lifestyle

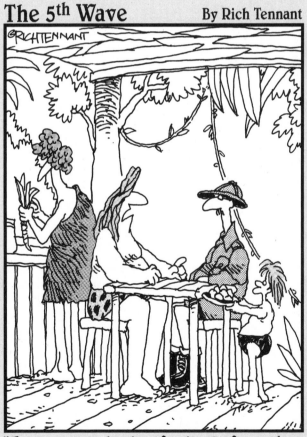

The 5th Wave   By Rich Tennant

"Jane start drying fruit. Before that we just eat cheetah. Too much fast food not good."

In this part . . .

Knowing which foods are superfoods is one thing; getting them into your diet is another. In this part, we give you tips and ideas for incorporating superfoods into your dietary routine and show you how to get your whole family involved.

We help you create a shopping list and tell you where and how to find the items on that list. And, for those interested in gardening, we show you how to grow some of your own superfoods right in your own backyard.

Chapter 11

Bringing Superfoods into Your Life

In This Chapter

▶ Getting superfoods into your diet

▶ Figuring out how much to eat

▶ Finding superfoods in restaurants

Choosing superfoods is beneficial no matter what the rest of your diet is like, but the results are magnified when those superfoods are incorporated into a diet that's healthful overall.

Getting started isn't all that difficult, and, once you get moving along, you'll want to keep your superfoods diet going, even at restaurants and parties. In this chapter, we show you how to incorporate superfoods into your lifestyle — at home, at work, or at play.

Transforming Your Diet into a Superfoods Diet

A superfoods diet isn't like a fad diet or crash diet that requires you to give up or severely restrict any nutrients. A healthy diet includes foods of all kinds, because when you eliminate certain food groups or nutrients (such as bread and cereals, carbohydrates, or fats), you feel deprived, and then you go off whatever diet you were on. By choosing a superfoods diet, you reduce the amounts of not-so-healthy foods you eat, and focus on adding lots of healthy (and delicious) foods from all the food groups.

The changes you make in your diet will last your whole life. You do need to sacrifice a little bit, like cutting way back on eating greasy processed foods and sugary snacks, but the payback is enjoying a healthy, youthful body. And when your superfoods diet has you feeling healthy and energetic, you won't really miss the junk foods at all.

Making the shift: Identifying the foods you should eat more or less of

Start with a basic healthy diet. Eat less of the foods that are bad for you and more of the foods that are good for you. First, restrict these foods:

- **Extra added sugar, including sucrose and high fructose corn syrup:** Replace regular soda with caffeine-free diet soda or water. Cut back on candy, pastries, and other sweets. Sweeteners add calories fast but don't add any nutrition, so don't consume more than 3 tablespoons of sugar, high fructose corn syrup, or honey per day (one can of soda has about $3^1/_2$ tablespoons of sweetener). Replace empty sugar calories with superfood fruits that are naturally sweet, and you won't miss the sugar.

- **Saturated and trans fats:** Cut back on fatty red meats, switch to nonfat milk, and avoid processed foods and stick margarines that have "partially hydrogenated oil" as an ingredient. Choose seafood, skinless chicken, turkey, lean beef, and pork, but avoid anything that's deep-fried. Substitute superfood fish and legumes for red meats in order to get the protein you need without the unhealthy saturated fats. Replace trans-fat-laden stick margarine with olive oil or with margarines made with olive oil, flax oil, or canola oil (without partial dehydrogenation).

- **Extra sodium:** It's okay to sprinkle some salt on your foods (some experts think unprocessed sea salt is best), but watch out for extra salt and sodium hidden in highly processed and canned foods and most boxed meal mixes. Superfoods in their natural forms are low in sodium. Look for low-sodium versions of canned foods (even superfoods), or opt for fresh or frozen whenever possible.

Replace the restricted items in the preceding list with healthier alternatives by eating more of these:

- **Healthy fats:** Eat foods rich in omega-3 fatty acids, such as fish, flax, chia, pumpkin seeds, and canola oil. Choose olive oil, avocado, and nuts for healthy polyunsaturated and monounsaturated fats.

- **Fiber:** Increase your intake of fruits, vegetables, and whole grains. Most days you should choose more vegetables than fruits. And consume whole-grain breads, cereals, and pasta to add much-needed fiber.

- **Healthy proteins:** The best protein sources include all meats, seafood, eggs, dairy products, nuts, and legumes. What makes a protein source healthful is not so much the type of protein, but how that source is prepared. For example, grilled shrimp is good, but shrimp scampi is high in saturated fat and bad for your heart and arteries. A skinless chicken breast is good, but deep-fried chicken is not so good because the batter adds extra fat and calories.

Keeping a food diary

People who keep track of the foods they eat in food diaries lose more weight than people who don't used food diaries, and the note-takers are more likely to keep off the weight. A food diary can be as simple as a little notebook you carry with you so you can write down all the foods you eat and the beverages you drink every day. Make a note of the portion sizes, too. Keeping a diary shows you whether you're getting enough fruits and vegetables, whole grains, and other healthful foods. You also know whether you're eating too many unhealthy foods.

You can get a little fancier with your food diary by keeping track of calories. (You can find calorie counts online at Web sites like `calorie count.about.com` or `www.nutrition data.com`, or pick up a calorie book at your local bookstore.) You also can keep track of the number of grams of fat, sugars, and sodium you consume. Go high-tech and use the pyramid tracker at `mypyramid.gov`, or join a group on a dieting Web site that allows you to enter the foods you eat and get the math done for you, instantly. Some sites even let you enter your foods from your cellphone, which is very convenient when you're on the run.

Calories matter. If you want to lose weight, you have to cut calories from your diet or exercise more — preferably both. If you want to gain weight, you need to add a few calories (from healthful foods) every day. Use a food diary to track your calorie consumption (see the sidebar "Keeping a food diary" for help).

Fitting in superfoods every day

We suggest that you eat at least two superfoods each day as you start your superfoods diet. Eat one at breakfast or as a snack, and eat another at lunch or dinner. When this becomes a habit, add a third superfood, and eventually a fourth. As you get used to choosing nutritious foods for every meal, many of your choices will automatically be superfoods.

Looking at your dietary needs for a typical day, you can see how easily superfoods can fit in. The United Stated Department of Agriculture (USDA) has designed a food pyramid to help you figure out how many foods you need to eat from each food group every day. Here's what the food pyramid calls for:

 ✔ **Six to eleven servings from the bread and cereal group:** At least half of these servings should be whole grains. Our superfoods grains — oats and quinoa — fit in nicely here. Other good choices include 100 percent whole wheat, spelt (which is similar to wheat), popcorn, cornmeal, brown rice, and barley.

 ✔ **Five to nine servings of fruits and vegetables:** All fruits and vegetables are good for you and can fulfill your daily need for this food group. It's best to choose a few more vegetables than fruits. For example, three servings of vegetables and two servings of fruit is fine for a smaller woman; a large man can eat five servings of vegetables and four servings of fruit. Our superfood fruits and vegetables are even better, because they're rich in extra nutrients and fiber.

✔ **Three servings of dairy or calcium-fortified foods:** Yogurt is really quite good for you because it contains *probiotics* (friendly bacteria that keep your gut healthy). Yogurt works with superfoods, too, because it goes very well with added fruit and nuts. Orange juice fortified with calcium is readily available, so it fits into this food group, too.

✔ **Two to three servings of meat and dry beans:** The best meats for this category are low-fat meats, so lean beef, pork, eggs, skinless chicken, turkey, fish, and seafood are good choices. Superfoods for this group include salmon, tuna, sardines, trout, and legumes.

✔ **Fats and oils:** You get the fats that you need from the foods you eat, including fish, meats, nuts, seeds, dressings, and any cooking oil you use. Here, fish does double duty as a superfood protein source and a healthful fat. Other good fats come from a variety of superfoods, including flax, pumpkin seeds, olive oil, avocado, and chia.

✔ **Discretionary calories:** This is where your treats — sodas, cookies, cakes, and candy — fit in, and the allotment is only about 100 to 200 calories per day. It's not much (we hate to break it to you, but a typical candy bar is 200 to 300 calories), but a little bit of these treats can keep cravings at bay so you don't feel deprived. Choose your superfood treats wisely. For example, enjoy 1 ounce of dark chocolate or one 5-ounce glass of wine, but don't overdo it.

Pump up the amount of fruits and vegetables you eat every day, because this is the easiest way to add more superfoods — almost automatically — given that many typical fruits and vegetables are superfoods.

Portion control: Determining what constitutes a serving

Understanding serving sizes is crucial for controlling portion sizes and getting enough (or avoiding getting too much) of certain foods. *Portion distortion,* or eating huge helpings of food, is one of the reasons people gain too much weight. Portion control is important for *energy-dense foods* (foods high in calories) such as nuts, seeds, and starchy foods like potatoes and pasta. It's even more important for snacks and junk food; one portion of tortilla chips is about 14 chips, not a whole big bag.

Servings are measured in ounces, cups, teaspoons, and tablespoons. We recommend that you purchase an inexpensive kitchen scale and some measuring cups and spoons to measure your daily servings. Also be sure to read the Nutrition Facts labels on packaged foods, which are sometimes a little misleading. For example, a can of condensed soup mixed with water is probably three servings, not just one. Even many "single-serving" microwavable soups actually contain two servings.

A serving and a portion are not necessarily the same. A *serving* is a measured amount, such as an 8-ounce glass of milk or ¹/₂ cup of sliced fruit. A *portion* is the amount of food that you choose to eat or that someone serves you. So while that giant bagel you buy at the coffee shop is only one *portion,* it may really be equal to four or five *servings* from the bread and cereal group. The following list identifies what constitutes a serving of some common foods:

- ✔ **Fruits:** One serving of fruit is equal to ¹/₂ cup of sliced fruit, or half of a large whole fruit. Half a cup is about the size of a baseball. One serving of dried fruit is smaller because it has been dehydrated. A serving of dried fruit is about the size of a golf ball.

- ✔ **Vegetables:** One serving of vegetables is also ¹/₂ cup, the size of a baseball. Because green leafy vegetables are so low in calories, one serving is about 1 to 2 cups.

- ✔ **Breads and cereals:** One slice of bread counts as a serving in the cereal group. A serving of rice or pasta equals ¹/₂ cup — again, about the size of a baseball (think of that plate of spaghetti — that's likely to be multiple servings).

- ✔ **Fats and oils:** One serving of oil or fat is 1 teaspoon, which is about the size of the tip of your thumb. Many of your fats are found in your protein sources, like nuts. One serving of nuts is 1 ounce. That's equal to 25 almonds or 9 walnuts.

- ✔ **Proteins:** One serving of protein is equal to 3 ounces of meat, fish, or poultry, which is about the size of a deck of cards (that big rib-eye at the steakhouse is about three servings). A serving of a thinner fillet of fish is about the size of a checkbook. One egg is equal to one protein serving, and one serving of legumes is ¹/₂ cup, about the size of a baseball.

When you're eating packaged foods, you can figure out how much of it constitutes one serving by taking a look at the Nutrition Facts label on the package. The USDA requires nutrition facts labeling on all packaged foods, based on servings per package. The Food and Drug Administration (FDA) allows common measurements to be used on the labels, such as cup, tablespoon, or teaspoon; or less specific measurements such as piece, slice, or fraction; or even to designate the containers themselves, such as a jar or bottle. Ounces may be used as a serving size, but only if a common household unit is not applicable and an appropriate visual unit is given, such as "1 oz chips = about 15 chips." See Chapter 13 for more in-depth info on deciphering package labels.

Think about these different serving sizes and how they vary from the portions you receive in restaurants (or maybe serve at home). When you're faced with a big plate of food at a restaurant, ask to have part of it wrapped up to go home with you. At home, you can control portion sizes by dishing up individual plates, rather than serving *family style* (with lots of bowls of food on the table), which leads to a lot of second and third helpings. Remember that calories count, and even too much of a superfood can lead to weight gain from extra calories.

Getting the right number of superfood servings

Getting the right number of servings is important for getting enough nutrition without getting too many (or too few) calories. Most of our superfoods are low in calories (fish, fruits, and vegetables), so that actually allows for more servings rather than fewer. However, you still need to be careful with some of our superfoods, such as the nuts and oils that can rack up the calories fast if you eat too much.

Volumes of veggies

Let's start with the foods you can eat a lot of — those delicious vegetables. All our superfood vegetables are low in calories because they're high in fiber (see Chapter 5). For example, one medium tomato has only about 25 calories, but it's packed with nutrients such as vitamin C and lutein (a powerful anti-oxidant). Green and other colorful vegetables are also low in calories, while being high in fiber and nutrients.

Eat several servings of vegetables every day. The USDA food pyramid suggests 2 cups at a minimum (at least three servings), but, for good health, you can eat much more than that — 4 cups each day of low-calorie vegetables are good for you and are a great way to eat your superfood vegetables.

Scores of fruits

You can also eat many servings of fruit as long as they're whole fruits or used as ingredients in healthy recipes. An apple is good for you; a piece of apple pie isn't, because pie has a lot of added sugar, fat, and calories. On the other hand, our Baked Apples (see Chapter 19) are a good option for getting more fruit in your diet with just a little extra sugar.

Fruit generally has a few more calories than vegetables, so you may want to keep that in mind if you're watching calories closely. An orange or an apple has about 80 calories. That's more than a tomato, but way less than a candy bar.

The USDA food pyramid includes about 1½ to 2 cups of fruit in a balanced diet (three to four of your daily five to nine servings of fruits and vegetables). That's about the same as eating one apple and half a banana. But because fruits are so good for you, feel free to eat 2½ to 3 cups every day.

Being smart with fish

Our superfood fish are rich in omega-3 fatty acids (see Chapter 7), and we agree with the American Heart Association recommendation that you should eat fish at least twice per week. Our superfood fish are all low in mercury, but there are valid concerns about mercury toxicity in fish, so it may be smart to limit your weekly intake to about 12 ounces, or three to four servings, each week.

Picking fats prudently

Nuts such as almonds and walnuts are so delicious that it's easy to get carried away when you eat them. Although the fats they contain are healthful fats, they also contain calories that need to be counted if you're watching your weight. If you want to lose weight, limit your servings of nuts and seeds to just one per day (about 25 almonds or 9 walnuts) and use them as one of your daily servings in the meat and beans category.

If you need to gain weight, eating extra servings of nuts is a good way to get extra nutritious calories — much better than choosing empty-calorie junk foods.

Olive oil is another one of our superfoods because the fats it contains are good for your heart (see Chapter 9). But olive oil is also high in calories. It's important to balance the healthful properties of good fats with the extra calories that can lead to weight gain, so measure olive oil carefully when you use it. Don't drench your salad with olive oil, for example; just give it a light drizzle.

Being cautious with two superfoods

Dark chocolate and red wine both contain beneficial phenols (see Chapter 9), but they need to be enjoyed in moderation. Cocoa is the magic ingredient in dark chocolate that makes it so good for you, but chocolate is usually eaten as that delicious confection called the candy bar, with added sugar and fats.

You don't need much dark chocolate — only about 1 ounce each day, or one small square of a dark chocolate candy bar. If you eat more than that, the calories and the sugar add up fast.

Red wine is another superfood that needs to be consumed wisely (see Chapter 9). We recommend no more than 5 ounces of red wine on any day. And if you don't drink alcohol, we don't want you to start. There are other ways to get those healthy phytochemicals.

Alcohol should not be consumed by women who are pregnant or nursing, people with a history or high risk of alcoholism, or people who are not of legal age to consume alcohol.

A little bit of alcohol may be beneficial, but more is definitely not better. Should you choose to enjoy red wine as a superfood, please do so responsibly.

Taking inventory

Look through your refrigerator, freezer, and cabinets and take an inventory of what's there. Dry beans, vegetables, fruits, seafood, and whole grains are good; you want to keep those. But do you also find lots of potato chips, pastries, ramen noodles, tortilla chips, candies, and ice cream? Those aren't so good. If you don't have the heart to throw them out, that's okay; just don't replace them with the same foods when they're gone. When that potato chip bag goes in the garbage, use the empty space to house a bunch of bananas or a few cans of tuna instead.

To remind yourself to buy foods that are good for you (and avoid the bad ones), make a shopping list. (You can find out lots more about shopping for superfoods in Chapter 13.) Using a shopping list keeps you on track with your superfoods diet and out of the junk food aisles.

Adding Superfoods to Your Meals

Another important step in getting started with a superfoods diet is getting those superfoods into your meals. Some of your favorite recipes may already have superfoods as ingredients (those are good to keep) and you can browse through our recipes in Chapters 16–19 to get more ideas.

So what do you do with the recipes that don't have any superfoods in them? Many recipes can be made healthier by substituting superfoods for ingredients that aren't so healthy. For example, many baked goods taste just as good when you replace some of the fat with applesauce. Or you can replace some flour with dry oatmeal (see our Salmon Cakes in Chapter 19). Another easy substitution is olive oil for regular vegetable oils.

If some of your favorite recipes just don't allow for substitutions, how about some additions? A plain muffin gets healthier when blueberries or dried cranberries and chopped pecans are added. Or sprinkle some chopped almonds on your favorite vegetable dishes. Top your oatmeal, vegetable side dishes, and salads with ground chia or flax seeds to add extra nutrition and nutty flavor.

Make superfoods a part of every meal: breakfast, lunch, and dinner. In the next three sections, we show you how.

Expanding the definition of breakfast

There isn't any reason why you need to eat "breakfast" foods in the morning — you can eat fish, chicken, or even whole-grain pasta if you prefer. A breakfast with plenty of protein (and much less sugar) keeps you feeling full and energetic all morning. So if you want to eat dinner foods at breakfast time, go ahead.

Starting your day with superfoods

Breakfast is a good time to get some superfoods into your stomach, which is a great way to start your day. Breakfast eaters tend to be more successful at watching their weight, and kids who eat breakfast do better in school. But remember, not any old breakfast foods will do. Typical breakfast foods usually include lots of sugar and fat. Pastries, sugary cereals, pancakes with syrup, sausages, and greasy eggs all taste good, but revising your menu to incorporate superfoods makes your breakfast much healthier.

If you're used to eating sweet stuff in the morning, reduce the sugar and get your sweetness fix from superfood fruits. Instead of sugar-frosted breakfast flakes, eat a bowl of whole-grain cereal topped with lots of berries or banana slices. (If you choose oatmeal to go with those berries, you already have two superfoods.)

You can make your omelets into superfood omelets when you cut back on the cheese and meats and add lots of vegetables like tomatoes, spinach, or broccoli. Check out Chapter 16 for our superfood breakfast recipes.

Need your morning caffeine fix? Switch out your coffee for green tea, which has antioxidants that may prevent cancer (see Chapter 9) and still has a little caffeine to perk you up.

If you regularly sleep in and skip breakfast, use the superfoods to get you into the healthy habit of eating something before work or school. You don't need to start eating a massive breakfast; just grab a banana and a handful of pecans, and you're ready to head out the door.

Packing healthier lunches

Lunch may mean eating at restaurants, cafeterias, or packing your lunch. We talk about restaurants later in this chapter; here we focus on lunches that you pack yourself.

Save money and get good nutrition by taking your lunch to work or school at least three days each week.

Sandwiches can be made with whole-grain bread (including oatmeal or nuts as ingredients), and you can add an extra slice of tomato or use spinach leaves in place of lettuce. Toss out the chips and pack crunchy vegetables instead.

When you want a change of pace from sandwiches, you can pack vegetable soup (use an insulated soup container if you don't have a refrigerator and microwave handy). If you have a refrigerator and microwave at work, then you can bring leftover salmon from dinner the night before. You can also pack a salad in a plastic container. Choose any of our superfood vegetables and fruits, plus some nuts (and maybe a little bit of cheese). Pour your salad dressing into a separate container or zip-top bag so your salad isn't soggy by lunchtime.

Round out your superfoods lunch with a healthy beverage. Dump the sugary soda and have 100 percent fruit or vegetable juice instead. Many varieties are available in single-serving bottles.

Keep healthy snacks at work so you won't find yourself raiding the vending machines. Dried fruits and nuts keep well and are very portable so you can take them wherever you go.

Remember that superfoods are good for kids, too, so send healthy lunches to school. Or, if your children eat in the cafeteria, urge them to choose some fruits and vegetables at lunchtime. Of course, we know kids don't always make the best choices on their own, so make sure they get their superfoods at breakfast and dinner.

Serving super dinner dishes

There are several ways to get superfoods into your dinners. Consider these options:

- ✔ Start your dinner with a healthy garden salad made with superfood vegetables on spinach leaves and topped with a few chopped nuts. You can even serve a big salad as a meal in itself.

- ✔ Serve a soup before dinner, like a vegetable stew.

- ✔ Choose superfoods as side dishes. A superfoods side dish can be as simple as steamed broccoli with a little lemon, or a bit fancier, like Creamy Feta Spinach (see Chapter 18). Make your side dishes colorful — it's the color in vegetables that adds so much of the extra antioxidant protection.

✔ Use superfood fish (see Chapter 7) for a variety of main dishes. Salmon is particularly good because of its high omega-3 fatty acid content. Tuna is good, and so is trout, so you can eat lots of fish and still have a variety of flavors.

✔ Bring superfoods to dinner with dessert. Our Baked Apples (see Chapter 19) are deliciously sweet with only a little added sugar. You can also serve berries and cream for a delicious and super-nutritious dessert.

When you plan dinner, divide your plate into four equal sections. One quarter is for your serving of protein, usually meat, poultry, or fish. Another section is for something starchy like potatoes or rice. The other half of the plate is for green and colorful vegetables, such as beets, carrots, and broccoli.

Facing objections from other family members? Many people have a natural resistance to change, even when it's for the better. See Chapter 12 for ideas on how to get everyone onboard.

Eating Out with Superfoods

Americans spend about half of their food dollars in restaurants. People eat out for convenience, because they travel a lot, and sometimes just for fun. While it's easy to go to a restaurant (or bring home take-out), it's important to remember two things: Many menu selections are high in calories, and they're served in huge portions.

Frequently dining out probably isn't the best way to maintain a healthy diet. But if you do eat many of your meals out, you can make better menu choices and even find a few superfoods in restaurants.

Finding fast-food superfood

Fast-food restaurants are everywhere, with a variety of specialties — hamburger places, hot dog stands, chicken places, ice cream stands, and sandwich shops, just to name a few. Usually, fast-food joints serve the meals with the most calories and the poorest nutrition.

So why do people eat them? Because they're cheap, convenient, and tasty. Our best advice is to avoid fast-food places when you can. When you need to eat fast food, choose small portions and look for superfoods. Finding superfoods at fast-food places is a little easier today than it was a couple of decades ago.

The best fast-food restaurants are the sub sandwich shops. There, you can choose lean meats, including tuna, and add tomatoes along with other vegetables. Opt for just a little dressing — sub shops usually don't use healthy oils.

Here are some tips for finding superfoods at fast-food restaurants:

- ✔ Choose a side salad or fruit, like apple slices, instead of greasy fries.
- ✔ Order apple or orange juice instead of soda.
- ✔ Eat a meal-sized salad for lunch.

Not all salads sold at fast-food restaurants are healthy. Taco salads are usually very high in calories and fat, as are salads topped with fried chicken strips. Look for salads with grilled, low-fat meats, or just fruits and vegetables.

Ordering superfoods at sit-down restaurants

Sit-down restaurants usually have more menu choices than fast-food restaurants. This is good because more healthy foods are available, but it's also bad because lots of unhealthy (but delicious) choices are offered too. The key to eating a superfoods diet in a sit-down restaurant is to choose wisely and not be tempted by the unhealthy foods.

Here are some tips for finding superfoods at sit-down restaurants:

- ✔ **Look for superfoods in the salads.** Many restaurants offer a variety of interesting and healthful salads. If the restaurant has a salad bar, be sure to take advantage of it by loading up on superfoods.
- ✔ **Ask what the vegetable of the day is when one is offered.**
- ✔ **Check out the soup of the day.** Vegetable soups are healthy and filling.
- ✔ **Order fish that has been baked or broiled.** Look for our superfood fish such as salmon, tuna, and trout, which are often sold at restaurants.
- ✔ **Look for vegetarian meals, which often include some superfoods.**
- ✔ **Ask for fruit for dessert.**

Many sit-down restaurants serve their meals in such large portions that it's easy to eat too much. When you eat out, ask to have half of your main meal wrapped to take home, or share your meal with a dining partner.

Seeking out superfoods at parties

Parties are a lot of fun and they usually include food and drink — sometimes a lot of food and drink — especially during the holiday season. Many people gain a pound or two each year between Thanksgiving and Christmas and never lose that extra weight. After a few years, that adds up.

Your superfoods diet will get you through parties. To ensure your success at staying the course, keep the following tips in mind:

✔ Avoid high-calorie sweets.

✔ Eat a small, high-fiber, superfood snack before you go, such as an apple, an orange, or a handful of nuts. Don't go to the party starving; you'll overeat and choose the wrong stuff.

✔ Don't stand by the buffet. Enjoy conversation with friends away from the food and the temptation.

✔ Look for foods that have lots of colorful fruits and vegetables, especially the fresh vegetables and dip.

✔ At a sit-down dinner party, don't take seconds of the turkey and gravy; have some extra broccoli or carrots if you're still hungry.

✔ Bring a superfoods side dish or appetizer (see Chapters 18 and 19) and show your friends and family that eating healthy foods doesn't mean you have to forfeit taste.

Chapter 12

Getting Your Family Onboard

Superfoods are good for family members of all ages, from kids to grand-parents. The growing bodies and minds of children need superfoods to feel good and do well in school. As parents and grandparents grow older, they don't need as much food, but the food they eat has to provide the right nutrients to age gracefully and stay healthy.

Getting your family to actually eat superfoods, though, can be challenging. Some members of your family may be excited about eating healthful foods, but others may not be quite ready for radical dietary changes. That's okay; there are ways to include everyone in a superfoods diet, even if just a little bit.

Fortunately, there are lots of superfoods, and they offer a bountiful variety of flavors and textures. That makes it easier to find superfoods that please everybody, even the pickiest kids and the grumpiest grandparents. Maybe getting your whole family onboard seems daunting, but don't worry. With a few tips, you'll have everyone eating better. In this chapter, we explain how to get superfoods into the diets of your family members.

Gathering for Family Meals

Many families have very demanding schedules with everyone heading in a different direction, so it may be difficult to monitor what foods everyone is eating all the time. Your family members may skip some meals or choose sugary snacks and sodas during the day. And that makes eating together even more important. When you share a family meal, you get the opportunity to provide healthful superfoods to everyone — at least for that meal.

Dinner may be the easiest meal for everyone to attend, or maybe breakfast time works better for your family. Either is fine, because it isn't the time of day that matters — it's the time together.

Ideally, you should have at least one meal together every day. In the real world, though, that isn't always possible. Don't worry if you can only get everybody together two or three times a week. Instead, focus on fitting in as many superfood-friendly family meals during your week as you can.

Understanding the importance of eating together

Families who eat meals together get more than nutritious meals with lots of superfoods — they also fare better emotionally. For many busy families, meals provide the only regular opportunity to catch up on each other's lives. Also, teenagers are less likely to suffer from eating disorders when the family shares meals. Family mealtime is a great time to reinforce table manners, how to share, and how to enjoy conversation with other people.

According to research done at the National Center on Addiction and Substance Abuse, kids who eat meals together with their family regularly have a lower risk of drug abuse, are less likely to smoke, and are less likely to be depressed.

Eating with friends and family is important for adults, too (especially for older adults). People tend to eat less when they're alone, which is one reason why malnutrition is more common in elderly people who live alone.

Adding superfoods to family meals

When you cook the family dinner, you get to decide what is served. What a great time to get some superfoods into everyone's diet! Here are some suggestions for adding superfoods to your family's menu:

- ✔ Start meals with a hearty soup, such as tomato bisque or bean soup.
- ✔ Serve a salad before a meal (or make it big and serve it as a meal). Salads are a great way to get lots of superfood fruits, vegetables, and nuts into a meal.
- ✔ Serve more fish and less red meat. Heart-healthy salmon, tuna, and trout are rich in omega-3 fatty acids and low in saturated fat.
- ✔ Add super side dishes such as kale, broccoli, carrots, or beets.
- ✔ Ditch the sugary desserts and enjoy fresh fruits and berries instead.

For more specific ideas, turn to Chapters 16–19 where we provide lots of delicious superfood recipes that are easy to incorporate into your menus and your lifestyle.

Planning Ahead for Your Family

It would be nice to be able to eat every meal together as a family, but that isn't possible. You may have different school and work schedules, and sports, clubs, and other activities may keep you busy at night. However, while you can't have everyone together for every meal, you can do your best to provide superfoods for everyone in your family.

Stocking your kitchen

You can help keep your family healthy by having good foods ready to go at any time, no matter how crazy your family's schedules are. That way, everyone gets good nutrition. Keep these foods ready for your family:

- ✔ **Oatmeal and oat cereals:** Your family can start the day with a healthful superfoods breakfast, even if you've already left for work. Hot oatmeal is easy to make, or you can buy cold cereals made with oats.

- ✔ **Fresh fruits:** Instead of a cookie jar, keep a fruit bowl on the counter for easy-to-grab, healthful snacks. Bananas, oranges, and apples keep very well at room temperature and are much healthier than greasy chips or sugary candy bars.

- ✔ **Superfoods lunches:** Pack superfoods lunches for family members to grab on their way out the door to work or school. Add tomatoes and avocado to sandwiches, and pack carrot sticks on the side. Include apple or orange juice as a superfoods beverage. Chapter 11 provides more healthy lunch ideas.

- ✔ **After-school snacks:** A lot of kids come home from school a few hours before dinnertime, and they're usually hungry. Keep a few superfoods around for your children. Canned tuna and almond butter are great for sandwiches (though not together!). Nuts and seeds are great for snacks. Guacamole and salsa make delicious dips.

- ✔ **Superfood beverages:** Cut out the sugary soft drinks and keep apple, pomegranate, and orange juice on hand. You can get some great new juice options that contain real fruit and vegetables, such as V8 Splash and V-Fusion (visit www.v8juice.com/products.aspx for more info). Each 8-ounce glass of V-Fusion equals one serving of fruit and one serving of vegetables! Also, kids (and adults) can make their own sodas by mixing fruit juice with club soda or sparkling water.

Preparing for traveling

Sometimes the family is together but too busy to focus on eating healthful foods, like when you're traveling or on vacation. Taking a vacation doesn't mean you have to give up your healthful superfoods diet. Whether you travel by car, bus, train, or plane, the trip will go better if everyone is well-fed.

Avoid the usual pitfalls of junk foods and fast foods that accompany most family vacations. Here are our tips for finding superfoods when you're away from home:

- ✔ **In the car:** Pack a cooler with crisp fresh vegetables and an assortment of veggie dips. Bring along some fruit juices in single-serving boxes and bottles.

- ✔ **At service stations:** When you stop to fill up your gas tank, the family may want to fill up on junk food. Help your family choose healthier alternatives, such as fresh fruits, granola mixes, nuts and seeds, and healthful beverages.

- ✔ **At airports and train stations:** Take a small bag of granola, nuts, seeds, and dried fruits such as cranberries, apples, and bananas so you aren't as tempted to stop for fast foods at the airport or train station.

- ✔ **At restaurants:** Choose vegetable-filled omelets for breakfast and start dinners with a fresh salad. Ask for cooked green or mixed vegetables as your side dish.

- ✔ **At hotels:** Bring along superfood snacks to eat at the hotel, or find the nearest grocery store where you can buy fresh superfood fruits and vegetables to keep in a cooler (or in a small refrigerator, if your hotel room has one).

Making Superfoods Kid-Friendly

Kids benefit from eating superfoods, especially the foods rich in omega-3 fatty acids such as fish, flax, chia seeds, walnuts, and soy. An article in the January 2008 issue of *Current Opinion in Psychiatry* states that omega-3 fatty acids may be valuable for treating depression in children. Research published in the June 2005 issue of *Physiology & Behavior* showed that children who ate oatmeal performed better on cognitive tests compared to children who ate regular ready-to-eat cereals.

Some kids enjoy healthful foods and are eager to try new things at mealtime. But if your children aren't ready for a lot of superfoods, don't worry. With a little patience and time, they'll eat superfoods on a regular basis. The following sections provide you with strategies to make eating superfoods painless.

Taking it one superfood at a time

Kids aren't always interested in foods that are good for them; they want foods that taste good. Salmon and broccoli may not be able to compete with cheeseburgers and fries. This can present a bit of a challenge at mealtime.

The key is to avoid overwhelming your kids by making an overnight transformation to the meals they normally eat. Instead, take it slowly and introduce the superfoods one at a time, starting with superfoods that are sweet or crunchy.

Children naturally prefer sweeter flavors, so start with the superfood fruits. Superfoods such as bananas, oranges, and berries are great because they're easy to eat and delicious. Although whole fruits are better than juice because they have pulp and fiber, 100 percent orange juice, apple juice, and pomegranate juice are still great beverages for kids. Juice has a lot of sugar, even if the manufacturer doesn't add any, so add some fresh spring water to dilute the juice. If you start children off on diluted juice early, they won't get used to the really sweet taste of straight juice; use a ratio of about two or three parts juice to one part water.

If your kids are big on peanut butter, you may find it quite easy to get them to eat nuts and seeds like walnuts, pecans, and pumpkin seeds. Nuts and seeds make great snacks and can be chopped and sprinkled on a number of foods.

Because of the risk of developing allergies, you should be cautious about introducing nuts to kids before the age of 2. If food allergies run in your family, you may want to wait until your child is at least 4 years old. Also, grind the nuts finely, as nuts are a choking hazard before the age of 4.

Vegetables may be a little more difficult. The flavor of vegetables doesn't appeal to a lot of children, which is unfortunate because they're so good for you. Try starting with carrots, which are a little sweeter than green vegetables. (See the "Disguising superfoods" section later in this chapter for more tips.)

If your kids don't like crunchy vegetables, go ahead and cook them until they're very tender. Even though overcooking tends to reduce some of the nutritional content, a serving of mushy broccoli still beats a bag of fries any day.

Truly picky eaters may need to be exposed to new foods dozens of times before they're ready to eat and enjoy them. (See the "Pleasing picky eaters" section later in this chapter.) Be patient, and keep serving superfoods along with your kids' regular fare.

Getting kids to help in the kitchen

Your kids may be more eager to try superfoods if they lend a hand in the kitchen. Learning how to cook can be a lot of fun for kids — as well as for the adult in charge.

Of course, you have to teach cooking skills that are appropriate for a child's age. You don't want to hand a 4-year-old a butcher knife, but he can help stir waffle batter, whereas a 12-year-old may be ready to learn how to peel and chop carrots. Here are some tips for teaching kids to cook:

- ✔ **Begin with safe and healthy habits.** Make sure everyone washes their hands. Teach your kids not to lick their fingers and hands; if they want a taste, have them use a clean spoon. Be sure that long hair is back in a ponytail and that no one is wearing any loose clothing that could pose a danger (such as catching fire from the stove or getting caught in an electric mixer).

Don't let your kids taste anything that contains raw meat or raw eggs; it could lead to your child contracting a food-borne illness. Thoroughly rinse your superfoods such as apples, berries, and carrots prior to eating to make sure there are no chemicals or debris on the skins. You can purchase produce rinses at your local supermarket, but you don't have to spend the money; washing them in tap water is fine.

- ✔ **Choose recipes together.** Grab a cookbook or go online to find some recipes, and have your children read the ingredients list. Ask them to search for recipes with a superfood or two and choose one they want to help you make.

- ✔ **Gather the ingredients.** With a little guidance, young children can help you collect the ingredients. Older children can help open cans and containers. In the process, you may take advantage of the opportunity to make a few discreet comments about the health benefits that the superfood ingredients you're using provide.

- ✔ **Let them help mix and cook.** Small children can help with stirring, although you don't want them to stir anything on the stove because it's too easy for them to burn themselves. But they can hand you things, like the pepper shaker or potholder, and learn by watching you. Older kids can learn to use mixers, blenders, and food processors. They can also help with some of the cooking under your watchful eye.

Give your kids lots of encouragement, and don't worry about the inevitable messes and mistakes. Learning to cook should be a fun experience.

Making superfoods fun

Use your child's interests, schoolwork, games, and hobbies to help introduce them to some of the superfoods. Find out what countries your kids are studying in geography class and look for superfoods from those regions. If they're studying the Middle East, for example, you can make Hummus and Pita (see the recipe in Chapter 19), or serve salmon when they're learning about Alaska.

You can also take your kids to the farmers' market when you go shopping and let them help you pick out the produce. You might even consider planting a garden with your kids. Just keep it simple: Most kids don't want to spend their whole summer weeding a garden, but they may be happy to tend to some tomatoes grown in flower pots.

Substitute superfoods in some of your kids' favorite recipes. If your kids like "ants on a log" (celery sticks with peanut butter, topped with raisins), for example, make them with dried cranberries and almond butter instead.

Kids also like foods they can dip. Serve apple wedges with warm caramel sauce or let them dip baby carrots in a sweet salad dressing or their favorite chip dip. Just make sure that they're actually eating the superfoods and not just licking off the dip!

Pleasing picky eaters

Some kids will eagerly try any new foods, but some kids (and even some adults) are just picky eaters. (Let's face it: There are plenty of adults who don't want to give up their meat and potatoes. Maybe you're one of them!) Feeding a picky eater can be very frustrating, and it takes a lot of patience.

Why are some kids so darned picky? It may be in their genes. According to an article in the March 1998 issue of *Pediatrics,* your genetics may influence your eating patterns, especially during childhood. For example, many people are born with a dislike of the bitter flavors found in many vegetables. They have a stronger preference for sweet flavors. Fortunately, most kids outgrow their picky eating stage and eventually eat a normal diet. But while you're waiting for your picky eater's taste buds to grow up, you can try these ideas in the kitchen to help them along.

As a parent or grandparent, you set an example for your picky eaters whenever you eat something new and healthful.

Being patient with youngsters

Dealing with a picky eater requires a lot of patience and understanding. Little kids can't control much of anything that happens in their lives, but they can control what they eat — sort of. So some picky eaters are going to give parents and grandparents a rough time. Many family dinners have been ruined by shouting matches between parents and kids who refuse to eat their carrots, string beans, fish, or something else.

Mealtime is important, so keep dinnertime comfortable by refusing to battle with your child. Avoid threats and punishment; they don't help. Instead, offer some foods you know your child likes alongside something new. If she refuses to eat it the first time she sees it, don't get mad. If she refuses to eat it the tenth time she sees it, don't get mad. Some experts believe it may take many exposures to a new food before kids are ready to try it.

As long as your children are healthy and growing normally, they're probably getting enough nutrition despite being picky about the foods they eat. However, you may want to give them a children's multivitamin, just to be sure.

Here's more help for picky eaters:

✔ Avoid snacks and high-calorie beverages before mealtime. Your child may be more willing to try something new if he's hungry.

✔ Offer new foods in small amounts. A spoonful of beets may not seem as daunting as a full serving.

✔ Don't withhold dessert as punishment or offer extra dessert as a reward.

✔ Have your child help you pick out fruits and vegetables at the grocery store. This may help build a positive association with a new food.

✔ Don't let your child play with toys, read a book, or watch television while eating. Picky eaters will use any excuse not to pay attention to their food.

✔ Let your picky eater experiment with condiments and toppings such as ketchup, mayonnaise, salad dressing, and mustard. He may find a combination that hits the spot.

Disguising superfoods

Sometimes picky eaters can be fooled if you disguise superfoods, especially vegetables, until they get used to the flavor and texture. One way to get your kids used to eating new foods is by topping them with something a little more familiar. Although this usually means adding a few extra calories with sweet or creamy sauces, it may be worth it to get your picky eater to enjoy something new.

Use a flavorful topping such as melted cheese, sweet-and-sour sauce, or a sweet glaze to enhance the flavor of vegetables. Another way to introduce your child to superfoods is by adding them to their favorite comfort foods.

Here are some ideas:

✔ Pour ginger sauce (or sweet-and-sour sauce) on cooked broccoli.

✔ Sweeten cooked carrots with a simple glaze. Cook one pound of carrots, add 1 tablespoon of canola oil and 2 tablespoons of maple syrup, and sauté for one or two minutes. Top with a dash of salt, pepper, and cinnamon.

✔ Sneak some spinach leaves into a salad along with the iceberg lettuce.

✔ Add cooked carrots or broccoli pieces to macaroni and cheese. Start with just a few pieces. Over time, add more vegetables to the mac and cheese.

✔ Top a pizza with tomato slices and spinach.

Some kids don't like the texture of vegetables, but can handle the flavor. Vegetable purées are easy to make by cleaning and chopping your vegetables into small pieces and steaming or simmering them in water until tender. Place about 2 cups of cooked vegetables into a blender with a small amount of liquid, and purée until smooth. Serve with salt and pepper or your favorite seasonings.

Pairing Superfoods to Suit the Meat-and-Potatoes Set

We usually associate picky eating with children, but there are plenty of grown-ups who aren't interested in changing the way they eat. Rather than making over an entire meal, just add a superfood or two. Your adult picky eaters can enjoy their usual meat-and-potatoes meal and still get the extra goodness of superfoods. Try these ideas:

✔ **Begin dinner with a superfood salad.** If your family isn't ready for spinach leaves, stick with the iceberg lettuce and add tomatoes, walnuts, almonds, raw broccoli, and berries.

✔ **Replace white bread with fine-textured whole-wheat bread.** Once your family accepts that bread, bring in whole-grain breads made with whole wheat plus oatmeal, nuts, and seeds.

✔ **Reduce the portion sizes for meat,** which is high in saturated fats and calories. Fill the rest of the plate with a helping of potatoes and a delicious superfood vegetable.

- ✔ **Turn mashed potatoes into a superfood side dish** by adding cooked spinach or garlic.

- ✔ **Add dried cranberries and walnuts to your favorite dressing or stuffing recipe,** or to a boxed stuffing mix.

- ✔ **Serve your baked potatoes with salsa as a topping** instead of saturated-fat-laden sour cream, butter, or gravy.

- ✔ **Serve glazed carrots as a side dish, or add shredded carrots to coleslaw and salads.**

- ✔ **Skip the sugary dessert.** Serve sliced bananas and berries with a little whipped topping and walnuts.

Almost any meat-and-potatoes meal can be made healthier by adding a superfood or two. Of course, the way you prepare and cook your meat counts, too. Avoid deep-fried meats, processed meats, and hot dogs and sausages that contain nitrates (a chemical that has been linked to some forms of cancer). Choose lean meats, poultry, and fish whenever possible.

Serving Superfoods to Your Extended or Far-from-Home Family Members

Your family may include parents, grandparents, aunts, uncles, and even some cousins who don't live with you, or you may have children in college or living on their own for the first time. Just because they aren't under your roof, though, doesn't mean you can't help them eat more healthfully.

Helping elderly family members

Getting good nutrition is important for all stages of life, including old age. Help improve the health of older family members, especially those who live alone, by bringing superfoods into their diets (along with a big dose of happiness).

- ✔ **Bring easy-to-heat meals.** When you prepare dinner at home, make some extra portions to take to family members or friends who live alone. Include an entrée, such as a healthful salmon dish, and some side vegetables, such as carrots, beets, or kale. Pack the portions into microwave-safe containers for easy reheating.

- ✔ **Make healthful snacks and fruit bowls.** Make sure your relative has fresh fruits and vegetables prepared and ready to eat. Provide a fruit bowl filled with fresh fruit, or bring along some fresh vegetables (already peeled and sliced) with dip.

✔ **Supply easy-to-prepare breakfast items.** Bring boxes of dry cereals made with whole grains (especially oats and quinoa) and fresh berries to add extra nutrition to breakfast. When you prepare our breakfast muffins (see Chapter 16 for the recipe), make a few extra to share.

✔ **Invite them over for dinner.** Elderly people who live alone often don't meet their nutritional needs because eating alone just isn't any fun.

Feeding college kids

Eating healthful foods may not be at the top of your college student's list of things to worry about. Either they've hit the dietary jackpot by signing up for a meal plan at the college dining hall, or they're living on their own, pinching pennies and trying to live off ramen noodles and peanut butter sandwiches.

Kids who go off to college are often victims of the *freshman 15* — the extra 15 pounds many students put on when they go to college. The weight gain may be due to buffet-style eating in the dining hall or just falling into a habit of buying and eating cheap junk foods like chips and cookies. Even though your kids may have had good eating habits while they were in high school, when they get to college, they don't have the same supervision (or restrictions) they had as younger teens.

Although you have to let your adult children make their own dietary choices, you can help them out a little. Send a superfoods care package with bags of mixed nuts and pumpkin seeds, cans of tuna and salmon, homemade granola, and oatmeal blueberry muffins (see Chapter 16 for granola and muffin recipes).

Fresh fruits, such as apples, oranges, and bananas, and nuts and seeds don't need refrigeration, so they're perfect as healthful snacks. No need to keep bags of greasy chips and candy bars around the dorm room.

Some kids find college to be a stressful time, and stress can lead to eating too much comfort food or junk food. Help stressed-out college students find relief by showing them how to set up schedules, making their dorm space comfortable, or helping them find some type of regular exercise. Less stress means they'll be less likely to load up on bad foods.

Share some easy superfood recipes with your college student, too. Superfood smoothie or protein shakes provide lots of nutrition and energy (see Chapter 19) and are simple to make. You can also pass along this easy superfood sandwich spread recipe: Mix some chopped hardboiled eggs, a can of tuna, fat-free mayo, and some other veggies if you choose, and spread it onto some whole-wheat bread.

Boil a dozen eggs at a time and you can eat the eggs alone for a quick, easy snack. Pull out the yolk for an even healthier option.

If your college student has roommates, encourage them to buy foods like eggs, chicken, and veggies as a group and stock the fridge and freezer. They can then grill a bunch of chicken, boil a pot of eggs, or cut up a bunch of veggies to have available for quick salads, sandwiches, and snacks. Suggest they take turns preparing meals, which increases their chances of getting a good meal by reducing the number of times each person actually has to prepare it.

Chapter 13

Shopping for Superfoods

- -

In This Chapter

▶ Planning healthy meals

▶ Finding and shopping for superfoods

▶ Fitting superfoods into your budget

- -

*F*inding and incorporating superfoods into your diet may seem a little daunting at first, but it isn't difficult once you have a game plan. Shopping for your superfoods diet may require a little more work, but with some simple strategies, you can streamline your shopping so that you can make fewer shopping trips, save money, and improve your health.

The best way to begin is by carefully creating meal plans around your superfoods. Then you can use that information to make a grocery shopping list and, finally, hit the stores. It also helps to know how to read those black-and-white Nutrition Facts labels you see on packaged foods so when you choose pre-packaged foods, you know how to choose the ones that are best for you and your family.

At the outset, you need to know which superfoods fit your needs best. Consumer Reports offers a number of free articles at www.consumerreports.org/cro/food/diet-nutrition/index.htm; the articles cover diet and nutrition, including summaries of recent research. You also can subscribe to the site's health newsletter for a small monthly or annual fee; a subscription gives you access to Consumer Reports product reviews and ratings.

In this chapter, we guide you through the maze of shopping for superfoods. We show you what to look for and what to avoid, and we give you tips for finding the best superfoods no matter where you shop.

Planning Meals and Preparing Your Grocery List

Shopping for your superfoods diet begins at home. The following sections help you plan healthy meals and prepare a grocery list that makes superfood shopping a breeze.

Deciding what to make

Planning meals in advance helps you avoid a last-minute rush, which too often means sacrificing nutrition for convenience. It also saves money, because you won't spend extra on take-out or at the drive-through.

Decide which meals you want to make for a week at a time, including breakfast, lunches you take to work or school, dinners, snacks, and any extras for weekends. Choose meals and snacks that are healthy and give you your daily servings of superfoods (we suggest two or more — see Chapter 11).

Keep these things in mind when planning your meals:

- ✔ **Choose healthful dishes.** Look for recipes that include healthful ingredients (especially our superfoods) and the best cooking methods. Baking, steaming, roasting, and stir-frying are good for you; deep-frying is not.

- ✔ **Save your favorite recipes.** You can mark the pages in your cookbooks, copy recipes on paper and keep them in a file, or use online cooking sites to collect recipes and store them on your computer.

- ✔ **Go for balance.** Each meal should contain some protein from lean meat, dry beans, eggs, poultry, or fish; some high-fiber carbohydrates from whole grains, fruits, and vegetables; and a little bit of healthy fat from nuts, seeds, and fish (that's why fish and nuts are so super).

- ✔ **If you have picky eaters, let them pick!** A meal or two each week, that is. Getting your family involved (especially kids) helps reduce that tendency they have to turn up their noses at anything new.

If your budget is tight (and whose isn't, right?), check out the "Saving Money on Superfoods" section later for more meal-planning advice that helps you save money on superfoods.

Making a list (and checking it twice)

After you have your meals planned for the week, you're ready to make your shopping list. A healthy superfoods shopping list should contain your every-day bulk and pantry-stocking items plus the packaged foods or ingredients you need to make the meals and snacks you've laid out — including the superfoods you want to incorporate.

Write your weekly meal plan on a sheet of notepaper (or use a spreadsheet program on your computer) so that making your grocery list is a snap. Referring to your meal plan when you make your list tells you exactly which foods and ingredients you need to buy.

Keep track of those staple items you need, such as flour (whole wheat), sugar (just a little), rice, coffee, tea (black, green, and herbal), herbs, and spices, by keeping a grocery list handy in the kitchen and jotting down items as they become depleted. You won't need to buy these goods every time you shop, but when you do, you can save money by buying them in bulk.

You may want to create a one- or two-page master, printable shopping list with all your basic pantry needs, to serve as a template for your weekly lists. Then, each week you can check off the basic items you need to restock, and add items that are specific to your weekly menus. This is much faster than starting a new list from scratch each time you need to shop.

So, which foods should be on your shopping list? Here are some ideas for you:

- ✔ **Buy lots of fresh fruits and vegetables.** Many fruits and vegetables qual-ify as superfoods because they have so many vitamins, minerals, and *phytochemicals* (natural compounds that keep you healthy).

 Everyone needs at least five servings of fruits and vegetables every day. Choose a variety of fresh fruits and vegetables to please everyone in your family.

- ✔ **Make at least half of your grains whole.** Whole grains are rich in fiber, so pick whole grains whenever possible — including bread and other baked goods, pasta, and cereals. Oatmeal is a superfood grain that you can find in some whole-grain breads and breakfast cereals.

 Read the labels on breads, grains, and pastas to be sure the products you choose are "100 percent whole grain."

- ✔ **Choose good protein sources.** The best options are fish, poultry, lean meats, nuts, eggs, seeds, and legumes. Fish contain omega-3 fatty acids, so they should be included in two or three meals each week. Legumes, nuts, and seeds also contain healthful fats and fiber. Skinless chicken and lean cuts of meat can round out your grocery list.

Limit fatty red meats, breaded meats, "fish sticks," processed lunch meats, sausages, and hotdogs, all of which contain fats and additives that are bad for your health.

✔ **Don't overlook beverages.** Instead of sugary soft drinks, add low-fat milk, fruit juices, and herbal teas to your shopping list. Orange, pomegranate, and apple juice are all superfood beverages as long as they contain 100 percent juice (check the labels). Sparkling water makes a healthful and simple beverage, too. Jazz it up with a wedge of lemon or lime, or make your own soft drink by mixing one part sparkling water with one part 100 percent fruit juice.

✔ **Include some dairy products.** Choose low-fat or nonfat milk, low-fat cheese, and yogurt. If you don't like dairy products or are lactose intolerant, you can choose calcium-fortified orange juice or soy beverages and soy/vegetarian cheese substitutes.

✔ **Add dressings, oils, and condiments.** Choose salad dressings made with olive or walnut oil, look for low-fat mayonnaise, and buy margarines made without trans fats (which can damage your arteries). Choose olive oil and canola oil for cooking. Both contain healthy fats that regular vegetable oils don't have.

✔ **Buy some sandwich fixings.** A sandwich can make a quick and healthy meal or snack, so include some healthy sandwich ingredients on your shopping list. Use whole-grain breads, with nut butters or low-fat turkey or chicken as your protein sources. Make your sandwiches super by adding tomatoes, spinach leaves instead of lettuce, or avocado slices.

✔ **Choose healthy dessert and snack foods.** Look for whole-grain crackers (low in sodium whenever possible), baked chips, yogurt cups, fresh or dried fruits, nut and seeds, string cheese, fresh raw vegetables, and a small amount of dark chocolate. Make sure all your snack choices are nutritious — or at least dip those chips in guacamole or salsa.

In addition to deciding which foods to buy, you have to decide which form to buy them in. Fresh foods are always best, but frozen and canned foods can serve as acceptable substitutes. Just keep these tips in mind:

✔ **Shop smart for frozen foods.** Buying frozen foods is a convenient way to keep vegetables, seafood, and poultry on hand. Some brands of frozen vegetables are super-convenient — you just toss the bag in the microwave, and they steam themselves in a few minutes.

Although some frozen foods are both convenient and healthy, don't rely on frozen meals to improve your health. Most are high in calories, fat, and sodium. A few brands of frozen meals are made with healthier ingredients, but they're typically very expensive and, in many cases, still high in sodium.

Instead of purchasing frozen pizza, buy whole-grain pizza crusts, a jar of pizza sauce (a great way to get lycopene-rich tomatoes), and cheese (experiment with flavorful cheeses such as feta or cheddar — you won't need as much). Top your pizza with spinach and tomato slices, and follow the baking instructions on the crust packaging for healthier pizzas that are almost as fast as their frozen counterparts.

✔ **Get the right kinds of canned and jarred food.** Some canned foods are better than others. Look for low-sodium soups, vegetables, and sauces. Choose canned fruits that aren't packed in sugary syrups. Avoid canned spaghetti, ravioli, and other high-calorie foods that aren't very high in nutrition. Healthful choices include legumes, tuna packed in water, canned salmon, tomato sauce, and applesauce. Don't forget about peanut butter (or, better yet, almond butter) and 100 percent fruit spreads.

Making Your Purchases

It's shopping time, so grab your grocery list and jump in the car. No, wait a minute. Make sure you eat a healthy snack (like an apple or peanut butter sandwich) before you go, because grocery shopping on an empty stomach often leads to buying too many treats and snacks you don't need. When your stomach is full, it's much easier to stick with your superfoods list.

Now you're ready to head out the door. But before you can begin shopping, you need to know where to go. It's also helpful to know how to make the best selections and how to interpret the package labels on the foods you'll encounter. The following sections give you the lowdown.

Checking out your store options

Wherever you do your shopping, you need to understand that not all superfoods are created, or sold, equally. Finding the best quality and prices for your superfoods may require you to get out there and shop around to see what's available.

Many superfoods are common, everyday foods, so finding them isn't that difficult (unless you're looking for a specific seaweed imported from Japan — that may require a bit of patience). Superfoods and other organic products are widely available in supermarkets everywhere, and this healthy trend doesn't show any signs of ending any time soon.

Consumers are increasingly demanding superfoods, so many conventional grocery stores are bulking up their inventories. A trip through the produce section of any grocery store offers many healthful fruits and vegetables, and you can always find fresh, frozen, or canned tuna or salmon.

You can also explore other sources for your superfoods, however. Established retail health food chains such as Whole Foods Market and Trader Joe's have set the standard as the go-to locations for superfoods. Small, local health food co-ops also offer superfoods, usually in a friendly and knowledgeable atmosphere.

Starting local

Everyone would love to have the superfoods marketplace epicenter within walking distance of their house, but for most people this just isn't the case. This doesn't mean you can't score big in your local community, though, so don't give up on superfoods too easily.

The first thing to do is identify all your local shopping sources. Small towns and neighborhoods may have only one grocery store or a convenience shop, while larger cities have many big-box retail chain stores and a handful of natural or organic stores to choose from, as well as a couple of farmers' markets. You can locate all of them through Web sites, newspaper ads, and the local Yellow Pages. Once you have a blueprint of the available resources, you can start your investigation.

Ask friends and neighbors where they find the best produce and selection of superfoods. They may know of places that aren't on your radar yet.

Don't worry if none of those big, fancy whole-foods stores are close by. Whether you live in a small town or a big bustling city, you can still find most of what you're looking for at your local grocery stores, even the small ones.

There are also plenty of small specialty shops owned by health-conscious individuals who have an interest in superfoods and go the extra distance to bring quality to their consumers. You might just have one of these health food stores right in your own neighborhood.

Finding value at the big-box stores

If you're looking for a greater selection at a lower cost, you may need to explore the larger retail chain stores. Just remember that while big stores can bring big savings, there may be a big cost in terms of quality. Sometimes freshness is lacking in the produce section, and some of the cheaper brands have less nutritious ingredients.

Retail chains usually have much bigger inventories than the smaller, privately owned "mom and pop" grocery stores. Sometimes known as "big-box stores," retail chains such as Super Target, Wal-Mart, Safeway, and Kroger routinely have better pricing because they can order in much larger quantities. But as we stated earlier, quantity doesn't always mean quality. Retail chains also like to move things off the shelves quickly, so, if superfoods don't sell, these stores won't stock them.

Discount clubs that require membership, such as Sam's Club and Costco, offer the biggest potential for savings. However, the best bargains at the store are not necessarily the most economical at home. For example, paying less for a huge bottle of olive oil may sound like a great deal, but if most of that oil goes to waste, you end up losing money. You also need to watch out for cheap, over-processed junk foods that contain too much sugar, saturated fats, trans fats, and sodium. Remember, low prices may not mean good nutrition.

When it comes to long-lasting items such as dry beans, oatmeal, frozen foods, and canned tuna, you may be able to save a lot of money by buying in bulk at the members-only clubs. Just be sure you know what the price is at your grocery store so that you can comparison shop before you make your purchases at places like Sam's Club or Costco.

Exploring the superfoods stores

The superfoods philosophy may not have hit your neighborhood market yet, but the trend is growing. This is evidenced by the rise of stores that cater to the health-conscious consumer, like Whole Foods Market and Trader Joe's (see the nearby sidebar for their stories). These two retailers account for a large percentage of the dollars being spent on health foods, including superfoods, and they're gaining new consumers daily. Leading the way are baby boomers looking for ways to improve their health and vitality.

You can find the locations of Whole Foods Market and Trader Joe's nearest you by checking their store locators online: www.wholefoodsmarket.com/stores/all/index.php and www.traderjoes.com/locations.asp. You can also search online for "natural foods markets" or "health food stores" along with the name of larger cites in your area to locate health food stores. Your phone book is another place to search for health food stores.

When you shop at the superfoods stores, be sure to read Nutrition Facts labels and ingredient labels, just like you would at a regular grocery store. Even some natural products are high in sodium. Also note which items are organic and which ones are not; you'll pay more for organic foods, but it may be worth the extra cost, especially for fresh produce that doesn't have pesticide residues.

Reaping the rewards of farmers' markets

Imagine getting all the supermarkets to bring their produce sections to a parking lot and display them so you could select the best available. Well, that's the exact setup of a farmers' market. Brilliant, isn't it?

Most consumers assume that if they go to a farmers' market, they'll have their choice of freshly picked produce. This may not exactly be the case — the produce may have been picked as much as a week earlier — but produce at farmers' markets is still likely to be fresher than what you usually find at your supermarket. In addition, many smaller farmers who sell their goods at farmers' markets grow organic produce and help save our soils by staying away from potentially harmful pesticides. What better way to support them than by buying their fruits and vegetables?

Some markets have grown into popular shopping grounds and can quickly become a regular pit stop in your morning routine. Often the weekend markets can provide excellent produce, but possibly more important is the information you can get if you talk to some of the seasoned vendors. You can count on finding fresh fruits and vegetables, but more and more markets are carrying additional superfoods like nuts, beans, herbs, and even fresh seafood.

Look in your local paper: Farmers' markets are usually advertised or listed. You can also check with local grocers, chefs, or even friends to find out whether they know of any quality markets. Other popular places for farmers to set up shop are flea markets and roadside stands. These are great opportunities to get their products in front of a large number of people.

Farmers' markets rarely have any problems regarding product safety, but you must understand that they are not regulated. Until you establish a good relationship with the vendors, you must exercise care in purchasing any products. Choose fresh-looking produce with no signs of mold or bruising.

Farmers have been feeling the crunch of economic decline. Buying directly from them is an excellent way to support your local community. Most of the time, you benefit from this buying arrangement too, getting fresh produce at a fraction of the price for which it's sold at the supermarkets. If you haven't been to a farmers' market, blow the dust off your old recipe books and plan some healthy meals with fresh, locally grown produce.

Check out www.farmersmarket.com or www.localharvest.org to find farmers' markets and other organic food growers near you.

Surfing for superfoods on the Web

It's easy to find apples, bananas, and spinach at any grocery store, but quinoa, wheat grass, and chia seeds may be more difficult to find, depending on where you live. Fortunately, you can turn to the Internet to order your superfoods and have them delivered right to your front door.

Dedicated to healthful eating: Whole Foods Market and Trader Joe's

Whole Foods Market was founded in 1980 as a small health food store and has become a fast-growing, all-natural retail giant. When Whole Foods Market first opened its doors, there were only a few natural food stores in the United States. Now Whole Foods Market alone has more than 250 locations in the United States, Canada, and the United Kingdom.

Whole Foods Market continues to pave the way for large corporations in the food and health industry. Whole Foods Market has established a strong presence with its dedication to healthy products, such as superfoods, as well as its attention to preserving the environment. It was the first supermarket to completely eliminate the use of plastic disposable bags to help protect the environment, and it hires employees whose sole purpose is to find ways to make the stores environmentally friendly.

Trader Joe's, another superfoods retailer, opened in 1958 as a chain of convenience stores and now has more than 300 stores in 23 states. The stores took on a new focus in 1967, aiming for an environmentally friendly atmosphere and a large selection of organic and gourmet foods. Today, Trader Joe's not only sells other manufacturers' great products, but also has more than 2,000 private-label products ranging from frozen goods to wine.

Many Web sites offer superfoods and dietary supplements. How do you know which Web sites to trust? Here are some things to think about when you're looking for superfoods online:

- **Look for contact information beyond an e-mail address.** Every good Web site will have phone numbers or a physical address. If you aren't comfortable with ordering products online, call the company and request a catalog.

- **Look for seals of approval.** The Better Business Bureau Online or the TRUSTe seals are prominently displayed by reputable Web sites.

- **Check out nutrition information and ingredients, just as you would in a bricks-and-mortar store.** If the site doesn't offer easy-to-find links to nutrition information, go to a different Web site.

- **Check shipping charges and estimated delivery times for your location.** Find out whether you need to sign for your delivery. *Note:* Some companies base their shipping charges on total price while others charge by the pound.

- **Check out the return policy.** In most cases, you won't be able to return a food product after you've opened the package, unless the product is somehow defective. If you're trying something new, order a small amount at first to see whether you like it.

Check out www.kalyx.com and www.sunfood.com. These two online stores offer a variety of superfoods and other healthful items.

Finding and choosing superfoods at the grocery store

If you opt to shop at a local grocery store, you can make the most of your shopping experience by taking the following notes into consideration:

- **Know that most of the superfoods are going to be found along the perimeter of the store.** Fruits and vegetables can be found in the produce section and fresh fish at the meat/seafood counter. The unhealthy, over-processed, sugary, and greasy stuff is usually in the middle aisles at eye level.

- **Choose fresh fruits and vegetables carefully.** Look for firm fruits with unblemished skins and no signs of mold or oozing fluids. Vegetables should be plump and firm. Find out whether the store stocks locally grown or organic produce.

Organically grown fruits and berries may be better for your health because they aren't treated with artificial pesticides. If your grocer doesn't carry organic produce, maybe it's because he doesn't know his customers want it. Try asking the owner or manager to stock a small supply of organic produce for you and your superfood-conscious neighbors.

Can't find the fresh fruits and vegetables you want in the produce section, or need to store your produce for more than a few days? Go to the freezer section where you can find a variety of fruits and vegetables, including some out-of-season fruits and delicious vegetable blends (just watch out for high-calorie sauces). What could be easier than buying a bag of perfectly prepared broccoli all ready to steam right in your microwave?

- **Select fish carefully.** Fresh fish should smell clean (not "fishy") and the flesh (both of whole fish or fillets) should be firm to the touch. The eyes should be clear and the gills should be bright. If you're in doubt, don't buy that trout.

If fresh fish isn't available, see whether the store carries frozen tuna or salmon steaks. Of course, all stores carry at least some variety of canned tuna, and some even carry canned salmon and sardines.

- **Don't consider meat color to be the best indicator of freshness.** You can tell more from the aroma and the feel of the meat, which should smell fresh and be firm to the touch — not slimy or sticky. Check the freshness date on the label.

Grass-fed versus corn-fed beef

Red meat such as beef is not considered a superfood, but some types of beef may be better than others. Organic beef comes from cattle that are not given growth hormones and are raised on grass. This beef has a higher omega-3 fatty acid content than traditional corn-fed beef. Other, healthier forms of red meat include bison, venison (deer), and elk, all of which contain much less fat than beef.

Prevent cross-contamination due to leakage that may occur with packaged fresh meats. Grab a couple of clear plastic bags from the produce section and slip your packaged raw meats into the bags to keep juices away from your other grocery items.

Reading food labels

The U. S. Food and Drug Administration (FDA) requires all packaged foods to carry Nutrition Facts labels that tell you about the nutritional content of the foods you're looking to buy (see Figure 13-1). These black-and-white labels are found on the back, side, or bottom of the package. Knowing how to read food labels will help you make healthier decisions when you're shopping for your foods — both superfoods and your regular groceries. It only takes a minute or two to find out what you need to know.

Figure 13-1:
Nutrition
Facts label.

Nutrition Facts

Serving Size 1 Tbsp (14g)
Servings Per Container 32

Amount Per Serving

Calories 100   Calories from Fat 100

	% Daily Value*
Total Fat 11g	17%
Saturated Fat** 4g	20%
Polyunsaturated Fat 3.5g	
Monounsaturated Fat 3.5g	
Cholesterol 0g	0%
Sodium 115mg	5%
Total Carbohydrate 0g	0%
Protein 0g	

Vitamin A 6%

Not a significant source of dietary fiber, sugars, vitamin C, calcium and iron

* Percent Daily Values are based on a 2000 calorie diet.

**Includes 2g trans fat.

Serving information

The top part of the Nutrition Facts label shows serving size and servings per container. Knowing how many servings are in a package is very important so you can decipher the rest of the nutritional information.

Serving sizes can be a little tricky. Look at the label on a can of condensed soup, for example. You may think that one can is one serving, but it's really two or three servings.

The nutrition information on the rest of the label is for one serving of the product. If you eat the whole can, bag, or box, you have to multiply all the nutrition information by the number of servings to get the whole story of what you're consuming.

Calories and nutrients

The largest section of the Nutrition Facts label shows you the number of calories per serving along with the amount of fat (information about saturated fat and trans fat is required if there's more than half a gram per serving; information about other fats is optional), carbohydrates (including sugars and fiber if there's more than 1 gram per serving of either), and protein each serving contains. It also shows the sodium content, which is very important to people who need to watch their blood pressure, and how much cholesterol the food contains, which is especially important for those with high cholesterol levels.

The information is stated in grams or milligrams and as a Daily Value percentage for a typical daily diet of about 2,000 calories. You don't need to take a calculator to the store with you to count every calorie or gram of fiber, but this part of the label gives you a good overall view of the general nutrition content of the product. For example, the Nutrition Facts label for one particular brand of macaroni and cheese shows that one serving has 400 calories, 15 grams of total fat (23 percent daily value), and 820 milligrams of sodium (34 percent daily value). So, this one serving of macaroni and cheese contains 20 percent of your daily calories (assuming you limit consumption to 2,000 calories a day), almost one-quarter of the fat you need for a whole day, and more than one-third of your recommended sodium intake. And this is for what is traditionally a side dish — not an entire meal. That doesn't mean you can't have macaroni and cheese. But it does mean you should watch how much fat and sodium, as well as total calories, you eat for the rest of the day.

Vitamins and minerals

The next part of the Nutrition Facts label gives a little more information on selected vitamins and minerals besides sodium. The FDA requires the amounts of calcium, iron, vitamin A, and vitamin C to be listed on the label, even if there aren't any. Sometimes you'll see information for other nutrients such as folic acid (a supplemental B vitamin) or thiamine (another B vitamin), if the food manufacturer chooses to show them.

Ingredients list

Packaged foods have to list the ingredients in order from greatest to least. This is helpful if you're looking to avoid, limit, or include specific ingredients. For example, some fruit juices contain water, sugar, or high-fructose corn syrup as additional ingredients. Of course, reading the ingredient list also points you to superfoods when you find ingredients like olive oil, soy, or garlic on the label.

What else you might see on the label

The Nutrition Facts label isn't the only source of information on packaged foods. Packages are often emblazoned with words like "natural," "organic," or "light," but they don't always mean what you think they do. Here are a few facts to think about when reading food packages:

- ✔ **How organic is "organic"?** Foods labeled as "100% organic" must contain all organically grown ingredients except for added water and salt. The word "organic" can be used on the label if more than 95 percent of the ingredients are organic, and the words "made with organic ingredients" can be used on the label if 70 percent of the ingredients are organic. (See the nearby sidebar for more on the meaning of "organic.")

- ✔ **What do words like "low," "reduced," or "-free" really mean?** Low-calorie foods contain less than 40 calories per serving. Low-fat foods contain less than 3 grams of fat per serving. Low-sodium foods contain less than 140 grams of sodium per serving. Foods with "reduced" on the label (like "reduced sugar" or "reduced calorie") must contain at least 25 percent fewer calories than the regular version of the same product. Calorie-free foods have less than 5 calories per serving, and fat-free foods can have up to 0.5 grams of fat per serving. The same holds for sugar: Foods can have 0.5 grams of sugar and still be labeled sugar-free.

- ✔ **Are those health claims real?** The FDA allows certain health claims to be made on food labels. In some cases, labels may state that certain ingredients may affect normal structure or function of the body, such as "fiber maintains bowel regularity," but may not state that an ingredient prevents or treats disease. Dietary supplement labels must state that the product "is not intended to diagnose, treat, cure, or prevent any disease" because their claims are not evaluated by the FDA. A few qualified health claims are allowed on labels, such as "Scientific evidence suggests but does not prove that eating 1.5 ounces per day of most nuts as part of a diet low in saturated fat and cholesterol may reduce the risk of heart disease." In these cases, the labels must adhere to strict wording that is determined by the FDA.

- ✔ **What's the difference between "made with" and "100 percent" labels?** When you buy whole-grain products and fruit or vegetable juices, be sure to look for the label "100%" (and double-check the ingredient list). If a bread label, for example, states, "made with whole grains," it may not contain many. Likewise, many fruit juice beverages contain as little as 10 percent actual juice — and often lots of sugar.

What is organic?

According to the United States Department of Agriculture,

"Organic meat, poultry, eggs and dairy products come from animals that are given no antibiotics or growth hormones. Organic food is produced without using most conventional pesticides, fertilizers made with synthetic ingredients or sewage sludge, bioengineering or ionizing radiation."

Organic foods may not contain more vitamins or minerals than traditionally grown or raised foods. However, going organic reduces your exposure to pesticide, antibiotic, and growth hormone residues.

Despite the FDA's intentions to control the wording on labels, some products still offer claims of amazing cures. Approach these with caution. Not only are the "cure" claims suspect; some of these products may actually harm your health rather than help it.

Saving Money on Superfoods

Eating healthfully can get expensive, but, with a little planning, you can enjoy healthy, superfood-rich meals without spending a fortune.

Here are some tips to get the nutrition you need without blowing your budget:

- ✓ **Look at grocery store ads and coupons when making out your weekly meal plan.** That way, you can select meals based on food items that are on sale. You can also find coupons online at sites like www.coupons.com. At www.smartsource.com, you can print out your coupons on your own. Some other sites, like www.grocerycoupons.net, have you place an "order" for the coupons you want, and then they're mailed to you. If you're not sure what you want, search for "grocery coupons" and tour various sites to see how they work.

- ✓ **Plan several uses for perishable ingredients so they're less likely to go to waste.** For example, if you plan to make our oatmeal blueberry muffins from Chapter 16 for breakfast on Monday, think about serving blueberries and whipped topping for dessert on Wednesday.

- ✓ **Buy the whole bird.** Chicken is a good source of protein and is low in fat when you remove the skin. Pre-cut chicken is convenient, but it's much more expensive than buying the whole bird and cutting it up yourself — unless you can catch the pre-cut stuff on sale at the grocery store.

✔ **Make plans for your leftovers.** Leftover baked salmon fillets (see Chapter 17) could be used to make salmon cakes (see Chapter 19). If you have a refrigerator and microwave at work, leftovers can also be part of a healthful and delicious lunch.

✔ **Make your own frozen meals.** Double your recipes and freeze half of them for use at a later time. Freeze the foods in microwave-safe containers or make aluminum foil pouches that can be warmed up in the oven.

✔ **Stock up on sale items.** Bulk items like dry beans and oatmeal and canned goods like black beans, tuna, and salmon have long shelf lives, so buy them when they're on sale and use them when you're ready.

✔ **Buy produce only when you plan to use it.** Check the sell-by dates on things like bagged spinach, and pass it up if you don't intend to use it by then. For all fresh produce, the general rule is to buy only as much as you'll use within a week, especially for items that don't freeze well.

✔ **Buy family-sized packages of lean meats, chicken, and superfood fish fillets when they're on sale.** Repack extra steaks, chops, chicken pieces, or fillets in freezing paper or freezer bags and freeze them for future use.

✔ **Substitute other protein sources for meat.** Black beans, pinto beans, lentils, and other legumes contain enough protein to take the place of meat in a meal and are far less expensive. Make your burritos with black beans instead of beef — you'll save money and get healthy at the same time.

✔ **Make your own snacks.** Combine whole-grain oat cereals like Cheerios with dried fruits and a variety of nuts (and even a few dark chocolate chips). Place individual portions in small snack-sized bags for portable, money-saving treats.

✔ **Buy fresh produce when it's in season.** Not only is it cheaper, but following the seasons is also a nice way to add variety to your meals. Many fruits and almost all vegetables can be frozen, so you can buy extra to enjoy during the off-season, too.

✔ **Grow your own superfoods.** Starting a home garden can be a great hobby and save you money on some of the foods that you use often. Even an herb garden can be cost-effective and convenient. (See Chapter 14 for more on starting your own garden.)

For more financial advice, see the earlier section "Finding value at the big-box stores" to find out about the pros and cons of shopping at large retail chain stores and buying in bulk.

Chapter 14

Growing Your Own Superfoods

. . . .

In This Chapter

▶ Seeing how you can benefit from growing your own superfoods

▶ Exploring different types of home gardens

▶ Tending your superfoods garden

▶ Reaping what you sow

. . . .

*N*aturally, you want your superfoods to be both healthy and safe — and, ideally, less expensive. A good way to achieve all these goals is to grow your own superfoods garden. In this chapter, we show you the advantages of growing your own superfoods, explore the different kinds of gardens you can cultivate, and share tips and tricks for tending and getting the most out of your superfoods garden.

We focus on superfoods gardening here, but we don't have the space to give you an encyclopedic knowledge of gardening. For that, we recommend *Gardening Basics For Dummies* by Steven A. Frowine and *Organic Gardening For Dummies* by Ann Whitman, both written in association with the National Gardening Association and published by Wiley. *Sustainable Landscaping For Dummies* by Owen E. Dell is another Wiley title that includes info about growing a healthy and safe garden.

Assessing the Advantages of Starting Your Own Superfoods Garden

Growing a garden that's bursting with healthy produce is a great accomplishment. Not everyone has the extra time to venture into a new hobby, but having at least one pastime is important to stimulate your mind and control stress levels. Besides the mental aspect, there are several other important reasons to grow your own superfoods. Not only can you fill your refrigerator and pantry with healthy foods, but you can also pad your pocketbook. That's right — starting your own garden can save you money. So read on to get everything you can out of a superfoods garden.

When you shop in any grocery store, you don't have control of the growing and processing of the foods you eat. But by starting your own superfoods garden, you can control growing and harvesting conditions so there are no questions about what your superfoods went through to get to your table.

Probably the most fun part of building your own garden is choosing what to grow. You can start a standard garden with a variety of veggies, fruit trees, and berries, or even an herb garden. Of course, the best superfoods gardens have a few of each.

When you plan your meals around all the superfoods you want to eat, shopping and cooking can get expensive, especially when you buy lots of organic foods and herbs. Starting your own garden can help expand your superfoods diet and save you money along the way.

You're likely to find a small section in the produce department for herbs, plants, and exotic superfoods, often with a limited selection. These isolated items can be expensive and are often bundled in amounts that are more than you can use, so you may end up throwing some of them away. Having an herb garden allows you to fresh-pick what you need without wasting money on leftovers. If your garden yields more produce than you can use, you can preserve your harvest or share it with friends. What a great way to introduce them to superfoods and home gardening!

When environmental factors disrupt the growing seasons for commercial farmers, prices of the affected produce can skyrocket or the amount available may be reduced. If you grow your own, you won't have to worry so much about those prices going up.

Planning Your Superfoods Garden

Building your superfoods garden can be a fun and exciting venture when you think about all the possibilities you have. Of course, growing takes time and you have to wait a little while to actually get a taste of your investment, but it's worth it in the end.

The easiest way to get started is to make a list of everything you'll need, because planning makes perfect. As with any do-it-yourself project, you may become a frequent flyer to your local gardening center, but starting with a detailed plan will help limit your driving time. The important thing to remember is that you can make your garden as big or as small as you want (you can even start with just one crop). Once you've decided which kind of garden you want, you can figure out what tools you'll need to make your garden flourish.

Deciding what kind of garden makes sense for you

Different types of gardens suit different needs and spaces. The best option for you and your family may end up being a combination of garden types, depending on how many superfoods you want to grow and how much room you have. Some types of gardens may be easier if you're a rookie, but as you gain experience and enjoy the great rewards of gardening, you may look to expand. We look at the most common options for home gardening to help you decide which type of garden best suits you.

Traditional backyard gardens

Go out in the backyard, mark off a large square, and start diggin' — you'll have a garden in no time.

Okay, it's not really that easy, but it's a common starting point, especially for new gardeners. When you picture a stretch of land at the back of your lot with rows of fresh produce neatly plotted, you're visualizing the typical backyard garden. To decide if this is a feasible option for you, here are a few things to consider:

- ✔ **Decide which superfoods you want to grow.** Some of the superfoods that do really well in backyard gardens are beans, tomatoes, broccoli, and spinach. You can also grow other great vegetables that didn't make the superfoods list successfully in a backyard garden, too. If you want to grow only one or two superfoods, a different type of garden may be better, such as a container garden (see the next section).

- ✔ **Find the right piece of land.** Look for a flat place that receives as much sun as possible. In the northern states, you need almost full sunlight — that is, sun exposure eight hours a day. In southern climes, you may be able to get away with half that many hours of sunlight.

- ✔ **Check the soil of the area you settle on.** Is it garden-ready, or will you have to adjust the soil? We provide information about soil types later in this chapter in the section "Understanding soil types."

- ✔ **Measure off the maximum area you can allocate to the garden.** Although you may have a large plot of land, it's best to start with a garden about 10 feet by 10 feet. You can always expand later, but you don't want to tear up a large plot of land in the beginning just in case you find that gardening isn't really your thing.

- ✔ **Make sure you have a water source for your garden location.** One example is a garden hose that reaches from the faucet to your garden. Rainfall is seldom consistent in most areas, so you'll need to supplement nature's moisture with a watering schedule.

If you're uncertain about your gardening abilities or interest, try starting with a single vegetable. Then, if you like, you can expand your garden — both in terms of size and variety of crops — in subsequent years.

Container gardens

Container gardens, as the name implies, use containers instead of a plot of land in which to grow produce. Container gardens are great if you're a beginner because they require less maintenance. They're also a popular choice for those who don't have the space for a traditional garden. Container gardens can be quite small, so most likely you can make room for one no matter where you live.

Container gardens allow you to plant a large variety of produce in a small area. They're a common choice for herb gardens, which can be planted in window boxes and on balconies.

For much more on container gardens, check out *Container Gardening For Dummies* by Bill Marken and the editors of the National Gardening Association (published by Wiley).

Hydroponic gardens

The whole premise of hydroponic gardening is to grow produce without soil. This obviously has to be a complicated system that takes months to master, right? Not at all! It may take a bit more time to master, but, when done right, hydroponics can be a very effective way to grow superfoods with high nutrient values indoors or outdoors. It's especially useful for people who don't have much outdoor space. You can grow a very diverse garden all within the confines of your home.

Hydroponic gardening also is useful when your climate isn't right for the kind of plants you want to grow — especially smaller crops like herbs. Hydroponics lets you create the right environment for these plants to thrive.

Another advantage of hydroponics is that you can maximize nutrient absorption through your fertilizer mixes and yield really healthy, nutrient-rich produce.

To find out more about hydroponic gardening, we recommend *Hydroponics for the Home Gardener* by Stewart Kenyon and Howard M. Resh (Key Porter Books).

Indoor gardens

Indoor gardening requires many of the same considerations as outdoor gardening, including soil and crop selection. The advantage to indoor gardening is that you don't have to contend with the vagaries of weather. You can establish much more consistent growing conditions, and you can grow your garden year-round. Indoor gardens usually have fewer pest problems, too.

Indoor gardens do require more attention to watering schedules and light exposure. Mother Nature won't destroy your indoor garden in a hail storm, but she also won't drizzle a gentle rain on it or soak it in abundant sunshine. If you tend to forget to water your houseplants or don't have a lot of natural light in your home, indoor gardening may not be your best option.

Figuring out which tools you need

Whatever type of garden you choose, you need an array of tools and supplies to make sure you can do it right the first time. Some standard tools are useful for all garden types, whereas some specific items are useful for certain types of gardens.

Starting with general gardening tools

You need some tools no matter what kind of garden you decide to start. Some of the smaller tools can be used for container and indoor gardens as well as traditional backyard gardens. If you have a large plot of land, you may want to invest in a rototiller (or rent one) to work up your soil before you plant your garden. Other must-haves include

- ✓ **Gloves:** Gloves aren't just to keep the dirt out of your fingernails. They also help prevent blisters on your hands when you're using gardening tools and protect your hands from cuts and scrapes.

  When working in soil, you have to be cautious about getting cuts and puncture wounds from thorns and other sharp objects. Tetanus bacteria can be found in soil, and it can get into your system through open wounds. Untreated, tetanus can lead to serious health conditions (including paralysis and lockjaw). Check with your doctor about your immunization status (you should have a booster shot every ten years), and be sure to cover any scratches or cuts with bandages before working in your garden.

- ✓ **A shovel or spade:** Both large and small shovels are convenient to have. You'll probably use small gardening shovels more frequently, but you'll need a larger one, too, for bigger jobs, such as planting superfood fruit trees. (See the nearby sidebar for the difference between a shovel and a spade and when you should use each tool.)

- ✓ **A hoe:** Hoes are designed to create troughs for planting seeds. They're also useful for removing weeds.

- ✓ **Rakes:** As with shovels, having both hand-held and full-length rakes is helpful for gardening. Rakes are used to churn the soil and manage weeds. (You won't need rakes for an indoor garden, and you may not even need one for a container garden.)

- ✓ **Garden snips or loppers:** These are bulky scissors for pruning plants, raspberry canes, and fruit trees.

✔ **A watering mechanism:** For smaller gardens, a simple watering can will do. For larger gardens, you'll likely need a hose and a spray nozzle that allows you to drench your garden in a gentle shower. You also may want to consider a sprinkler, but be sure you can control the force of the water flow. Plants of all kinds do best with a slower, gentler flow of water that gives the soil time to absorb the moisture. High-pressure water flow often runs off the surface and can damage tender plants. For hydroponic gardens, you can get simple watering pumps that will recirculate and keep the water levels adequate.

✔ **A cart:** Unless you just get a kick out of running back and forth between your garden and your shed or garage (or wherever you store your gardening tools and supplies), you'll want to invest in a wheelbarrow or small wagon for your outdoor garden (obviously you won't need one for indoor or container gardens). It's much easier to cart your soil, fertilizer, seeds, and tools all at once. It comes in handy at harvest time, too.

Choosing containers

If you opt for a container garden, you don't have to spend a lot on fancy containers. Consider using household items that you would normally throw out or recycle, such as coffee cans or cut-down milk cartons. These are ideal for small plants such as herbs, or to start seedlings that you'll transplant outdoors later in the spring, like tomatoes or peppers.

You can also purchase containers for your garden practically anywhere. Gardening centers, nurseries, and even discount retailers carry a variety of plastic, ceramic, or wood containers in season.

Plants grown in pots need good drainage to prevent being over-watered. If you use coffee cans or milk cartons, punch a few holes in the bottom to allow for drainage. Remember to place each container on a plate or tray to catch any overflow. If your containers don't come with water trays, you can make your own with sturdy paper or Styrofoam plates, or you can look for a plastic serving platter or tray at your local dollar store. Just make sure that whatever you use has at least slightly raised sides to prevent leaks, and don't over-water your container garden.

Add a layer of gravel to the bottom of your containers before adding your potting soil. This improves drainage. Don't use dirt from your backyard in your containers or flowerpots because it probably won't be the right texture for container gardening. Potting soil has better texture and nutrients for container plants.

Be sure to choose plants that will fit the container you're using and not grow too big. The full-size orange tree that you've always wanted isn't likely to thrive in your container garden, but miniature varieties of oranges, lemons, and limes are bred specifically for small spaces.

Should you use a shovel or a spade?

Shovels are designed to move dirt; spades are designed to loosen it. Shovels have pointed tips and a gooseneck handle, which help you lift dirt and deposit it somewhere else. Spades have square blades and straight handles, which make them ideal for prying and loosening. But you'll work a lot harder if you try to use a spade to move dirt. If all you want to do is pry up sod and loosen the topsoil for your garden, use a spade. If you need to dig a large hole, use a shovel. For smaller holes, use a small gardening shovel (the kind that often comes with a hand-rake for breaking up clumps of dirt).

Considering light sources

Some indoor gardens can survive on indirect sunlight that comes in through the windows, but if your home doesn't allow for adequate light, you may need a grow light. These are easy enough to buy and install, and they can be placed on timers to keep the plants from burning or drying out.

Choose fluorescent light bulbs made especially for growing plants. Incandescent (regular) light bulbs won't give your plants the type of light they need. Many garden centers and home improvement stores carry kits for growing plants indoors.

Keeping growing seasons in mind

In some ways, plants are like people. Some like it hot and sunny, some prefer shade and cooler temperatures, some do best in dry conditions, and some need more moisture to thrive. Some plant varieties are very sensitive to certain climates, and they may not deliver optimal taste or nutritional value in other settings. Think about grape vineyards. The farmers search for not only the best soil, but also the best climate to grow their grapes. This can spell the difference between a good wine and a great wine.

Keep growing seasons in mind when you plan your superfoods garden. Spinach and kale need to grow in the cooler temperatures of spring or later fall. Tomatoes may need to be started indoors (plant the seeds in small pots) and transplanted when the weather is warm enough (or you can buy plants that are ready to be transplanted).

The *Farmer's Almanac* is an excellent source to determine the best time to grow your superfoods. You can go to www.farmersalmanac.com and pull up information specific to your area. Most commonly, growing charts are divided by north and south, but you may find specifics for east and west as well. Your local gardening center should be able to provide a growing chart that shows you the best times to grow specific superfoods in your area.

Selecting Your Superfood Seeds

Getting delicious superfoods from your garden starts with finding quality seeds, which is easier than ever. You can find seeds online, in catalogs, or at your local gardening center or big-box store, or you can ask vendors at your local farmers' markets where they get their seeds.

Try to find *organic seeds,* which haven't been exposed to chemicals or to genetic modification. Many companies such as High Mowing Seeds (www. highmowingseeds.com) and Yardlover (www.yardlover.com) offer them. Note that international companies often offer a better variety of fruits, vegetables, and herbs. Check out the Organic Consumers Association Web site at www.organicconsumers.org. Click on Find Organics on the home page, and then select Organic Non-GMO Seeds under the Food menu for state-by-state and international listings of companies that sell organic seeds.

Here are some more things to think about as you choose your super seeds:

- ✔ **Decide what you want to grow.** Many of the superfoods come in many varieties, including different sizes, shapes, and colors. Choosing the right seeds can make a big difference. For instance, if you're salivating over large, voluptuous tomatoes, you don't want to plant cherry tomato seeds.

- ✔ **Choose the right seeds for your garden type.** Container, hydroponic, and indoor gardens impose some limitations on the seeds you choose. It will be difficult to grow large tomatoes in these garden formats, but they do great in backyard gardens. Herbs and some of the smaller vegetables like cherry tomatoes, beans, and broccoli do well in container gardens, although they may require larger containers to flourish. Larger produce requires even larger containers. You may also try growing some sprouts such as chia and flax. If you're interested in growing fruit, containers are great for growing strawberries.

- ✔ **Consider your garden's location.** Some plants, like tomatoes, grow best in full sun, and some, like spinach, need a little shade. You also need to think about your soil type and the temperature. Carrots can stand heat but need lighter soil. Kale and spinach need cooler temperatures. If you're confused by soil types, temperatures, full sun, partial sun, and drainage, talk to an expert at a garden center or contact your county extension office.

- ✔ **Match crops with your climate.** Ordering your plants and seeds from catalogs or online is convenient, but you need to exercise a little care. First, you need to locate your hardiness zone (every reputable catalog will have a map of the United States with the hardiness zones labeled in different colors). When you browse the catalog, be sure to read the description for the plants you want to grow to make sure they'll grow and flourish in your zone. If you're not comfortable ordering seeds online or from a catalog from some faraway place, shop locally. A local garden shop will only carry the seeds for plants that grow in your area.

Enriching the Soil

Soil is a dynamic environment that needs to be monitored and protected if you expect it to produce the food that nourishes your body. Pesticides (chemicals that kill or repel insects, microorganisms, and even rodents) and herbicides (chemicals that kill unwanted plants) often leave residues on fruits and vegetables that may build up in your body. The great news is that you can have a successful garden without these chemicals.

The potting soil used for your container and indoor gardens is different from the soil in your yard. Potting soil is designed to allow roots to grow easily and to retain the right amount of water. Remember to use a layer of gravel at the bottom of your container to help extra water drain away so your roots don't rot. If you have questions about potting soil, go to a local nursery or garden center and ask for some help.

For a backyard garden, you need to understand a bit more about soil and how it can impact the way your superfoods are grown.

Peeking into an underground ecosystem

To the naked eye, soil looks like . . . well, dirt. But there's a busy, underground system of life, or *ecosystem,* in those clumps of earth that works to keep the soil — and all that springs from it — healthy.

- ✔ **Microorganisms,** tiny living creatures that live in the ground, continuously break down all the wastes and chemicals in the dirt and turn them into nutrients, creating a rich environment for farming.
- ✔ **Macro-organisms,** such as worms and larger bugs, make tunnels through the ground, giving the nutrients room to disperse into the soil.

Billions of organisms inhabit the soil, including bacteria, algae, and fungus. They use air, water, minerals, and heat from the sun, and cause reactions that make soil functional. They all play a role in creating the right environment for planting.

Ever wonder what happens to leaves, chewing gum, paper bags, and even engine oil when it gets into the soil? Macro- and microorganisms team up to decompose these and other substances, magically converting them into an enriched environment for plants to grow. These organisms are impressively effective at breaking down even the most extreme substances and repairing soil damage, although this can take quite a while to accomplish.

One way to judge whether you have good soil is by the number of large earthworms you find when you dig down beneath the topsoil. They may be a little slimy, but they can be a good guide to good soil. Large, plump earthworms indicate a soil environment rich in nutrients.

Understanding soil types

Soil types are made up of the gradual breakdown of rock and the decomposition of plants, manure, and decaying animal matter. There are three main categories of soils that can support plant growth, but they have very different nutrient content. Differences in soil can make a major difference in the nutrient content of the crops. The primary soil types are

- **Clay soil.** Clay soil is a good, fertile soil, but it can be difficult to work with because it's hard to separate and can trap air and water, creating an unpleasant environment for plants. Clay soil tends to either dry out quickly or retain too much water, and either extreme presents a challenge for gardening.

- **Sandy soil.** Sandy soil is composed of mostly large particles that allow air and water to move relatively freely. But the nutrients can also drain right out of the soil, leaving little for the root systems of the plants to absorb. As with clay soil, sandy soil also can dry out quickly.

- **Loamy soil.** Loamy soil is the most desirable because it has a good mixture of all particle sizes, allowing for good air circulation and water drainage. This soil type has a higher percentage of organic matter and therefore offers the most natural fertile environment to grow in.

Many garden centers and home improvement centers offer soil testing as a service. Alternatively, you can buy a simple pH testing kit. To collect a soil sample, check with the garden center for instructions, which will be similar to this:

1. **Collect a spade, some newspaper (or other clean paper), and a bucket.**

   Clean the spade and bucket thoroughly to remove any type of residue that may alter the test results.

2. **Dig four or five holes (about 8 inches deep) in different parts of your planting area to get a good sample of the soil in your garden.**

3. **Use the spade to slice out a portion of soil along the side of each hole. Place the slices of soil into your bucket.**

4. **Mix the soil in the bucket and spread the soil on newspaper to dry out.**

5. **Collect about a pint of soil (or whatever amount the garden center or home improvement store requires) as a sample.**

Once you know the pH of your soil, you can adjust it as needed. You can add sulfur to the soil to lower the pH or you can add lime to the soil to increase the pH.

The soil test may also tell you other information about your soil, such as the amounts of phosphorus, potassium, and nitrogen. An expert can help you choose the best products for improving your soil.

Caring for Your Superfoods Garden

Your garden will need regular maintenance to keep your superfood plants healthy. All plants need the right amount of water, and you need to remove weeds so they don't use up nutrients or choke out your plants. A little boost of the right type of fertilizer will help your superfood plants grow big and healthy, too.

With the right kind of TLC, your garden will reward you with a bounty of superfoods at harvest time. You'll have plenty of fresh produce for your kitchen, and probably enough to give to friends and family besides. Of course, you can also freeze or can the extra produce to enjoy during the winter. Enjoying the fruits of your labor in January can be great motivation to plant a garden again the following spring.

Watering wisely

This seems like a no-brainer, but the correct balance of water is important for plant growth. If you've ever had houseplants die (or you've failed at previous gardening attempts), don't give up on your green thumb yet. Maybe you just put your plants on the wrong watering schedules.

Farmers deal with watering problems on a large scale, but changes in water quantity, whether too much or too little, can ruin crops on any scale. A general rule of thumb for watering is to give a deep watering once a week. Sprinkling your plants every day doesn't have the same beneficial effect as a deep soaking that gets down into the root systems.

Watering needs depend on a number of factors, including your climate and the type of soil you use. Soil types that don't drain well can fool you into overwatering, which can damage your plants. Sandy soils, on the other hand, may dry out quickly, so you may have to water more than once a week.

Water responsibly. If you water at the wrong time of day, much of the water is wasted to evaporation. The best time to water is either early in the morning or around dusk. If you water too much, run-off can steal nutrients and excess moisture can damage your plants by promoting fungi growth. And if you water too often, you may promote disease that encourages the use of more herbicides, which in turn can damage the soil.

Controlling pests

Anyone who has tended a garden knows that insects can cause your rose-ate dreams of a bountiful harvest to crash down in ruins. What about those pesky weeds that seem to be growing taller than your tomato plant? The quick thing to do is grab pesticides and herbicides to eliminate these pests, but there are much better ways to fight them. One reason farmers pay so much attention to the soil is to prevent potential hazards before they occur. Keeping damaging weeds, insects, and organisms to a minimum comes from solid watering habits, proper fertilization, and mechanical options, such as crop covers that keep the weeds in the dark and the pests away. The main thing to remember is to try to leave the chemicals on the shelves.

Plenty of earth-friendly solutions exist for controlling weeds and pests. You'll have to consider using pesticides unless you're one lucky gardener, but think green and choose environmentally friendly options.

Whipping weeds

Weeds are more than unsightly plants that give your garden an unkempt appearance. An overgrowth of weeds causes problems for your garden by competing with your garden plants for water, nutrients, and (if the weeds are large enough) sunlight.

The most eco-friendly way to control weeds is to pull them out of the ground as they grow. You don't need any chemicals, but it can take a lot of time (and hard work) if you have a large garden. An easier way to control weeds is with herbicides. Many chemical herbicides either prevent seeds from sprouting or kill growing plants by contact. These chemical herbicides are very effective, but you need to know exactly how to use them so you don't destroy your garden plants. Plus, they're poisonous, so you'll probably want to use something safer.

You can prevent weed growth by using *mulch* (material such as shredded bark, grass clippings, straw, and shredded leaves that you can spread over the top of your garden). You simply spread mulch around your garden plants once they're up and growing. The mulch prevents weeds from growing by blocking sunlight.

Don't spread mulch over your garden seeds right after you plant them. You'll smother your seeds and your garden plants won't grow. Wait until all your plants are growing before you mulch them.

Using mulch on your soil may help to keep in moisture, so you may have to water less frequently, depending on the location of your garden.

Another option is to use a weed-barrier cloth between your rows of garden plants. The cloth blocks weeds from growing but allows water into the soil. Many people cover the weed-barrier cloth with attractive mulch.

Beating bugs

Gardens attract a lot of bugs. Many of them are beneficial, especially for fruits that need to be pollinated. However, some pests, such as cabbage worms, aphids, and borers, damage crops. You can spray chemical insecticides on bugs, but these pesticides are poisonous.

To avoid the poisons of chemical pesticides, you can choose one of the following available insecticides that are safe for your organic garden:

- **Rotenone** is made from the roots of legumes and deprives insects of oxygen.

- **Horticultural oil** is refined petroleum oil that is mixed with water and sprayed onto the insects. The oil causes the insects to suffocate. The oil evaporates and doesn't leave any toxic residue.

- **Insecticidal soap** can be sprayed on insects to kill them. Insecticidal soap is the safest type of natural insecticide.

- **Bt (Bacillus thuringiensis)** contains bacteria that can be dusted on plants. The bacteria kill insects but are non-toxic to humans and animals.

You can buy an inexpensive sprayer at any garden or home improvement store to spray these insecticides on your garden.

Blocking bunnies and other four-legged critters

Many four-legged creatures, especially rabbits and deer, may want to dine on your delicious garden plants. Skunks and raccoons may be attracted to grubs in the soil and will think nothing of ripping up your garden to get to them. Even your cat and dog may take pleasure in a good dig in your garden. Thus, you may need to use barriers to protect your garden.

If small animals are a problem, you can build a small fence around your garden using posts and wire fencing that will block most animals. If deer are a problem, you may need a larger fence. Go to your home improvement store for help in choosing the right fencing materials (or maybe hire someone to install a fence for you).

If building a fence isn't a good option, try spraying a mixture of water and hot sauce, such as Tabasco sauce, on your plants. A mixture of 2 tablespoons of Tabasco sauce to 1 gallon of water should make your plants less attractive to animals. Of course, you'll have to reapply the mixture after rains.

Using superfood-friendly fertilizers

Fertilizers are intended to supplement your soil; they really aren't the main source of nutrition for your garden. But they do help boost the natural nutrient content of your soil. To grow healthy crops, soil must contain three main nutrients:

- ✔ **Nitrogen:** Considered the most important of the three main nutrients, nitrogen plays a role in chlorophyll development and photosynthesis, making it at least partly responsible for the bright colors in superfood fruits and vegetables.

- ✔ **Phosphorous:** This nutrient is the major contributor to root systems and other structural strength. Phosphorous tends to be a bit more stable in the soil when compared to nitrogen. When plants are not growing as big or they drop their produce too fast, a phosphorous deficiency may be the culprit.

- ✔ **Potassium:** As with phosphorous, potassium works to make crops strong, but it also helps with flavor. Potassium doesn't deplete as fast as nitrogen, so it doesn't have to be added as frequently. In fact, some soils maintain good potassium levels without any additives.

Fertilizers generally supplement the soil's supply of these three main nutrients, and some toss in other nutrients, such as iron, copper, zinc, and manganese.

There are two types of fertilizers, inorganic and organic.

- ✔ **Inorganic:** *Inorganic fertilizers* use chemicals to provide the nutrient boost soil needs. A standard mix is called 10-10-10, which indicates an equal mix of each of the three main nutrients.

- ✔ **Organic:** *Organic fertilizer* is made from dead plant material and animal components. It doesn't contain any chemicals, which makes it much more earth-friendly. You can make your own organic fertilizer by starting a compost pile where organic matter, such as yard waste, fruits, vegetables, lawn clippings, and manure, is allowed to decompose. This process takes about eight to ten weeks. Organic matter helps add all the beneficial organisms that the soil needs to create nutrients and protect it from harmful organisms. Animal manure has been a farmer's favorite for creating great soil environments.

 It's important to use the recommended amount of fertilizer. Use too much, and the excess can drain off into water supplies or pool in your garden and damage your crops. Even organic matter such as manure can harm your crops if it isn't aged properly before you apply it; fresh manure can contain too much nitrogen, which can damage crops just as inorganic fertilizers can.

Farmers regularly use crop rotation to help keep soil fresh and revitalized, and it's a technique you can use, too. Say your garden has ten rows — two rows of spinach, two rows of carrots, two rows of beets, two rows of tomatoes, and two rows of strawberries. Next year, you may want to plant the tomatoes where this year's carrots were and the strawberries where you had the spinach this year. Crop rotation can help the soil recover from nutrient depletion, and it can prevent pests from building permanent homes near their favorite plants.

Harvesting Your Superfoods

You grew your crops, cultivated your herbs, and pruned your fruit trees to branches full of fruit, but when is the absolute best time to actually harvest the goods? You don't want to pick, pull, or cut produce too early because you might disrupt the nutrients that you're looking to get out of these superfoods. You also may sacrifice texture and flavor by harvesting at the wrong time: Think about how the texture and taste of a banana differs when the peel is green from when it's mottled.

Once disconnected from the nutrient system that feeds it (the stem), fruits and vegetables go through a different type of processing that ultimately determines how long you can wait before you eat them. The chart in Table 14-1 provides tips on optimal harvesting time for various superfoods.

Once the color and size seem to be adequate, you should plan to harvest in the morning when it's cool. Make sure you don't leave the produce in direct sunlight or heat for too long; transfer it to a cool place for storage and continued maturing.

By picking only the produce that's ready, you may get several harvests out of a single plant. But if you pick too much of the produce early, the plant may stop producing and you'll have to start again.

Rely on your senses and take a taste of the harvest to see whether it tastes ready. As you gain more experience gardening, you'll discover how your superfood crops change with age. Then, you can harvest based on your desired taste and texture. You may want to pick some for eating and let some of your crop mature more for cooking (or vice versa). So use the guidelines shown in Table 14-1, but let your taste buds be the leader in your harvesting schedule.

The timing of harvesting can also affect next year's crops. If you let some vegetables fully mature, it may reduce the production of next year's crops.

Table 14-1	Harvesting Common Superfoods	
Produce	*Harvesting Tips*	*Other Information*
Beets	Harvest when they reach 1–2 inches in diameter or when the tops of the beets are popping out of the soil.	You can also use the tops of the beets as a green for cooking.
Broccoli	Cut the broccoli buds when they're grouped together, and make sure to leave about 5 inches of stalk. Pick them before they turn yellow or flower.	Harvest once the individual bulbs in the buds are about the size of a match head.
Carrots	Harvest when the carrots appear to be at least $3/4$ inch in diameter and bright orange, about 60 days after planting.	If you harvest early, you should taste the carrots to see whether you like the slightly different texture and flavor.
Cauliflower	Pick when the buds look full, compact, and smooth.	Don't wait too long to harvest; the head will start to come apart.
Garlic	Pick bulbs when the tops start to turn brown/yellow. Make sure you dig them out; don't pull on the tops, as this can damage the bulb.	After picking, dry the bulbs on a screen. Once they've dried, cut the roots back to the edge of the bulb, and they're ready to use.
Kale	Harvest the outer leaves once the plant has 6–8 leaves.	Once they bloom, pull the pods and throw them away.
Lima Beans	Pods should be full and bright green. Harvest before the beans turn yellow.	The ends of the bean should feel spongy.
Spinach	Harvest from the outside in, once the plant is fully green. Take the outer 3–4 leaves. Spinach needs a cooler climate. If you live in a hot climate, you may want to grow chard instead.	If you take only a few outer leaves at a time, the plant will continue to grow and produce. Pick the outer leaves but try to leave 3–4 along the center.
Strawberries	Strawberries usually are ready to pick about 30 days after the plant blossoms.	Strawberries don't ripen after they're picked, so be sure to wait until they're fully red.
Tomatoes	Harvest when most of the tomato is full color. Let the tomato ripen on the plant as much as possible.	Focus on color rather than size in deciding when to harvest. Do not refrigerate after harvesting.

Part IV
Putting Superfoods on Your Table

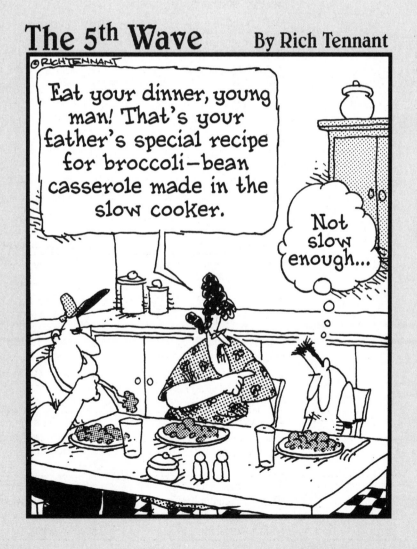

In this part . . .

The nutritional value of any food can be affected by the way you prepare it, and superfoods are no exception. In this part, we describe the best cooking and storage methods for various superfoods to make sure they're as healthful as they can be.

Then we offer our favorite superfood recipes for every meal, as well as appetizers, snacks, and desserts. Some of these recipes could be called super-duper, because they include several superfood ingredients.

Chapter 15

Preparing and Preserving Superfoods without Sacrificing Nutrition

Superfoods are super because they contain lots of nutrients, healthy fats, phytochemicals, and/or fiber. You want to make sure you keep your superfoods healthful by choosing the best cooking methods (or sometimes, not cooking them at all). Once any food has been harvested, it begins to lose some of its nutritional value — especially fruits and vegetables. You can't do much about this natural loss of vitamins (other than growing your own garden — see Chapter 14), but you can choose preparation and cooking methods that help to preserve the nutrients that are left.

You may want to stock your freezer and shelves with superfoods you've grown in your own garden or purchased in bulk when the price has been right, or you may want to save leftovers for lunch the next day. It's important to follow the rules of food safety for the proper storage of superfoods.

So remember to keep your foods super by cooking them right and storing them properly. You'll save money because you won't waste food, and you'll enjoy all your superfoods year-round. In this chapter, we talk about how to prepare your superfoods, how to cook them, and how to save them for later.

To Cook or Not to Cook

Should you eat your superfoods raw or cooked? Raw fruits and vegetables are good because the nutrients aren't lost in cooking. But eating most raw fish, for example, just isn't a good idea (unless you're a real sushi aficionado).

Fruits and vegetables offer the most nutrients just after they're harvested. As soon as they're picked, some of the vitamins that are sensitive to heat or light begin to degrade. When you expose these foods to the heat of cooking, you reduce some of the nutrient content even more.

Sometimes, preparation is just a personal preference. One person may love crunchy carrots, while another may prefer a purée. Or maybe you love spinach leaves in a salad, but not cooked. In these cases, our superfoods are perfectly healthy either way.

Sometimes it's a toss-up for the nutritional benefit, too. The anthocyanins in the blue pigment in blueberries and the lycopene in the red pigment of tomatoes are more concentrated by cooking, but the amounts of vitamins C and B in both foods are decreased by cooking.

Dealing with superfoods that can't take the heat

While most of our superfoods can be eaten either raw or cooked, some of them are best eaten (or stored) in their fresh, raw form as the following list explains.

- **Oranges and strawberries:** Cooking oranges and strawberries doesn't make them unhealthy. However, it decreases the amount of vitamin C, folate, and other B vitamins dramatically. These two superfood fruits should be eaten raw to maintain their nutrient content. Also, keep strawberries whole and leave the peel on the oranges until you're ready to eat them. Once you cut into your fruits, the vitamin C starts to diminish.

- **Nuts and seeds:** Raw nuts and seeds may be better than roasted nuts and seeds. They last much longer, and you don't have to watch for any excess salt or unhealthy flavorings that are often added during roasting. While roasted nuts and seeds contain the same nutritional content as their raw counterparts, they become rancid more quickly, so don't roast them until you're ready to eat them, or buy the amount of roasted nuts and seeds that you can eat in a few days and store them in an airtight container in the refrigerator.

✔ **Flax seeds and flaxseed oil:** The oils in flax are delicate, and cooking and heat exposure destroy flax's health properties. The fats will go bad if the flax isn't stored properly. Buy unmilled flax seeds in small bags and keep them refrigerated. When you're ready to use the seeds, grind a spoonful in a coffee grinder. Add flaxseed oil to foods that have already been cooked, and always store bottled flaxseed oil in the refrigerator.

✔ **Wheat grass:** Wheat grass is usually consumed in powdered form or as a juice. In either case, wheat grass is processed without high heat because heat destroys the enzymes that are believed to be beneficial to health.

The fact that some foods are best raw doesn't mean proper storage isn't a concern. Apples, bananas, and oranges keep at room temperature for a few days, but should be refrigerated for longer storage. Raw vegetables, super-food oils such as olive oil and flaxseed oil, and raw nuts should be refrigerated in covered containers.

Olive oil starts to spoil as soon as you open the container. It's okay to keep small amounts of oil in a cool dark space away from your oven or other sources of heat, but if you buy large containers of oil, keep most of it refrigerated until you need it.

It's important to keep your raw superfoods safe from cross-contamination of bacteria that may be found in raw meats or unwashed food:

✔ **Use separate utensils for cutting raw meats.** Say you're serving a salad with raw tomatoes, carrots, and spinach leaves, along with baked chicken for dinner. If you use a knife and a cutting board to cut raw chicken, don't use that same knife and cutting board for preparing your raw salad vegetables.

✔ **Wash your hands thoroughly.** Wash your hands before you prepare a meal and after you handle any raw meats or unwashed produce. This helps to stop the spread of bacteria.

✔ **Rinse fruits and vegetables before preparing them.** Even if you throw away the peels, you should rinse your produce first to remove any bacteria from the surface. Rinse pre-packaged greens such as spinach leaves, too.

✔ **Store raw produce away from raw meats.** Keep raw meats in plastic bags to prevent leakage of fluids, and, when you store them in the fridge, don't put them above any foods that you'll eat raw, such as fruits and veggies.

Sprouting lentils

Lentils can be sprouted just like alfalfa seeds or beans, and you can eat the raw sprouts in a salad or stir-fry. Sprouting lentils at home is a fun project and very easy to do by following these steps:

1. Place ½ cup lentils in a glass jar with 2 cups water. Cover the jar with cheesecloth, secure with a rubber band, and let sit overnight.

2. The next morning, drain the water, rinse the lentils, and cover with fresh water. Repeat this process for two days.

3. On the third or fourth day, you'll see ¼- to ½-inch sprouts peeking out of the lentils. When you see the sprouts, they're ready to go. Drain the sprouted lentils and refrigerate them in a jar or plastic bag.

Cooking when cooking is best

Some superfoods need to be cooked (or processed in some manner) before you eat them, as the following list explains. Don't worry: Cooking doesn't harm the nutritional value of these foods.

- **Dry beans and soybeans:** Dry beans such as black beans and soybeans must be cooked before you eat them. Raw dry beans will cause stomachaches because they contain phytohaemagglutinin (a type of protein known as a lectin that causes red blood cells to bind together) and are difficult to digest.

- **Lentils:** Like the dry beans, lentils need to be cooked before you eat them. Alternatively, lentils can be sprouted and you can eat the raw sprouts, as the nearby sidebar explains.

- **Fish:** Our superfood fish should be cooked, too, unless you're very skilled at preparing raw fish dishes such as sushi and sashimi, and you can find the best sources for purchasing healthful raw fish. Cooking fish doesn't ruin protein, nutrients, or omega-3 fatty acids. We have several recipes for salmon dishes (see Chapter 17), and pre-cooked salmon and tuna are available in convenient cans and pouches that can be used for delicious superfood sandwiches and salads. Fish doesn't need to be overcooked, and fish like tuna and salmon can be served medium-rare. According to the United States Department of Agriculture (USDA), fish should be cooked to an internal temperature of 145 degrees Fahrenheit.

Using the Healthiest Cooking Methods

Cooking changes the foods we eat. Think of an egg: a fried or hard-boiled egg bears little physical resemblance to a raw one. Likewise, the color and texture of meat changes when you cook it. And even the toughest vegetables and grains become soft and tender with cooking.

We cook the foods we eat for a variety of reasons:

✔ **To change the temperature.** Some foods are more appealing when they're served hot (not many people can enjoy a bowl of cold chicken noodle soup, for example). Other foods are good either hot or cold, like green tea: Served hot, it's a cup of steaming comfort on a damp, gray day. Served cold, it's a refreshing break on a sunny, warm afternoon.

✔ **To change the flavor.** Cooking changes the flavor of many foods, and not only because of the heat. Seasoning a food you cook with luscious herbs and spices can transform a dull vegetable into something delicious.

✔ **To change the texture.** Cooking makes vegetables soft, so someone who doesn't like crunchy carrots might just love a cooked carrot purée. The flesh of fish becomes flaky when it's ready to eat, rather than rubbery. Legumes and grains start out as hard seeds and become soft and tender morsels when they're cooked.

✔ **To kill bacteria.** The foods in your kitchen have probably been in quite a few different places and may have been exposed to bacteria and molds that can make you sick. This is especially true for meat, poultry, and fish that may be contaminated with bacteria such as salmonella and E. coli. Exposure to high temperatures wipes these little bugs right out.

Cooking foods also changes the nutritional content. Some nutrients like vitamin A, lycopene, and some other phytochemicals become more concentrated, but vitamin C and the B vitamins are usually greatly reduced with cooking. Of course, the cooking methods you choose make a difference in the amount of nutrients lost. Generally, methods that use shorter exposure to heat result in less nutritional loss.

Boiling is a poor cooking method for vegetables because the heat and cooking time cause nutrients to be destroyed or leached into the cooking water. If you do boil your vegetables, use the cooking water whenever possible in soup, stew, or sauces. Deep-frying and pan-frying are even worse because they introduce extra unhealthy fats and calories. Some methods, like grilling and slow-cooking, can be good or bad, so we give you some tips on how to do them right.

Steaming

Steaming vegetables retains more of the nutrients that would normally get washed away in boiling water. Steaming also allows for a wonderful crisp-tender texture compared to boiled vegetables that often get mushy.

Steaming is easy. Even if you don't have a fancy countertop steamer, you can steam your vegetables in a pot on the stove using an expandable vegetable steamer:

1. **Add 1 inch of water to a cooking pot and place on high heat. Place an expandable vegetable steamer into the pot.**

   The bottom of the steamer will be just above water level.

2. **When the water is boiling, place your vegetables into the steamer and steam them until they're crisp-tender.**

   This takes about three to five minutes, depending on the size of the pieces.

3. **Serve your vegetables with a sprinkle of lemon juice, salt, and pepper.**

Electric steamers are very convenient. Add water to the steamer (follow the manufacturer's instructions) and place your vegetables in the steamer basket. Steam until vegetables are crisp-tender. These electric steamers usually work very well as rice-cookers, too.

Expandable vegetable steamers are inexpensive and easy to find in most grocery stores and retail stores that carry home goods. Electric steamers vary in cost depending on size and additional features, such as the ability to cook two separate vegetables at the same time or program the steamer's timer. Black and Decker makes several styles of electric vegetable steamers for any budget or need.

Stir-frying and sautéing

Shorter cooking time makes stir-frying and sautéing better for superfoods than other types of frying because most of the nutrient content is preserved. Both methods use high heat with just a small amount of oil. To stir fry, you use a spoon or spatula to stir the foods as they cook. To sauté, you keep the pan moving and use a flipping motion to toss the foods so they don't burn. Use a large nonstick skillet or a wok and oils that can take the heat (peanut, olive, and canola oils are good choices), and cook vegetables only until they're crisp-tender. Follow these steps for both cooking methods:

1. **Prepare your vegetables and ingredients before you start cooking — you don't want to overcook one vegetable while you're slicing another. Wash and cut vegetables into bite-sized pieces.**

   If you're adding meat to your stir-fry, be sure to cook it thoroughly before you cook your vegetables. Don't put raw meat on your cooked vegetables.

2. **Heat the wok or sauté pan to a high temperature and then add a small amount of oil.**

3. **For a simple stir-fry, add garlic or onion and stir for one minute.**

4. **Add other vegetables and cook them (stirring constantly) until they're crisp-tender.**

5. **Add any sauces, such as soy sauce, ginger sauce, or teriyaki sauce, about halfway through the cooking time.**

When you sauté foods, control the temperature. Otherwise the oil may get too hot and start to smoke.

A sauté pan has a wide, flat bottom and should be made from high-quality, heavy-gauge metal, such as stainless steel, with a copper core or aluminum bottom. This type of pan conducts heat evenly for the best cooking. Calphalon and All-Clad make high-quality and affordable sauté pans.

Traditional woks are made with thin carbon steel, but they must be seasoned, so many people prefer stainless steel woks. Joyce Chen makes carbon steel and nonstick woks that are terrific for stir-frying at home.

Poaching

Poaching is cooking a food in a liquid. One well-known example is a poached egg, which is cooked in water. You can simmer your foods in wine, vinegar, or low-sodium broth to add flavor. Add even more flavor by sprinkling some herbs and spices into the poaching liquid.

Poaching isn't the same as boiling. You use low heat so that your liquid just simmers (you'll see a few small bubbles rise to the surface of the liquid).

Poaching is typically used to cook meats, poultry, and fish (it's perfect for salmon), but you can also poach vegetables and fruits. Following are a couple ideas:

- ✔ Poach salmon fillets in a broth of equal parts white wine and low-sodium chicken broth, with some lemon juice and a dash of salt and pepper. Simmer the fillets for about 10 minutes or until the flesh is flaky. Serve with some slices of lemon and roasted vegetables on the side.

- ✔ Poach apples for a healthful sweet treat. Wash and cut two Granny Smith apples into halves and poach in apple cider with a cinnamon stick and $1/4$ teaspoon of nutmeg. Simmer apples until they're tender, about 10 to 15 minutes. Serve with a sauce of $1/2$ cup of plain yogurt and 1 tablespoon of honey, and sprinkle with chopped almonds.

Choose a saucepan that is just a bit bigger than the food you're poaching, and use enough liquid to just cover your food. The pan should be made of a heavy-gauge stainless steel with a copper core or aluminum bottom. Copper and aluminum conduct heat well, but you don't want these two metals to come in direct contact with your food because they can interact negatively with foods; stainless steel does not. All-Clad and Calphalon produce high-quality saucepans at a good price.

Roasting and baking

Traditionally, roasting was done over open flames and baking was done in an oven, but today the two terms are almost interchangeable. You can roast or bake meats and vegetables in your oven, but you bake desserts, breads, and pastries.

Roasting and baking reduce vitamin content, but they're still considered healthful cooking methods because neither requires additional fat (although adding a little olive oil to roast vegetables adds a nice flavor).

Roasting brings out the natural flavors in vegetables, especially the sweetness, so it may be a great way to please picky eaters who don't like the bitter taste of vegetables.

To roast vegetables:

1. **Preheat oven to 400 degrees Fahrenheit, and place one layer of washed and sliced vegetables on a roasting pan or foil-lined baking dish.**

   For best results, cut the vegetables into pieces that are about the same size.

2. **Drizzle a small amount of olive oil over your vegetables (you don't need much).**

   You can also use an olive oil spray.

3. **Add your favorite seasonings, such as rosemary, oregano, nutmeg, and salt and pepper.**

4. **Roast until the vegetables are tender (pierce them with a fork) and slightly browned — about 20 to 35 minutes.**

Serve roasted superfood carrots and beets (see Chapter 5) topped with toasted nuts for a delicious side dish. You can also bake fish fillets (see our salmon recipes in Chapter 17) or whole fish in your oven. You can roast your own pumpkin seeds; however, you should do so at a much lower temperature: about 300 degrees Fahrenheit.

Choose high-quality roasting and baking pans for best results. Look for heavy aluminized steel, which is important for even cooking. A nonstick surface is also necessary. Some roasting pans come with a metal rack so meat and poultry can cook without wallowing in grease. Chicago Metallic makes high-quality, affordable lines of cookware.

How microwaves work

Microwave ovens cook food when the radio waves emitted in the oven are absorbed by the water, fat, and sugar in the foods. The microwaves are converted to heat, which cooks the food. Plastic, glass, and ceramic materials don't absorb microwaves, so they stay cool (until the heat from the food warms them up). The air surrounding the food isn't warm at all (unlike the inside of a conventional oven), so foods don't brown or get crusty when you cook them unless you use special foils that can brown the edges of breads and pastries by exposing the surfaces of these foods to extra heat.

Slow-cooking

Preparing dinner with a slow cooker, or crockpot, is easy. Simply add your ingredients to the cooker before you go to work, and when you get home, dinner's hot and ready. Slow cookers cook foods at lower temperatures but for very long periods of time. You lose some of the vitamins, but if you need the convenience, using a slow cooker can still be very healthful.

Make a simple vegetable soup by using low-sodium chicken broth and your choice of vegetables. You can also cook dry beans in a slow cooker with water, onions, garlic, salt, and pepper.

To get the healthiest meals from your slow cooker, follow these guidelines:

✔ Choose recipes that are low in saturated fats (avoid using high-fat red meats) and low in sodium, and use the liquid as part of the final dish (think pasta sauce, soup, or stew), because some of the vitamins that are cooked out of the foods will be found in the broth.

✔ Keep perishable ingredients refrigerated until you're ready to start the slow cooker.

✔ To make sure your food reaches the right temperature, fill the slow cooker at least half full, but not more than ²/₃ full.

Grilling

You probably think of grilling as a way to cook hamburgers, steaks, and hot-dogs on a warm summer day. But you can also grill many superfoods, such as fish, vegetables, and even some fruits. You'll keep your kitchen cooler and enjoy healthful foods with a grilled flavor.

You can buy a charcoal grill, which is preferred by many cooks for the charcoal flavoring, or you can buy a gas grill, which is more convenient. Either grill works just fine.

Cut vegetables in long slices so they won't fall through the grates of the grill. Brush them with olive oil or marinate them in a seasoned dressing. Place the vegetables on the grill and cook until tender. Add some salt and pepper, and they're ready to serve.

Follow these steps to cook fish on the grill:

1. **Lay two sheets of aluminum foil flat (or use heavy-duty aluminum foil to prevent accidental tearing of the foil).**

2. **Place one fish fillet in the center of the foil and fold up all four sides slightly; add a splash of white wine, olive oil, lemon juice, and a clove of garlic.**

3. **Fold the foil over the fish and crimp the sides together to seal the pouch.**

4. **Place the pouch on a grill over medium heat and cook until fish is tender and flaky, about 15 to 20 minutes.**

Grills come in a broad range of sizes and prices, from small portable tabletop grills to very large grills. Weber makes high-quality grills, both charcoal and gas varieties.

Microwaving safely

Almost every kitchen has a microwave oven, and they're wonderfully fast and convenient. Microwave radiation may sound scary, but that part of microwaving is very safe. The problem with using a microwave oven is that it may cook unevenly, which can leave cold spots in foods that don't reach a high enough temperature for thorough cooking.

Your microwave works best for heating foods that have already been cooked or only need to be warmed. However, you can buy accessories that allow you to cook some foods nicely, such as microwave steamers and turntables that allow for more even cooking.

Follow these tips to use your microwave safely:

- ✔ Arrange foods to be heated evenly in your microwave-safe container. Cover loosely with plastic wrap or a lid to trap heat from the foods (and protect your microwave oven from the inevitable splatters).

- ✔ Use containers that have been approved for microwave use. Some soft plastics give off toxic substances when they're exposed to hot foods. Glass and ceramic are safe and stand up to the heat of microwaved foods better than thin plastic containers. Don't cook (or reheat) foods in Styrofoam containers.

- ✔ Stir soft foods and liquids frequently while cooking to avoid hot and cold spots.

✔ If you use a microwave to thaw foods, follow the manufacturer's instructions that accompany your microwave and cook the thawed foods right away. Be especially careful with thawed meats, poultry, and fish. They're still raw, and improper handling can result in cross-contamination of other foods.

Some frozen vegetables are packaged in special steamer bags made from microwave-safe plastics. These are quite convenient, but be careful when you open the bags because the vegetables inside will be very hot.

Storing for Later Use

It would be wonderful to start every meal with fresh, in-season superfoods, but that isn't practical. Some of your superfoods will need to be kept in storage for a while. Or, if you make a big meal, you may have some leftovers to keep for lunch the next day.

Some people like to prepare a week's worth (or more) of meals at one time to keep in the refrigerator or freezer until needed. Then these meals can be popped into the oven or microwave for easy cooking at the end of a busy day.

To keep your superfoods healthful, you need to follow a few simple rules to keep them safe and delicious. This is important for storage of leftovers, for long-term freezing of foods, and for canning and preserving.

Keeping cold foods cold and hot foods hot

Keep your foods at the proper temperature to reduce the risk of spoilage and bacterial contamination. Your refrigerator should be kept at 40 degrees Fahrenheit or lower, and your freezer should be kept at 0 degrees Fahrenheit. Hot foods need to be kept at 140 degrees Fahrenheit or higher to prevent bacterial growth. Perishable foods should only remain at room temperature for two hours (or only one hour if the air temperature is about 90 degrees or higher). Leaving food out in the open air longer than that may lead to spoilage and food-borne illness.

To ensure food safety, heed the following tips:

✔ When you buy your groceries, choose the cold and frozen foods last and drive straight home after shopping. Don't leave your food in a hot car.

✔ Remove leftovers promptly after a meal and keep them in resealable containers in your refrigerator. Use them within three or four days.

✔ Keep picnic foods cold in coolers with ice. Keep raw meats in a separate cooler to prevent cross-contamination with other foods.

✔ Keep hot picnic and party foods (like a buffet) at 140 degrees or warmer.

✔ Transport cold foods in portable coolers and hot foods in insulated containers.

✔ Pack lunches in insulated bags with frozen cold-packs to keep beverages and perishable foods cold and sandwiches safe. Keep soups, hot foods, and warm beverages in insulated containers, like the ones made by Thermos.

Freezing superfoods for later

You can keep most foods in the freezer for several months. However, improperly frozen foods will show signs of *freezer burn,* which appears as white, dried-out patches on your food. You can freeze raw and cooked foods as long as they're in separate containers.

✔ **Wrap your superfoods fish (and low-fat meat and poultry) in heavy-duty freezer paper.** The plastic wrap used at the meat counter in stores can't withstand freezing for long periods, and your food will be ruined.

✔ **Retain the color and texture of vegetables by blanching them before freezing.** Simply place small amounts of the vegetables (about the amount you want to store in a freezer container) in boiling water for a short time (usually 3 to 5 minutes) to partially cook the vegetable. You can test doneness by biting into a piece — it should still be crunchy. Plunge the vegetables into a bowl of ice water as soon as you remove them from the boiling water to stop the cooking process and bring the temperature down. When the vegetables are cold, place them in freezer containers and freeze.

✔ **Use freezer bags, some of which are even microwave-safe and specially treated to prevent freezer burn.** Remove as much air as possible from each bag before zipping it shut.

If you freeze a lot of food, you may want to buy a vacuum sealing machine and rolls of freezer bag material. These machines remove all of the air, which means you can store the foods longer with less chance of freezer burn.

✔ **Thaw your foods in the microwave or in a large pot of cold water in the refrigerator.** Don't set them out at room temperature because this can invite bacterial growth.

✔ **Most superfood fruits can be frozen without any special preparation (see Chapter 5). However, you may want to use sturdy containers to prevent the fruit from getting crushed in the freezer.**

Try once-a-week (or once-a-month) cooking if you have a big freezer. Spend a day preparing meals with your fresh ingredients and freeze them to be cooked and served during the subsequent days or weeks. For example, you can place four raw, skinless chicken breasts in a large freezer bag with ¹/₂ cup olive oil, your favorite dry herbs, and salt and pepper, and pop it in the freezer. When you want to eat them, thaw them in the refrigerator or microwave and bake in an oven preheated to 350 degrees Fahrenheit until cooked through. Heat a bag of superfood vegetables for a side dish, and add a salad made with pre-washed greens and fresh vegetables.

You can also cook your meals in large amounts and freeze extra portions that you simply heat and eat later (think vegetarian lasagna).

Canning and preserving

People have canned and preserved foods for home use for quite some time. While freezing is probably the easiest method for long-term storage of foods, there's something nice about a cabinet full of home-canned vegetables, fruits, sauces, and pickled foods. When you can foods, you heat them to a temperature that will kill bacteria and allow the jars to seal.

Canning your superfoods

There are two types of canning methods: a water bath and pressure canning. The water bath method uses hot water to heat jars that have been filled with foods. This works fine for fruits, pickles, and tomatoes, but not for other vegetables.

All other vegetables need to be canned with a pressure canner. Vegetables are low in acid, so they're likely to become contaminated with *botulism* (a food-borne illness caused by a toxin that can withstand high temperatures).

To properly can foods, start with scrupulously clean jars to ensure your foods don't get contaminated with bacteria or other substances. Also make sure the jars don't have any cracks or chips, especially on the rims, as that may prevent the lids from sealing. Then follow these steps:

1. **Prepare the vegetables you want to can by cleaning them, cutting them into pieces, placing them in a large pot, and covering them with water.**

2. **Boil the vegetables for five minutes.**

3. **Add vegetables and boiling water to your jars, leaving about 1 inch of headspace. Add 1 teaspoon of salt to each jar.**

4. **Place the canning lids on the jars and secure with the rings.**

   Follow the instructions that come with your pressure canner for processing.

   Be sure that all canning jars seal properly. Any unsealed jars need to be kept in the refrigerator or reprocessed.

Beets can be pickled or canned with vinegar, similar to pickling cucumbers or peppers.

Water canners are simply large pots with wire racks. They're inexpensive and easy to find in stores. Presto makes pressure canners that you can use for your low-acid vegetables.

Dehydrating your superfoods

You may want to try drying some of your superfoods (like apples, bananas, and strawberries) in a dehydrator. Prepare your fruits and layer them on the drying racks; then place the racks in the dehydrator. Your fruits are dehydrated and preserved when they appear shriveled with a leathery texture.

Use dried fruits in breakfast cereals, or make your own granola (see Chapter 16). Make fruit leathers by puréeing fruit and spreading it on special fruit leather paper.

Dehydrators vary by capacity and amount of airflow. Look for a dehydrator that offers lots of drying space and heats with an even temperature. Excalibur makes affordable dehydrators for home use.

Smoking superfood fish

Many people enjoy smoked salmon and smoked trout, and, if you own a smoker, you'll enjoy making your own smoked fish. A smoker is similar to a grill, but you cook with smoke that carries the flavor of the wood that's burned in the smoker.

The best part of smoking your own fish is that you control the ingredients used in the preparation. Some commercial brands of smoked fish contain *nitrates,* chemicals found in smoked foods, lunchmeats, and sausages that have been linked to a higher risk of some cancers.

To smoke your own fish:

1. **Prepare your salmon or trout by soaking it in a brine (salt water) before smoking.**

2. **Choose wood that complements the flavor of your fish.**

   Alder is often used for salmon. Other woods that work well with fish include apple and oak.

3. **Follow the manufacturer's instructions for using your smoker.**

Serve your smoked fish as an appetizer with whole-grain crackers, or top a healthful pizza with some smoked salmon, sun-dried tomatoes, and basil.

Smokers vary greatly in price, and you can choose from charcoal or electric units. Weber makes terrific charcoal smokers at lower prices. Old Smokey makes inexpensive electric smokers that perform very well.

Chapter 16

Starting the Day Right: Superfood Breakfast Recipes

In This Chapter

▶ Understanding why you need to eat breakfast

▶ Making breakfast quick and easy

▶ Indulging on the weekends

Is eating breakfast all that important? Yes, absolutely. Kids have an easier time learning in school and people who eat breakfast every day have an easier time watching their weight. This doesn't mean that just any food will do. A couple of glazed donuts with a can of high-caffeine soda isn't a good breakfast. Cold cereal from a box is better, but still may have too much sugar that you don't need. There are much healthier alternatives, and breakfast time is a great time to start with some superfoods.

In this chapter, we give you some delicious and easy breakfast ideas, tips, and recipes so you can start every day with a super breakfast.

Understanding the Importance of the Most Important Meal of the Day

When you eat breakfast, you *break* the *fast* your body went through during the night. You need breakfast to refuel your body and your brain. A study reported in the journal *Pediatrics* found that high school students who eat breakfast are more alert and have better cognitive function. The same goes for adults, too. When you eat breakfast, you replenish the glucose (a type of sugar) that your brain needs to function, so you feel better and think better.

Unfortunately, many people mistakenly believe that skipping breakfast will help them lose weight, but it doesn't work. According to the Mayo Clinic, eating breakfast is actually good for weight loss. People who eat breakfast every day are much more likely to be at a healthy weight. When you skip breakfast, you end up eating too much when you do finally eat.

That doesn't mean you have to eat the instant you get out of bed. You can wait to eat until you feel hungry. Just remember to eat something nutritious.

Not any old breakfast will do. You need to eat a healthful, balanced breakfast to start your day. Choose a variety of foods that will give you plenty of nutrients and fiber, such as whole grains, low-fat dairy products, protein sources, and fruits and vegetables. Here are some examples of simple but healthful breakfasts:

- ✔ A slice of whole-grain toast with almond butter, a fresh piece of fruit, and a glass of nonfat milk

- ✔ A small bowl of whole-grain, high-fiber cold cereal with blueberries and nonfat milk, and calcium-fortified orange juice

- ✔ One hard-boiled egg, a small whole-grain bagel, and low-fat cream cheese with a cup of green tea

- ✔ Hot oatmeal topped with strawberries and walnuts

Making Super Breakfast Recipes

When you add superfoods to your breakfast lineup, you take breakfast to a higher level. Breakfast is a super time to get these superfoods into your day:

- ✔ **Oats:** Enjoy oatmeal, whole-grain bread, muffins, or cereal, or add oats to pancake and waffle recipes.

- ✔ **Fruits and berries:** A piece of fresh fruit, such as an apple, banana, or orange, can be added to any breakfast. Sliced fruits and berries can be added to cereal or to crepes, pancakes, or waffles.

✔ **Nuts and seeds:** Top oatmeal with walnuts, pecans, or almonds, or sprinkle flax or chia seeds on your cereal.

✔ **Green tea:** Replace one cup of coffee with hot green tea.

✔ **Vegetables:** Include spinach, broccoli, or tomatoes in egg dishes.

The following recipes can help you get some of these superfoods in your breakfast. We have "breakfast-on-the-go" recipes for foods that you can grab just before you head out the door. We also have some easy recipes that take a little more time, but not much effort. They'll be ready about the same time your coffee's done. There are also delicious recipes that are perfect for weekends or whenever you have a little extra time.

Eating on the go

These recipes are perfect for anyone who has a habit of skipping breakfast because "there just isn't enough time." Breakfast doesn't need to be a full-sized, sit-down meal, with lots of dirty pots, pans, and dishes to wash.

The secret is to have your breakfast foods ready to go so they don't need much preparation. Make our muffins or granola on the weekends and use them for breakfast during the week. Your breakfast-on-the-go items may also include hard-boiled eggs, whole-wheat toast with nut butter, and single-serving cups of yogurt (but avoid extra sugar).

Some of our superfood breakfast recipes may not be as sweet as the cereal and pastry items you may be used to eating. But cutting back on sugar allows you to taste the flavors of the fruits, nuts, and grains. If you're used to a sugary breakfast, you can add a little sugar, honey, 100 percent fruit spread or artificial sweetener — just not too much.

Ready-to-eat cereals

Grocery stores devote entire aisles to ready-to-eat cereals that are convenient and tasty, and some are quite healthful. Just about all cereals are fortified with extra vitamins and minerals. The problem is that some are overloaded with sugar, especially kids' cereals. Too much sugar means too many calories.

Read the labels. Choose cereals that are low in sugar (even the non-frosted cereals can be sugary) and high in fiber. Look for the words "100 percent whole wheat" or "100 percent whole grain" on the label. Shredded wheat, toasted oat rings, and puffed wheat bran flakes are all excellent choices. Dress them up with berries, sliced bananas, raisins, or peaches. Still need a little more sweetness? Add just one teaspoon of sugar or honey, or a little sucralose (known best as Splenda).

☺ Oatmeal Blueberry Muffins

Make these muffins the night before, so they're ready to go in the morning. These muffins aren't as sweet as the muffins you find in bakeries and coffee shops, but they're delicious plain. You can also spread a little 100 percent fruit spread or honey on them for extra flavor and sweetness. These muffins are healthy because they incorporate two superfoods — blueberries and oatmeal — and because they're 100 percent whole-grain.

Prep time: *About 10 minutes*

Cooking time: *25 minutes*

Yield: *8 servings*

³/₄ cup whole-wheat flour	*¹/₂ cup plain nonfat yogurt*
³/₄ cup old-fashioned rolled oats	*¹/₄ cup low-fat or nonfat milk*
¹/₄ cup firmly packed dark brown sugar	*2 tablespoons canola oil*
1¹/₂ teaspoons baking powder	*1 large egg, beaten lightly*
¹/₂ teaspoon salt	*³/₄ cup fresh or frozen blueberries*

1 Preheat oven to 400 degrees Fahrenheit.

2 In a bowl, stir together the flour, oats, brown sugar, baking powder, and salt.

3 In second bowl, combine the yogurt, milk, oil, and egg. Stir the yogurt mixture into the flour mixture until just combined. Fold in blueberries.

4 Divide the batter among 8 paper-lined cupcake tins and bake on the middle rack of oven for 25 minutes.

Per serving: *Calories 152 (From Fat 45); Fat 5g (Saturated 1g); Cholesterol 27mg; Sodium 245mg; Carbohydrate 23g (Dietary Fiber 3g); Protein 5g.*

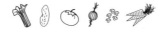

☺ Make-Your-Own Granola

Make this granola to keep handy as a quick snack, or eat it as a cold cereal with milk. This granola has a toasty, nutty flavor and is a delicious way to enjoy almonds, oats, and cranberries.

Prep time: *About 10 minutes*

Cooking time: *20 to 30 minutes*

Yield: *6 servings*

2 cups rolled oats

½ cup raw unsalted slivered almonds

¼ cup raw unsalted sunflower seeds

¼ cup raw unsalted pumpkin seeds

¼ cup honey

½ cup canola oil

½ cup dried cranberries

1 Preheat oven to 300 degrees Fahrenheit.

2 Mix together oats, almonds, and sunflower and pumpkin seeds in a bowl.

3 Mix the honey and oil together in a separate bowl, then pour onto dry mixture. Stir well.

4 Spread onto a greased baking pan and bake for 20 to 30 minutes, or until golden in color, stirring occasionally.

5 Pour into bowl and add cranberries. Let the granola cool, then store in a covered container.

6 At breakfast time, pour ³/₄ cup cereal into bowl and add milk, or pack in individual snack bags.

Per serving: Calories 458 (From Fat 275); Fat 31g (Saturated 3g); Cholesterol 0mg; Sodium 3mg; Carbohydrate 42g (Dietary Fiber 5g); Protein 9g.

☽ Simple Peanut Butter and Banana Smoothie

Smoothies are delicious and very good for you when you use healthful ingredients. This breakfast smoothie is a good source of protein and is super with the addition of the banana. You could make it even more super by using plain soy beverage instead of milk.

Prep time: *About 5 minutes*

Yield: *1 serving*

1 banana (for best texture, peel, break into chunks, and freeze ahead of time)

²/₃ cup low-fat or nonfat milk

2 tablespoons peanut butter

1 tablespoon honey

3 to 4 ice cubes

1 Combine banana, milk, peanut butter, and honey in blender. Blend at high speed until smooth and creamy.

2 Add ice and blend until smooth. Pour in a tall glass to serve.

Per serving: Calories 431 (From Fat 168); Fat 19g (Saturated 5g); Cholesterol 7mg; Sodium 235mg; Carbohydrate 59g (Dietary Fiber 5g); Protein 15g.

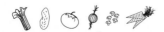

Easy breakfast recipes

Maybe you aren't in a big rush in the morning, but you still don't want to spend time cooking extravagant breakfast foods. Not to worry. These recipes are easy to make and taste great.

These recipes feature fresh fruits that are rich in nutrients and fiber, plus whole grains whenever possible. Oats are our favorite whole grain, and we also include a recipe for hot quinoa, which is perfect to warm up with on a cold morning.

⌾ Banana Cream Oatmeal

A bowl of hot oatmeal is so good on a cool morning. Oatmeal is already a superfood, but we add a banana to make it even more super. This is a little sweeter than our other breakfast recipes, so it's a great choice for kids (or grown-ups) who have grown accustomed to sugary breakfast cereals.

Prep time: About 2 minutes

Cooking time: 4 minutes

Yield: 2 servings

1 cup rolled oats

1³/₄ cups water

1 tablespoon brown sugar (or substitute artificial sweetener)

¹/₈ teaspoon salt

¹/₂ cup banana slices

2 tablespoons half-and-half (or substitute nonfat milk, soy beverage, or rice milk)

¹/₄ cup walnuts (optional)

1 Stir the oats, water, brown sugar, and salt together in a microwave-safe bowl.

2 Microwave on high for 2 minutes. Remove from microwave, add bananas and stir. Return to microwave and cook for additional 2 minutes.

3 Divide oatmeal into two serving bowls. Drizzle with half-and-half and top with walnuts if desired.

Per serving: Calories 234 (From Fat 40); Fat 4g (Saturated 2g); Cholesterol 6mg; Sodium 156mg; Carbohydrate 43g (Dietary Fiber 5g); Protein 7g.

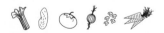

☕ Fruit and Yogurt Parfait

This beautiful breakfast packs a nutritional punch with fresh fruit, yogurt, and granola. The recipe is versatile, too. You can choose one type of fruit or use a mixture of different fruits and berries. Use our Make-Your-Own Granola (see the preceding section) or any whole-grain cereal.

Prep time: *About 5 to 10 minutes*

Yield: *2 servings*

1 cup plain nonfat yogurt

¼ cup honey (optional)

1 cup fresh cherries, strawberries, blueberries (or these fruits can be frozen, thawed, and drained) and/or banana slices

½ cup granola or whole-grain cereal

1 Mix yogurt and honey in a small mixing bowl.

2 Spoon half of the fruit or berries into the bottom of each parfait glass.

3 Add half of the yogurt to each glass.

4 Top with half of the granola or cereal.

Per serving: *Calories 233 (From Fat 47); Fat 5g (Saturated 2g); Cholesterol 3mg; Sodium 104mg; Carbohydrate 39g (Dietary Fiber 3g); Protein 10g.*

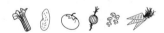

🍓 Strawberry Breakfast Pizzas

Fresh strawberries are rich in vitamin C and phytochemicals that help to keep you healthy, and they're the featured ingredient in this breakfast pizza recipe. This is very easy to make and fun for kids to assemble with a little help.

Prep time: About 10 minutes

Yield: 4 servings

2 whole-wheat English muffins

⅓ cup plain nonfat yogurt

1 tablespoon honey

¾ cup fresh strawberries, sliced (frozen strawberries may be too soft and mushy)

2 tablespoons strawberry all-fruit spread

1 Split and toast English muffins.

2 In a small bowl, mix together the yogurt and honey.

3 Spoon ¼ of the yogurt and honey mixture onto each English muffin half. Place a layer of strawberry slices on each half.

4 Warm the fruit spread in the microwave oven in 5-second bursts (up to 15 seconds), until it's similar in consistency to syrup.

5 Drizzle the warm fruit spread over the muffins and serve.

Per serving: Calories 125 (From Fat 8); Fat 1g (Saturated 0g); Cholesterol 0mg; Sodium 228mg; Carbohydrate 27g (Dietary Fiber 3g); Protein 4g.

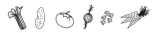

🍓 Hot Quinoa with Cinnamon and Fruit

Quinoa is actually a seed, but we use it like a grain in cooking. It has a light fluffy texture and a slightly nutty flavor. In this recipe, we combine quinoa with berries and bananas for a hot breakfast dish that's high in fiber and nutrients.

Prep time: About 10 minutes

Cooking time: About 15 minutes

Yield: 4 servings

1 cup nonfat milk

1 cup water

1 cup quinoa, rinsed

1½ cups fresh blueberries and/or strawberries

½ cup bananas

½ teaspoon ground cinnamon

2 tablespoons honey

Pinch of salt

1 Combine milk, water, and quinoa in saucepan. Bring to a boil over high heat.

2 Reduce heat to low, cover, and simmer for about 15 minutes, or until most of the liquid is absorbed.

3 Remove from heat and let stand for 5 minutes. Stir in berries, bananas, and cinnamon.

4 Serve immediately in four bowls. Add a drizzle of honey and pinch of salt to each bowl.

Tip: *Instead of fresh berries, you can use frozen blueberries, thawed and drained, but frozen strawberries may be too mushy and should be avoided.*

Per serving: *Calories 229 (From Fat 26); Fat 3g (Saturated 0g); Cholesterol 1mg; Sodium 44mg; Carbohydrate 45g (Dietary Fiber 5g); Protein 8g.*

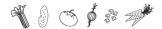

Living lavishly on the weekends

Start your weekend mornings with these healthful and delicious breakfast recipes that are worth the little extra time they take to prepare. Get a jump-start on your daily superfoods intake with recipes that will satisfy your sweet tooth (with less sugar) plus two savory egg dishes.

The lowdown on natural sweeteners

What is the nutritional difference between regular sugar and high-fructose corn syrup? *Almost nothing.* What about between regular sugar and turbinado (raw sugar)? *Just the color.* What about honey — is that better? *Maybe a little, but very little.* Nutritionally, honey and sugar are the same. Some experts claim some honey has some health benefits, but research to support those claims isn't clear. What is clear, however, is the delicious flavor of honey that you won't find with sugar, which really only tastes sweet. But don't give honey to children under 1 year of age, as it can cause botulism in babies.

Americans really like sweet stuff. Sodas, candies, and pastries are obviously high in sugar, but sugar is creeping into our diet in lots of processed foods. According to the U.S. Department of Agriculture, consumption of sweeteners added to processed foods has gone up 23 percent since the 1980s. Increased consumption of sugar has resulted in increased calorie intakes. Combine that with less physical activity, and the result is unwanted weight gain that leads to chronic diseases such as heart disease, diabetes, and some cancers.

Does this mean you should eliminate all sweeteners from your diet? No. A small amount of sugar or honey or even high-fructose corn syrup every day is okay. You can cut back a lot of the sweeteners in your diet just by being aware of what you eat. Read labels, opt for whole foods, and choose recipes wisely.

Many of these recipes feature superfood fruits and whole grains, especially oats. We've cut back the sugar and brought out the flavor of the fruits. Our egg dishes contain superfood vegetables and nuts. Don't want to eat eggs? Our egg dishes will work with substitutes such as Egg Beaters.

☉ *Whole-Wheat and Oat Pancakes*

Homemade pancakes are a favorite breakfast food, but typical pancakes are low in fiber and high in sugar. These pancakes are better for you because they're made with whole grains and nonfat milk and have the additional goodness of applesauce.

Prep time: *About 10 minutes*

Cooking time: *About 4 minutes for each pancake*

Yield: *4 servings*

1 egg	¹/₂ cup unsweetened applesauce
¹/₂ cup oat flour	2 tablespoons canola oil
¹/₂ cup whole-wheat flour	2 teaspoons baking powder
¹/₂ cup nonfat milk	Canola oil or nonstick cooking spray

1 Whisk the egg in mixing bowl until beaten.

2 Add flours, milk, applesauce, oil, and baking powder; mix well.

3 Heat skillet over medium heat and coat with oil or nonstick cooking spray.

4 Pour ¹/₄ cup of batter into skillet, cook until batter bubbles, about two minutes, turn and cook for two more minutes.

5 Repeat for the rest of the batter.

6 Serve with light syrup or fruit spread.

Per serving: *Calories 201 (From Fat 84); Fat 9g (Saturated 1g); Cholesterol 54mg; Sodium 223mg; Carbohydrate 24g (Dietary Fiber 4g); Protein 7g.*

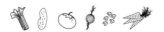

☙ Cinnamon Blueberry Whole-Grain Waffles

These waffles include oats and blueberries to make them into superfood waffles. We also use whole-wheat flour for a hearty flavor and more fiber.

Prep time: *About 15 minutes*

Cooking time: *About 5 minutes for each waffle*

Yield: *8 servings*

1¼ cup whole-wheat flour

½ cup quick-cooking oats

3 teaspoons baking powder

¼ teaspoon salt

½ teaspoon cinnamon

1½ cups reduced-fat milk

2 tablespoons canola oil

1 large egg, lightly beaten

1 cup fresh blueberries, or frozen blueberries, thawed and drained

1 Heat waffle iron following manufacturer's instructions.

2 In a large bowl, combine flour, oats, baking powder, salt, and cinnamon.

3 In a separate bowl, stir together milk, canola oil, and egg.

4 Combine wet and dry ingredients and stir until large lumps disappear, but don't over-mix.

5 Fold in blueberries.

6 Make waffles according to your waffle iron's instructions. Serve with light syrup or nonfat whipped topping and more blueberries.

Per serving: *Calories 153 (From Fat 48); Fat 5g (Saturated 1g); Cholesterol 28mg; Sodium 249mg; Carbohydrate 22g (Dietary Fiber 3g); Protein 6g.*

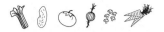

☺ Blueberry Yogurt Crepes

These crepes are made with whole-wheat flour, yet they're still nice and light. The filling is made with yogurt and honey for a sweet and tangy flavor that goes nicely with blueberries. Don't have any blueberries? Try our crepes with strawberries instead.

Prep time: *About 15 minutes*

Cooking time: *About 2 minutes for each crepe*

Yield: *4 servings (2 crepes each)*

1 cup low-fat milk	*1 cup plain nonfat yogurt*
³/₄ cup whole-wheat flour	*2 tablespoons honey*
2 eggs	*¹/₄ teaspoon vanilla*
¹/₄ teaspoon salt	*1¹/₂ to 2 cups fresh blueberries or frozen blueberries, thawed and drained*
Canola oil or nonstick cooking spray	

1 Combine milk, flour, eggs, and salt. Whisk until smooth.

2 Heat a nonstick 11-inch skillet over medium heat, and then spray it with nonstick spray or give it a quick swipe with an oiled paper towel.

3 Pour ¹/₄ cup crepe batter into the skillet. Pick up the skillet and swirl it around gently to spread the batter. Cook for 40 seconds.

4 Carefully turn crepe over and cook for another 40 seconds. Repeat for each crepe, remembering to spray or oil the skillet again for each crepe.

5 Combine yogurt, honey, and vanilla in mixing bowl and blend thoroughly.

6 Spoon about 1 tablespoon of yogurt mixture and ¹/₄ cup blueberries onto each crepe. Roll and serve.

Per serving: Calories 237 (From Fat 35); Fat 4g (Saturated 1g); Cholesterol 110mg; Sodium 260mg; Carbohydrate 41g (Dietary Fiber 4g); Protein 12g.

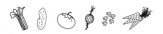

☺ Low-Fat Apple Cranberry Cobbler

Apples and cranberries are two of our superfood fruits, and this apple cranberry cobbler can be served at breakfast or as a delicious dessert. Leave the peelings on your apples for extra nutrition and fiber.

Prep time: *About 20 minutes*

Cooking time: *About 25 to 30 minutes*

Yield: *8 servings*

3 apples, cored and cut into bite-sized chunks

¹/₂ cup fresh cranberries or frozen cranberries, thawed and drained

¹/₂ cup honey

¹/₄ cup water or apple juice

¹/₂ teaspoon cinnamon

¹/₄ teaspoon nutmeg

³/₄ cup whole-wheat flour

¹/₂ cup rolled oats

1¹/₂ teaspoon baking powder

1 teaspoon sugar

¹/₄ teaspoon salt

²/₃ cup skim milk

2 tablespoons canola oil

Nonstick cooking spray

1 Preheat oven to 325 degrees Fahrenheit.

2 Place apples, cranberries, honey, water or apple juice, cinnamon, and nutmeg in a saucepan and cook over medium heat until apples are tender and cranberries pop and open, about 20 minutes.

3 In a mixing bowl, combine flour, oats, baking powder, sugar, and salt, and blend thoroughly.

4 Add milk and canola oil to the dry mixture; stir just until dry ingredients are moistened.

5 Spray a 9-inch pie plate with nonstick spray, and then fill it with the warm apple mixture.

6 Drop dough by spoonfuls onto top of apple mixture, covering evenly.

7 Bake in oven for 25 to 30 minutes, until topping is golden brown.

Per serving: Calories 143 (From Fat 17); Fat 2g (Saturated 0g); Cholesterol 0mg; Sodium 156mg; Carbohydrate 31g (Dietary Fiber 4g); Protein 3g.

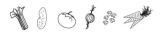

○ *Vegetable Omelet*

Eggs are a favorite part of breakfast. Enjoy this omelet for breakfast served with whole-grain toast and a glass of orange juice on the side. This omelet contains garlic and tomatoes as superfoods, along with other healthful vegetables.

Prep time: *About 15 minutes*

Cooking time: *About 7 to 8 minutes*

Yield: *4 servings*

3 eggs (or equivalent amount of egg substitute, such as Egg Beaters)

¹/₄ cup nonfat milk

Canola oil or nonstick cooking spray

3 green onions, chopped

1 clove garlic, chopped

¹/₄ cup mushrooms

¹/₄ cup chopped red or green pepper

¹/₄ chopped tomato without seeds

¹/₄ cup grated cheddar cheese

Salt and black pepper to taste

1 Whisk eggs and milk in mixing bowl.

2 Spray nonstick skillet with nonstick cooking spray, or coat lightly with canola oil. Heat skillet over medium heat.

3 Add onions, garlic, mushrooms, peppers, and tomatoes to the skillet and cook until onions are translucent, stirring continuously.

4 Transfer the vegetables to a bowl. Wipe the skillet and re-apply nonstick spray or oil.

5 Add eggs to the skillet. As the eggs cook, loosen the edges and let the raw egg slide underneath. Cook for about 1 minute.

6 When eggs appear to be nearly cooked, add onions, garlic, mushrooms, peppers, tomatoes, cheese, salt, and black pepper to one half of the omelet.

7 Fold the other side of the omelet over the filling. Turn off heat, and cover. Serve after the cheese has melted, about one minute.

Per serving: *Calories 98 (From Fat 48); Fat 5g (Saturated 2g); Cholesterol 163mg; Sodium 290mg; Carbohydrate 5g (Dietary Fiber 1g); Protein 8g.*

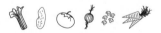

○ *Spinach Quiche with Pecans*

Quiche is a Sunday brunch staple, although many people think it's high in fat and calories. Our version has a little less cheese, no high-fat crust, and no greasy bacon, and it includes the superfoods spinach and pecans.

Prep time: *About 20 minutes*

Cooking time: *About 40 to 45 minutes*

Yield: *4 servings*

Nonstick cooking spray

4 eggs

1 onion, chopped

10-ounce package frozen chopped spinach, thawed and drained

¹/₂ cup grated Monterey Jack cheese

¹/₂ cup grated Parmesan cheese

¹/₂ cup low-fat cottage cheese

¹/₃ cup chopped pecans

¹/₂ teaspoon salt

¹/₄ teaspoon ground black pepper

¹/₈ teaspoon ground nutmeg

1 Preheat oven to 325 degrees Fahrenheit.

2 Spray a 9-inch glass pie pan with nonstick cooking spray.

3 Add eggs to mixing bowl; whisk until beaten. Mix in the rest of the ingredients, and pour into pie pan.

4 Bake for 35 to 40 minutes, or until a knife inserted into center of the quiche comes out clean.

Per serving: *Calories 293 (From Fat 180); Fat 20g (Saturated 7g); Cholesterol 234mg; Sodium 798mg; Carbohydrate 9g (Dietary Fiber 3g); Protein 21g.*

Chapter 17

Gathering for the Family Meal: Superfood Main Dish Recipes

In This Chapter

▶ Planning main dishes: Good food and good conversation

▶ Understanding the importance of a healthy family meal

▶ Making superfoods dishes to share

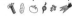
*W*hen you and your family are on the go, tracking what everyone is eating and whether you're getting the right balance of foods during the day can be hard. That's why it's important to plan and prepare healthy superfoods dinners for your family. Family dinners are a great opportunity to get everyone to eat healthily and gain back some ground from the poor eating habits that both children and adults may indulge in during the day.

When preparing dinner, you can get superfoods in everything from salmon to pizza. After you get some creative meal ideas, you'll see how fun and easy it is to make healthy (and delicious) main dishes. In this chapter, we offer some easy recipes that cover a variety of superfoods — and will surely keep your family coming back for more!

Making the Most of Family Mealtime

Turn off the TV, let the phone go to voice mail, and disconnect from the World Wide Web, because it's time to sit down for an hour devoted to food and companionship. It just happens that dinner is the most consistent time for family gathering. Dinnertime is the perfect time to get in touch with your family and find out what's going on in everyone's day. Getting everyone together for dinner may be a challenge, but try to enjoy every chance you get.

Several studies have looked at the importance of family mealtimes, for both children and adults. A study in the *Journal of the American Dietetic Association* showed that both children and parents strongly value family meals. Columbia University researchers found that children who ate more than five meals per week with their families had higher grades. Other studies have looked into school and work performance, drug use, and language skills, and have found similar positive outcomes associated with families who share several meals a week. A study published in the *Archives of Pediatric and Adolescent Medicine* claims that eating family meals may reduce the number of teens afflicted with eating disorders. Wow — all this from spending some quality family time around the table enjoying good food.

Obviously, dinner is a time to feed both your bodies and your relationships. People who eat alone tend to eat less and may therefore suffer from malnutrition — an important fact to remember if you have friends and family members who spend most of their mealtimes alone. Invite them to join you when you can.

If you have trouble getting your family to the dinner table without simultaneously watching TV or attempting to scarf down the food and scram, you may have to get creative to get them into main meal festivities. One way to keep the attendance up is to get the family involved in meal planning and preparation. Young children often love to cook, and they'll jump at the chance to help in the kitchen.

Putting together a meal is a great accomplishment, especially when you're new to the kitchen, so be sure to compliment the chef.

Making a Statement with the Main Dish

The recipes for the main dishes in this chapter have a nice mix of superfoods that are sure to tantalize your taste buds! These recipes are easy to follow and a perfect way to get friends and family involved in the planning, cooking, and, most important, eating of healthy meals. You also find easy tricks for adding and substituting ingredients to get more nutritious superfoods into the recipes.

Too many of us are set on the idea that food that tastes good usually isn't good for you. Dinner is a perfect time to direct everyone's attention to the fun aspects of putting together a healthy meal. Let everyone know that they're eating superfoods. Tell your family how the foods and ingredients contribute to good health. With these delicious superfoods meals, both young and old can discover that healthy eating can also taste good.

When you cook for friends, offer them recipes for the dishes you prepare. Friends may often want the recipe, but may be afraid to ask. Make it easy for them, and they can leave with a full belly and a fresh new superfoods dish for their own repertoire!

In this section, we have a few fish recipes that are always a great choice for tasty main dishes. However, we also include a nice mix of other meal options. Whether you want a zesty burger, stir-fry, or a hot bowl of super stew, we provide a lot of flexibility here for your main meal.

Baked Salmon Fillets

Salmon is one of the fish that are packed with the most omega-3 fatty acids. Even people who don't like fish are likely to enjoy salmon when you prepare it this way. Salmon is also low in saturated fat and a great source of protein, and it has high concentrations of B vitamins and magnesium.

Prep time: *About 15 minutes*

Cooking time: *Approximately 20 minutes*

Yield: *4 servings*

4 salmon fillets, 4 ounces each	1 white onion, finely chopped
3 tablespoons olive oil, divided	2 tablespoons chopped fresh dill
Salt and pepper	1 teaspoon fresh lemon juice

1 Preheat oven to 425 degrees Fahrenheit.

2 Rinse the salmon fillets under water and pat dry. Brush salmon fillets with 1 tablespoon olive oil, and sprinkle with salt and pepper.

3 Place fillets in baking dish. Bake for about 15 to 20 minutes, or until salmon is firm and flakes easily with a fork or knife.

4 Remove the salmon from the oven and cover to keep warm.

5 Heat a sauté pan to medium high, and add the remaining olive oil, onion, and fresh dill. Cook until the onions are soft and translucent.

6 Stir in fresh lemon juice.

7 Spoon sautéed sauce over salmon and serve.

Per serving: Calories 257 (From Fat 130); Fat 15g (Saturated 2g); Cholesterol 65mg; Sodium 230mg; Carbohydrate 6g (Dietary Fiber 1g); Protein 25g.

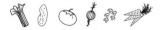

Baked Salmon with Sour Cream

The addition of garlic and onion give a great, savory taste to this fresh fish. You get healthy fats from the salmon and antioxidants and immune-boosting power from another superfood, garlic.

Prep time: *About 15 minutes*

Cooking time: *Approximately 20 minutes*

Yield: *4 servings*

4 salmon fillets, about 4 ounces each	*2 teaspoons finely chopped onion*
1 tablespoon olive oil	*1 clove garlic, minced*
Salt and pepper	*1 cup low-fat sour cream*
2 tablespoons fresh lemon juice	*1 bunch of parsley*

1 Preheat oven to 425 degrees Fahrenheit.

2 Rinse the salmon fillets under water and pat dry, and then place the salmon fillets in a baking dish. Lightly brush with olive oil, season with salt and pepper, and then sprinkle with lemon juice.

3 In a separate bowl, mix the onion and garlic together.

4 Spread sour cream on top of the fillets, and then sprinkle the onion and garlic over the sour cream. Bake 15 to 20 minutes until firm, or until the salmon flakes easily when tested with a knife or fork.

5 Garnish with parsley and serve.

Per serving: Calories 395 (From Fat 161); Fat 18g (Saturated 6g); Cholesterol 117mg; Sodium 358mg; Carbohydrate 14g (Dietary Fiber 1g); Protein 42g.

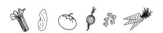

Black Bean Cilantro Lime Salmon

The last of our superfood salmon recipes offers another option for preparing a healthy salmon dish. Adding black beans increases the fiber content and adds to the already healthy benefits of the salmon.

Prep time: *About 15 minutes*

Cooking time: *Approximately 20 minutes*

Yield: *4 servings*

4 salmon fillets, about 4 ounces each

2 tablespoons olive oil, divided

Salt and pepper to taste

1 lime

1 lemon

1 onion, chopped

¹/₂ cup black beans (canned beans are a suitable substitute, but we prefer fresh beans)

1 to 2 tablespoons chopped fresh cilantro

1 to 2 tablespoons chopped fresh basil

1 Preheat oven to 425 degrees Fahrenheit.

2 Place salmon fillets in a baking dish. Brush fillets with 1 tablespoon olive oil and season with salt and pepper.

3 Cut lime and lemon into wedges for squeezing.

4 Bake for 10 to 15 minutes, or until the salmon flakes when tested with a fork.

5 While salmon is baking, add remaining tablespoon olive oil, chopped onion, and black beans to small sauté pan. Sprinkle with salt and pepper to taste. Sauté on medium heat for 5 to 7 minutes until onions soften and beans are soft but not mushy.

6 Top salmon fillets with beans and onion mixture, and squeeze fresh lime and lemon wedges over top.

7 Finish with chopped fresh cilantro and basil, and serve.

Per serving: Calories 375 (From Fat 122); Fat 14g (Saturated 2g); Cholesterol 97mg; Sodium 273mg; Carbohydrate 19g (Dietary Fiber 6g); Protein 43g.

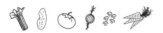

⏱ Black Soybean Quesadillas

This is a great low-carb meal with both soybeans and garlic. Black soybeans have a milder flavor than regular yellow soybeans. These quesadillas are a tasty treat for those trying to lose or maintain their weight. The soybeans are a great source of protein, healthy fatty acids, and plenty of vitamins and minerals. Garlic adds great flavor and has immune and antioxidant benefits.

Prep time: *About 20 minutes*

Cooking time: *10 to 15 minutes*

Yield: *4 servings*

Nonstick cooking spray

4 low-carb or whole-grain tortillas

³/₄ cup (3 ounces) shredded reduced-fat Monterey Jack or cheddar cheese

¹/₂ cup black soybeans, rinsed and drained (fresh soybeans are preferable, but you may use canned)

2 green onions, chopped

¹/₄ cup chopped fresh cilantro

1 clove garlic, minced

¹/₂ teaspoon ground cumin

¹/₂ cup chunky salsa

Chopped fresh cilantro, for garnish (optional)

1 Preheat oven to 425 degrees Fahrenheit.

2 Place two tortillas on a large, nonstick baking sheet. (If you use a regular baking sheet, spray it with nonstick cooking spray first.) Sprinkle half the cheese on the two tortillas.

3 In a small bowl, combine soybeans, green onions, cilantro, garlic, and cumin. Mix lightly, and then spoon this bean mixture evenly over the cheese on the tortillas.

4 Sprinkle the remaining cheese on top of the beans, top with the remaining tortillas, press down on the top of each tortilla slightly, and spray each top tortilla with cooking spray.

5 Bake for 10 to 12 minutes, or until the tortillas are lightly browned and the cheese is melted.

6 Remove from oven and cool slightly. Cut the tortillas into quarters and serve salsa on the side for dipping. Top with fresh cilantro if desired.

Per serving: Calories 195 (From Fat 68); Fat 8g (Saturated 3g); Cholesterol 15mg; Sodium 408mg; Carbohydrate 18g (Dietary Fiber 10g); Protein 15g.

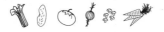

⏱ Vegetable Pizza

A typical pizza is dripping with grease from processed meats and too much cheese. Our pizza is leaner with less cheese and no greasy meat, so it has fewer calories than a regular pizza. Our pizza is better for you, too, because the crust is made with whole grains and the toppings include superfood vegetables.

Prep time: *About 20 minutes*

Cooking time: *15 to 20 minutes*

Yield: *16 servings (2 pizzas)*

4 cups whole-wheat flour

2 tablespoons active dry yeast

1¹/₂ teaspoons salt

2 cups warm water (about 120 degrees)

2 tablespoons olive oil, divided

1 teaspoon sugar

6-ounce can tomato paste

8-ounce can tomato sauce

1 clove garlic, minced

1 teaspoon salt

¹/₂ teaspoon sugar

¹/₂ teaspoon dried oregano

¹/₄ teaspoon dried marjoram

¹/₄ teaspoon dried basil

¹/₈ teaspoon ground black pepper

¹/₈ teaspoon cayenne pepper

¹/₂ medium onion, thinly sliced

¹/₂ green pepper, thinly sliced

¹/₂ red pepper, thinly sliced

1 large tomato, sliced and seeded

1 cup sliced mushrooms (any variety)

1 cup chopped sun-dried tomatoes

10-ounce package frozen spinach, thawed and drained

1 cup chopped green olives

1 cup chopped broccoli

16 ounces shredded part-skim (low-fat) mozzarella cheese

1 Preheat oven to 425 degrees Fahrenheit.

2 Pour flour into a mixing bowl. Stir in yeast and salt. Add water, oil, and sugar, and mix well. Cover the bowl with a damp cloth and place it in a warm area for 30 to 40 minutes to rise.

3 While the crust is rising, combine tomato paste, tomato sauce, garlic, remaining tablespoon of olive oil, salt, sugar, oregano, marjoram, basil, black pepper, and cayenne pepper in a mixing bowl; stir to mix thoroughly.

4 Punch down the dough, remove it from the bowl, and divide it in half. With a rolling pin, roll each half out until it's about 12 to 13 inches in diameter. Transfer the dough onto two greased, 14-inch pizza pans, and press out the edges.

5 Divide the sauce mixture between the two crusts, ladling it out and spreading it to within ¹/₂ inch of the edges.

6 Spread the veggie toppings evenly over the crusts. Sprinkle cheese over the top of each pizza.

7 Bake on the bottom rack of the oven for 15 to 20 minutes, or until crust is golden brown and cheese is melted. Slice into eight pieces.

Tip: *Depending on the size of your pizzas, you may need to bake them one at a time.*

Per serving: *Calories 285 (From Fat 93); Fat 10g (Saturated 4g); Cholesterol 16mg; Sodium 1,094mg; Carbohydrate 37g (Dietary Fiber 7g); Protein 15g.*

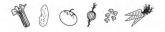

Trout Amandine

Trout has a mild flavor and is rich in omega-3 fatty acids; almonds are rich in healthy fats. Our version of trout almandine calls for poaching, which is a very healthful way to prepare fish.

Prep time: *About 10 minutes*

Cooking time: *17 to 19 minutes*

Yield: *2 servings*

¼ cup slivered almonds	*¼ cup chopped green onions*
½ cup dry white wine	*¼ teaspoon salt*
⅓ cup lemon juice (or 2 to 3 fresh lemons, squeezed)	*⅛ teaspoon pepper*
	2 fillets of trout (6 to 8 ounces each)
¼ cup chopped fresh parsley	*1 fresh lemon*

1 Place almonds in small, nonstick skillet and toast over medium heat. Stir frequently until the almonds are slightly brown, about 3 to 5 minutes. Remove from heat.

2 Pour wine, lemon juice, parsley, green onions, salt, and pepper into a large, nonstick skillet over medium heat and cook until the mixture begins to boil, about 4 minutes.

3 Reduce to low heat and then add trout fillets. Cover the skillet to poach the fish until the flesh is opaque and flaky, about 10 minutes.

4 While fish is poaching, slice lemon.

5 Top trout fillets with almonds and a small amount of poaching liquid, and serve with lemon slices.

Per serving: *Calories 298 (From Fat 131); Fat 15g (Saturated 2g); Cholesterol 97mg; Sodium 237mg; Carbohydrate 4g (Dietary Fiber 1g); Protein 37g.*

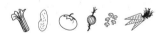

Tuna Melt Wraps

This sandwich recipe contains five superfoods — tuna, spinach, tomato, olive oil, and avocado. These warm wraps are easy to make and go nicely with a side salad or cup of soup. If you don't want to use a broiler, you can use your microwave oven.

Prep time: *About 10 minutes*

Cooking time: *2 to 3 minutes*

Yield: *2 servings*

2 whole-wheat tortillas

5 ounces canned tuna (regular or albacore), drained

¹/₂ cup shredded part-skim mozzarella cheese

1 cup fresh spinach leaves

¹/₂ cup diced tomato

¹/₄ cup diced avocado

2 teaspoons extra-virgin olive oil

1 teaspoon balsamic vinegar

Salt and pepper to taste

1 Preheat broiler to high.

2 Place tortillas on a baking sheet. Place half the tuna in the middle of each tortilla, and sprinkle with cheese (divide the cheese between the two tortillas).

3 Place in the broiler until cheese is melted and tuna is warm, about 2 to 3 minutes. Remove from the broiler.

4 Transfer the tortillas to a clean cutting board. Add half of the spinach leaves, tomato, and avocado to each tortilla. Drizzle about 1 teaspoon of olive oil and balsamic vinegar over each. Add salt and pepper.

5 Fold up one quarter of each tortilla to form the bottom. Roll the sides in to form a cone shape, with the top open.

Tip: *You can make these melts in the microwave instead of the broiler if you prefer. To do so, place a tortilla on a microwave-safe plate and top with tuna and cheese. Cook on high until cheese is melted, about 1 to 1¹/₂ minutes (microwave oven times can vary greatly).*

Per serving: *Calories 312 (From Fat 118); Fat 13g (Saturated 4g); Cholesterol 38mg; Sodium 852mg; Carbohydrate 25g (Dietary Fiber 4g); Protein 29g.*

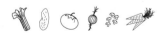

☞ Tomato and Lentil Stew

Canned tomatoes are an excellent source of lycopene, which is good for your heart and prostate. Lentils are rich in fiber, folate, and protein. This superfood stew can be served as a meal with a small side salad and a slice of hearty, whole-grain bread.

Prep time: *About 20 minutes*

Cooking time: *40 minutes*

Yield: *4 servings*

1 tablespoon olive oil	½ teaspoon crushed red pepper
1 medium onion, finely chopped	½ cup dry red wine
4 medium carrots, diced	15-ounce can chopped tomatoes
4 medium celery ribs, diced	¾ cup dry red lentils
2 to 3 garlic cloves, crushed	4 cups low-sodium chicken or vegetable broth
¾ teaspoon dried basil	Salt and pepper to taste
¾ teaspoon dried thyme	

1 Heat oil in a Dutch oven or large soup pot. Add onion, carrots, celery, and garlic, and cook over low heat for about 5 minutes until soft, stirring occasionally.

2 Stir in basil, thyme, red pepper, red wine, tomatoes, and lentils. Cook for another 5 minutes, stirring constantly.

3 Add broth and bring to a boil. Reduce to low heat and simmer gently for 25 to 30 minutes, or until lentils are soft. Add salt and pepper to taste.

Vary It!: *If you want a slightly thicker or creamier soup, stir the soup with a whisk for about 30 seconds to break up the lentils, thickening the soup.*

Per serving: *Calories 255 (From Fat 46); Fat 5g (Saturated 1g); Cholesterol 4mg; Sodium 491mg; Carbohydrate 40g (Dietary Fiber 11g); Protein 14g.*

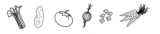

⌁ Southwestern Black Bean Burgers

Hamburgers are a family favorite; however, they're high in saturated fat, and that's not good for you. Our Southwestern Black Bean Burgers are rich in antioxidants, vitamins, and fiber, and low in calories. These burgers can also be cooked ahead of time and reheated when you're ready to eat.

Prep time: *About 10 minutes*

Cooking time: *10 minutes*

Yield: *4 servings*

15- to 16-ounce can black beans, rinsed and drained

⅓ cup chopped red onion

¼ cup chopped fresh cilantro

¼ cup dry, whole-wheat bread crumbs

2 tablespoons chunky salsa or green chili sauce

1 teaspoon ground cumin

½ teaspoon hot pepper sauce (such as Tabasco)

Salt and pepper to taste

Canola oil or nonstick cooking spray

4 whole-wheat hamburger buns

1 In a large bowl, mash the beans. Stir in the onion, cilantro, bread crumbs, salsa, cumin, and hot pepper sauce. Add salt and pepper.

2 Moisten your hands with water. Shape the bean mixture into four 3-inch burgers.

3 Oil or spray a large, nonstick skillet and place over medium heat. When skillet is hot, add the burgers and cook until lightly browned on the bottom, about 5 minutes. Turn and cook for 5 minutes longer, or until heated through.

4 Serve on whole-wheat hamburger buns.

Tip: If you can't find ready-made whole-wheat bread crumbs, you can easily make them with 1 slice of whole-wheat bread in a food processor.

Per serving: Calories 199 (From Fat 23); Fat 3g (Saturated 0g); Cholesterol 0mg; Sodium 617mg; Carbohydrate 38g (Dietary Fiber 9g); Protein 9g.

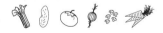

Basil Pesto and Broccoli Pasta with Chicken

Broccoli is one of our favorite superfood vegetables. Pesto is rich in antioxidants that are good for your health. You can buy pesto at most grocery stores, or try your hand at making your own. Our pesto contains walnuts, which are a superfood, along with healthful olive oil and garlic. Make this dish even more healthful by using whole-grain pasta.

Basil Pesto

Prep time: *About 10 minutes*

Yield: *1¹/₂ cups*

3 tablespoons walnuts

1¹/₂ tablespoons pine nuts

4 garlic cloves

3 cups fresh basil leaves, packed

³/₄ cup extra-virgin olive oil

¹/₃ cup grated Parmesan cheese

1 Place the walnuts, pine nuts, and garlic in a food processor. Process for 15 seconds.

2 Add the basil leaves, olive oil, and Parmesan cheese. Process again until the pesto is thoroughly puréed, about 10 seconds. Use right away or refrigerate in an airtight container for up to one week.

Per serving: *Calories 307 (From Fat 290); Fat 32g (Saturated 5g); Cholesterol 4mg; Sodium 95mg; Carbohydrate 3g (Dietary Fiber 1g); Protein 4g.*

Broccoli Pasta with Chicken

Prep time: *About 15 minutes*

Cooking time: *20 to 25 minutes*

Yield: *6 servings*

12 ounces dry penne or rigatoni pasta

3 tablespoons olive oil, divided

1 pound skinless, boneless chicken breast, cut into bite-sized pieces

1 red bell pepper, cut into bite-sized pieces

4 cups broccoli florets

1 tablespoon minced garlic

1 cup chopped tomatoes

³/₄ cup prepared basil pesto (see preceding recipe to make your own)

¹/₃ cup freshly grated Parmesan cheese

Salt and pepper to taste

1 Cook the pasta in a large pot of water for 8 to 10 minutes until tender but firm.

2 While pasta cooks, heat 2 tablespoons olive oil in a large, nonstick skillet over medium heat. Add chicken and red pepper, and cook for 5 to 10 minutes, or until chicken is cooked through. Remove from heat and transfer the chicken and pepper mixture to a large serving bowl.

3 Fill medium saucepan with water and bring to boil over medium-high heat. Blanch broccoli florets for 3 minutes, and then drain.

4 Pour remaining tablespoon of olive oil in the skillet used for the chicken and peppers. Add garlic, tomatoes, and pesto, and sauté for 2 minutes.

5 Add the pasta, broccoli, pesto mixture, and Parmesan cheese to the chicken and peppers. Toss to combine and add salt and pepper to taste.

Per serving: Calories 544 (From Fat 233); Fat 26g (Saturated 5g); Cholesterol 47mg; Sodium 290mg; Carbohydrate 51g (Dietary Fiber 6g); Protein 30g.

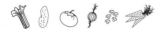

🍎 Tofu Stir-Fry

Tofu is made from soybeans and works well as a substitute for meat in stir-fry dishes. Our tofu stir-fry also contains olive oil, broccoli, and carrots, along with other healthful vegetables, which make it a delicious superfoods meal.

Prep time: *About 20 minutes*

Cooking time: *10 minutes*

Yield: *4 servings*

1 tablespoon olive oil

¼ cup cornstarch

16-ounce package extra firm tofu, drained and cut into cubes

½ medium onion, sliced

2 cloves garlic, finely chopped

1 tablespoon minced fresh ginger

2 cups broccoli florets

1 carrot, peeled and sliced

1 green bell pepper, seeded and cut into strips

1 small head bok choy, chopped

1 cup sliced fresh mushrooms

1 cup chopped canned bamboo shoots, drained

½ teaspoon crushed red pepper

½ cup water

¼ cup rice wine vinegar

2 tablespoons honey

2 tablespoons soy sauce

1 In a large skillet or wok, heat oil over medium-high heat. In a small bowl, toss tofu cubes in cornstarch to coat. Add tofu to the skillet or wok, and sauté until golden brown, about 2 to 3 minutes, stirring only occasionally.

2 Stir in onion, garlic, and ginger, and sauté for 1 minute.

3 Stir in broccoli, carrot, and bell pepper, and sauté for 2 minutes. Stir in bok choy, mushrooms, bamboo shoots, and crushed red pepper. Heat through, about 5 minutes, stirring continuously. Remove from heat.

4 In a small saucepan, combine water, rice wine vinegar, honey, and soy sauce, and bring to a simmer, stirring constantly. Pour over stir-fry mixture, toss, and serve.

Per serving: Calories 235 (From Fat 103); Fat 11g (Saturated 2g); Cholesterol 0mg; Sodium 508mg; Carbohydrate 21g (Dietary Fiber 5g); Protein 18g.

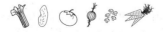

Chicken or Beef Fajitas with Avocado Sauce

This is a great recipe if you're hosting a party and aren't sure whether the guests would prefer beef or chicken. The key is the superfood avocado sauce that tops the meats and goes great with either one. This sauce combines both garlic and avocado — two great superfoods.

Prep time: *About 20 minutes*

Cooking time: *10 to 15 minutes*

Yield: *6 servings*

Six to eight 8-inch or larger whole-grain tortillas	2 medium avocados, peeled, seeded, and sliced
1 tablespoon olive oil	¹/₂ medium onion, chopped
2 yellow or red bell peppers, cut into thin strips	2 tablespoons lemon juice
1 medium onion, thinly sliced	1 clove garlic, minced
2 tablespoons fajita seasoning	¹/₄ teaspoon dried cilantro or 1 tablespoon chopped fresh cilantro
¹/₄ cup water	¹/₂ teaspoon salt
4 boneless, skinless chicken breasts cut into thin strips, or 1 to 2 pounds of flank steak or other steak of choice sliced into thin strips, or half beef and half chicken	¹/₄ teaspoon pepper
	Shredded cheese and lettuce (optional)

1 Preheat oven to 425 degrees Fahrenheit.

2 Wrap the stack of tortillas in foil and place them in oven for 10 to 15 minutes.

3 Heat a large, nonstick skillet on high; add olive oil, peppers, and sliced onion, and sauté until vegetables begin to soften, about 3 minutes.

4 Mix fajita seasoning and water in a small bowl, and then pour the mixture into the skillet. Add the meat and sautéed vegetables, and cook for about 5 to 10 minutes until the meat is cooked through.

5 Make the avocado sauce by placing avocados, chopped onion, lemon juice, garlic, cilantro, salt, and pepper into a food processor; cover and blend until well mixed.

6 Serve the meat and vegetables on individual tortillas, and spoon avocado sauce on top. Top with shredded cheese and lettuce as desired.

Vary It!: *Instead of whole-grain tortillas, try low-carb spinach wraps.*

Per serving: *Calories 338 (From Fat 133); Fat 15g (Saturated 3g); Cholesterol 49mg; Sodium 373mg; Carbohydrate 33g (Dietary Fiber 8g); Protein 23g.*

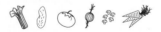

Turkey Chili

This recipe features the superfoods tomatoes, kidney beans, and garlic. The lean ground turkey keeps it low-fat and good for you.

Prep time: *About 15 minutes*

Cooking time: *40 to 55 minutes*

Yield: *8 servings*

1½ teaspoons olive oil	½ teaspoon salt
1 medium onion, chopped	½ teaspoon ground black pepper
1 pound lean ground turkey	16-ounce can kidney beans, rinsed and drained
2 tablespoons chili powder	1 cup water
1 tablespoon chopped fresh cilantro	1 cup beer
½ teaspoon paprika	28-ounce can crushed tomatoes
½ teaspoon dried oregano	4-ounce can green chiles, undrained
½ teaspoon ground cayenne pepper	1 tablespoon minced garlic

1 Heat the oil in a large soup pot over medium heat. Add the onion and cook for about 3 to 4 minutes.

2 Add the ground turkey to the onions, and then stir in the chili powder, cilantro, paprika, oregano, cayenne pepper, salt, and black pepper. Cook until the meat is evenly browned, about 5 minutes.

3 In a small bowl, mash approximately half of the beans.

4 Add the water and beer to the pot, and stir in the tomatoes, mashed and whole kidney beans, green chiles, and garlic. Stir until combined.

5 Reduce heat to low, cover, and simmer 30 to 45 minutes before serving. Stir occasionally.

Per serving: Calories 158 (From Fat 16); Fat 2g (Saturated 0g); Cholesterol 37mg; Sodium 456mg; Carbohydrate 18g (Dietary Fiber 4g); Protein 18g.

Pork Chops and Apples

Pork chops are a good source of selenium and B vitamins. This superfoods recipe adds the goodness of apples and pecans, plus some raisins and honey for a touch of sweetness.

Prep time: *About 10 minutes*

Cooking time: *10 to 15 minutes*

Yield: *4 servings*

Nonstick cooking spray

Four 4-ounce boneless pork chops, ½ inch thick, trimmed of fat

½ cup finely chopped onion

1 large tart apple, such as Macintosh, Yellow Delicious, Rome, or Winesap, cored and finely chopped

¼ cup raisins

¼ cup chopped pecans

½ cup low-sodium chicken broth

½ cup apple juice

3 tablespoons honey

2 teaspoons Dijon mustard

¼ teaspoon dried thyme

¼ teaspoon cinnamon

1 tablespoon water

1 teaspoon cornstarch

1 Spray a large skillet with nonstick cooking spray and place over medium-high heat. Add the chops and cook until done, at least 4 to 5 minutes per side, or to an internal temperature of 180 degrees Fahrenheit. Transfer the pork chops to a plate and cover with foil to keep warm.

2 While the chops are cooking, spray a medium saucepan with nonstick cooking spray and place over medium-high heat. Add the onion to the pan and sauté 2 to 3 minutes, until it starts to soften, stirring continuously.

3 Add the apple slices to the onion and sauté until the apples start to become tender, about 3 to 5 minutes, stirring continuously.

4 Add the raisins and pecans to the onion and apple mixture. Stir in the broth, apple juice, honey, mustard, thyme, and cinnamon; cook for 5 minutes.

5 Mix water and cornstarch in a small bowl, and add to the apple mixture. Stir until thickened and glossy, about 1 minute. Serve over chops.

Tip: *Serve leftover sauce over brown rice.*

Per serving: *Calories 349 (From Fat 116); Fat 13g (Saturated 3g); Cholesterol 67mg; Sodium 241mg; Carbohydrate 36g (Dietary Fiber 3g); Protein 25g.*

Chapter 18

Filling Your Plate: Super Salad and Side Dish Recipes

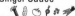
Salads and sides dishes are perfect for introducing superfoods into your lifestyle. In this chapter, we offer some tips for making delicious and healthy salads and side dishes, along with some of our favorite recipes.

Making Sides and Salads Super Healthy

We suggest that you eat five to nine servings of fruits and vegetables of different colors every day to get a variety of antioxidant-rich phytochemicals, fiber, and nutrients (see Chapters 4 and 5). You can get several of those servings by making salads and side dishes that include some of the fruit and vegetable superfoods.

The ingredients and cooking method called for in a recipe determine how healthy the resulting side or salad will be. When you page through your cookbooks (or surf online) to find healthy salads and side dishes, look for recipes that include

✔ Fruits, vegetables, or legumes as main ingredients

✔ Healthful oils such as olive, walnut, or canola oil

    ✔ Only small amounts of sugar (or, better yet, none at all)

    ✔ Cooking methods that don't add extra fat and calories — baking, roasting, sautéing, and stir-frying

If your favorite recipes don't include superfoods as ingredients, you can make them a little bit healthier by making substitutions like these:

    ✔ Use dried cranberries instead of raisins in slaws and salads.

    ✔ Substitute albacore tuna for chicken in salads.

    ✔ Start your salad with raw spinach leaves instead of iceberg lettuce.

    ✔ Top your salad with pecans or sunflower seeds instead of croutons.

    ✔ Replace vegetable oil with olive oil.

Making Super Salads and Sides

These recipes are all created with superfoods, along with other ingredients that are good for you. Many of them don't require any cooking time — all you need are a few ingredients and a few minutes to prepare them. And several of them are easy enough that you can enlist the help of your children.

Serving up super salads

Serve up a healthy salad to go alongside a sandwich at lunch or in place of a vegetable at dinner. You can also enjoy one of these salads as a delicious and healthy afternoon snack — say, when you're hungry and dinner is still three hours away.

⌣ Apple Carrot Salad

Apples, carrots, and cranberries are rich in nutrients and antioxidants. This recipe calls for a light mayonnaise to keep your fat intake down. Alternately, you could use a mayonnaise made with an omega-3-rich oil such as canola oil.

Prep time: *About 5 to 15 minutes*

Yield: *6 servings*

3 medium sweet-tart apples, such as Gala or Fuji, rinsed, cored, and chopped into ¹/₂-inch chunks

1 cup shredded carrots

¹/₂ cup dried cranberries

¹/₄ cup walnuts (optional)

1 tablespoon lemon juice

¹/₃ cup low-fat mayonnaise

In a large bowl, combine apples, carrots, cranberries, walnuts (if desired), lemon juice, and mayonnaise, and stir thoroughly. Store in an airtight container in the refrigerator until you're ready to serve.

Tip: You can add more grated carrots to this recipe, if you like.

Per serving: Calories 102 (From Fat 11); Fat 1g (Saturated 0g); Cholesterol 0mg; Sodium 130mg; Carbohydrate 25g (Dietary Fiber 3g); Protein 0g.

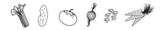

☕ *Tomato and Avocado Salad*

Tomatoes, avocados, and olive oil offer a delicious combination of vitamins, antioxidants, and healthful oils — truly a heart-healthy dish!

Prep time: About 5 to 15 minutes

Yield: 4 servings

1 avocado, peeled, pitted, and sliced

2 small tomatoes, each cut into 8 wedges

1 small sweet onion, thinly sliced

¹/₂ cup olive oil

2 tablespoons lime juice

2 tablespoons chopped fresh cilantro

Salt and pepper to taste

1 Arrange avocado, tomatoes, and onion on a serving plate in alternating fashion.

2 Whisk together the olive oil, lime juice, and cilantro. Pour the dressing over the salad, and add salt and pepper to taste.

Vary It!: If fresh cilantro isn't available or isn't to your liking, you can use parsley instead.

Per serving: Calories 322 (From Fat 301); Fat 33g (Saturated 5g); Cholesterol 0mg; Sodium 150mg; Carbohydrate 7g (Dietary Fiber 5g); Protein 2g.

⏲ Refreshing Bean Salad

This salad packs a lot of punch with antioxidant-rich vegetables. Red onions are a good source of quercetin, a powerful bioflavonoid antioxidant. The beans add plenty of protein and fiber to keep you feeling full without adding lots of calories.

Prep time: *About 15 minutes*

Refrigeration time: *At least 3 hours*

Yield: *4 servings*

1 red onion, peeled and chopped	1 sprig parsley, chopped
1 red bell pepper, chopped	¹/₂ fresh lemon, squeezed
2 15-ounce cans cut green beans, drained	3 tablespoons olive oil
15-ounce can soybeans, rinsed and drained	¹/₂ cup balsamic vinegar
1 cup red kidney beans, rinsed and drained	

1 Toss beans, onion, pepper, and parsley in a large bowl, mixing well.

2 In a small bowl, whisk together the lemon juice, vinegar, and olive oil. Poor over the bean mixture, and toss to combine. Cover and refrigerate for a minimum of 3 hours prior to serving.

Tip: *You can use rice vinegar instead of balsamic to preserve the coloring of the vegetables.*

Per serving: *Calories 271 (From Fat 129); Fat 14g (Saturated 2g); Cholesterol 0mg; Sodium 578mg; Carbohydrate 29g (Dietary Fiber 8g); Protein 11g.*

⏲ Cucumber and Tomato Salad

Tomatoes shine as the superfood star of this recipe, and they're combined with two other superfoods — garlic and olive oil. The rest of the ingredients are good for you, too. Cucumbers add vitamin C and minerals, and feta cheese adds protein and calcium.

Prep time: *About 15 minutes*

Yield: *4 servings*

2 cucumbers, peeled and thinly sliced

¹/₂ cup red onion, thinly sliced

2 large tomatoes, cut into small wedges or diced

¹/₄ cup crumbled feta cheese

¹/₂ teaspoon minced garlic

¹/₃ cup red wine vinegar

2 tablespoons olive oil

1 teaspoon chopped fresh oregano

Salt and pepper to taste

1 In a large mixing bowl, combine the cucumber, onion, tomato, and feta cheese.

2 In a small bowl, whisk together the garlic, vinegar, oil, oregano, salt, and pepper. Add to the cucumber and tomato mixture, and toss to combine. Cover and refrigerate until you're ready to serve.

Per serving: *Calories 126 (From Fat 84); Fat 9g (Saturated 2g); Cholesterol 8mg; Sodium 263mg; Carbohydrate 9g (Dietary Fiber 2g); Protein 3g.*

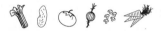

☞ Caribbean Bean Salad

Make any meal a super meal with this salad — it contains four of our superfoods. The nutrients and phytochemicals come from tomatoes, oranges, black beans, and soybeans. Romaine lettuce is rich in vitamins and minerals and super-low in calories.

Prep time: *About 15 minutes*

Yield: *4 servings*

4 cups chopped romaine lettuce

1 medium red onion, diced

1 tomato, chopped

1 cucumber, peeled, seeded, and sliced

1 orange, peeled and sliced

¹/₂ cup canned black beans, rinsed and drained

¹/₂ cup canned soybeans, rinsed and drained

1 tablespoon olive oil

3 tablespoons red wine vinegar

1 teaspoon dried oregano

Black pepper to taste

1 In a large bowl, combine the lettuce, onion, tomato, cucumber, orange, and beans.

2 In a small bowl, whisk together the olive oil, vinegar, and oregano. Pour over the vegetable and bean mixture, and toss to combine. Add pepper to taste.

Per serving: *Calories 143 (From Fat 49); Fat 6g (Saturated 1g); Cholesterol 0mg; Sodium 157mg; Carbohydrate 20g (Dietary Fiber 7g); Protein 7g.*

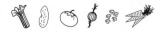

Tuna Bean Salad

Soy and tuna both contain fats that are good for your heart. This light salad is delicious and filling enough to make a meal by itself. Plus, the celery and parsley add vitamins C, A, and K to your daily intake.

Prep time: *About 20 minutes*

Refrigeration time: *2 hours*

Yield: *4 servings*

12-ounce can solid white tuna, drained	*2 cups chopped romaine lettuce*
15-ounce can soybeans, rinsed and drained	*$\frac{1}{4}$ cup lemon juice, or the juice of 2 lemons*
1 cup chopped green onion (about 8 scallions)	*2 tablespoons olive oil*
$\frac{1}{2}$ cup finely chopped white onion	*$\frac{1}{2}$ teaspoon dried oregano*
2 tablespoons chopped fresh parsley	*Salt and pepper to taste*
$\frac{1}{2}$ cup diced celery	

1 In a large bowl, place the tuna, soybeans, green and white onions, parsley, and celery, toss to combine.

2 In a small bowl, whisk together the lemon juice, olive oil, oregano, salt, and pepper. Stir into the tuna and soybean mixture. Cover and refrigerate for 2 hours.

3 Place romaine lettuce into individual serving bowls. Add the dressed tuna and soybean mixture to the lettuce, and mix well.

Per serving: *Calories 171 (From Fat 62); Fat 7g (Saturated 2g); Cholesterol 20mg; Sodium 396mg; Carbohydrate 12g (Dietary Fiber 4g); Protein 17g.*

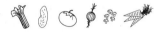

⟳ *Soybean Arugula Salad*

This salad contains lots of nutrients, antioxidants, fiber, and healthy fats. Arugula is an aromatic salad green that's low in calories and high in vitamins A and C.

Prep time: *About 20 minutes, plus 2 to 3 hours for flavors to combine*

Cooking time: *5 minutes*

Yield: *4 servings*

Two 15-ounce cans of soybeans, undrained	*3 tablespoons sherry vinegar*
1 teaspoon salt, divided	*⅓ cup olive oil*
1 teaspoon ground black pepper, divided	*3 diced Roma tomatoes*
1 teaspoon garlic powder	*¼ cup chopped black olives*
2 garlic cloves	*1 large bunch (about 5 ounces) of arugula, stems removed, and chopped*
¾ teaspoon dried rosemary	*¼ cup grated parmesan cheese*
1 teaspoon dried oregano	
1 tablespoon red wine vinegar	

1 Heat the beans in medium saucepan over medium heat, and add ½ teaspoon salt, ½ teaspoon black pepper, and garlic powder. Remove from the heat when the beans start to bubble. Strain the beans after cooking.

2 In a blender or small food processor, place garlic cloves, rosemary, oregano, vinegars, ½ teaspoon salt, and ½ teaspoon pepper. Blend while slowly adding olive oil until the mixture is emulsified.

3 In a large bowl, combine the beans, tomatoes, and olives. Pour the desired amount of dressing over it, and toss to combine. Cover and let sit for 2 to 3 hours to let the flavors come together. Serve at room temperature.

4 Immediately before serving, mix in chopped arugula and add freshly grated parmesan.

Per serving: *Calories 318 (From Fat 206); Fat 23g (Saturated 3g); Cholesterol 4mg; Sodium 754mg; Carbohydrate 16g (Dietary Fiber 7g); Protein 13g.*

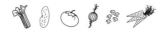

℧ Strawberry and Spinach Salad

Strawberries, spinach, and almonds give this salad a lot of nutrients, including vitamin C and calcium. Sesame seeds add trace minerals copper and manganese that help keep your bones healthy. The sweet taste of the strawberries in this recipe helps introduce kids to superfoods.

Prep time: About 30 minutes

Yield: 4 servings

2 tablespoons sugar	1 quart strawberries, hulled and sliced
½ cup olive oil	10 ounces fresh spinach, rinsed and dried
¼ cup balsamic vinegar	¼ cup sliced almonds
¼ teaspoon Worcestershire sauce	3 tablespoons toasted sesame seeds

1 In a small bowl, whisk together sugar, olive oil, balsamic vinegar, and Worcestershire sauce.

2 In a large bowl, combine the strawberries, spinach, almonds, and sesame seeds. Just before serving, add the dressing to the salad, and toss to combine.

Per serving: Calories 783 (From Fat 302); Fat 34g (Saturated 4g); Cholesterol 0mg; Sodium 125mg; Carbohydrate 124g (Dietary Fiber 9g); Protein 5g.

Creating super side dishes

These side dishes are loaded with nutrients and antioxidants. Serve them alongside grilled salmon or tuna steaks for super-duper healthy meals.

℧ Roasted Kale

Kids love crispy foods, so this side dish is a good way to introduce picky eaters to green vegetables. Kale is a great source of vitamins A and C, plus kale has lots of calcium and iron. This recipe is so easy, even little kids can help.

Prep time: About 10 minutes

Cooking time: 15 to 20 minutes

Yield: 2 servings

1 bunch kale (about 1 pound)	2 cloves garlic, crushed
1 tablespoon olive oil	Sea salt and pepper to taste

1 Preheat oven to 375 degrees Fahrenheit. Rinse the kale under running water and shake to dry. Tear the leaves into smaller pieces, and remove and discard tough rib sections.

2 In a small bowl, whisk together the olive oil, garlic, salt, and pepper.

3 In a large bowl, toss the kale leaves with the olive oil mixture. Spread leaves on a baking sheet. Bake for 15 to 20 minutes, turning the kale every 7 to 8 minutes. It's done when the leaves are crispy and bright green with just a little brown around the edges.

Tip: Roasted kale keeps well in an airtight container for two days.

Per serving: Calories 132 (From Fat 70); Fat 8g (Saturated 1g); Cholesterol 0mg; Sodium 346mg; Carbohydrate 15g (Dietary Fiber 5g); Protein 5g.

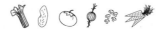

Roasted Beets

Red beets are rich in antioxidants and vitamins. Roast the beets in your oven to serve as a simple side dish with a little salt and pepper. For extra flavor and variety, add a sprinkling of goat cheese on top of the roasted beets.

Prep time: About 10 minutes

Cooking time: 45 to 50 minutes

Yield: 5 servings

1 bunch small, fresh beets (3 to 4 beets)   Salt and pepper to taste

3 tablespoons olive oil

1 Preheat oven to 400 degrees Fahrenheit. Wash beets and remove tops.

2 Place beets on a large sheet of aluminum foil, and drizzle with olive oil. Fold the foil over and seal the edges to make a pouch. Use a knife to make a small slit in the foil to allow steam to escape.

3 Put the pouch on a baking sheet and bake for 45 to 50 minutes, or until tender (when a knife slides easily into a beet).

4 Remove from the oven and carefully open the pouch. Let the beets cool at least 20 minutes before sliding the skins off and serving with salt and pepper.

Per serving: Calories 98 (From Fat 74); Fat 8g (Saturated 1g); Cholesterol 0mg; Sodium 164mg; Carbohydrate 6g (Dietary Fiber 2g); Protein 1g.

◔ Orange Ginger Baby Carrots

Carrots and oranges give this side dish a lot of vitamins and antioxidants. Ginger has been used as a digestive aid for centuries. This recipe is great for kids who are still learning to love vegetables, and it's so easy to make that your kids can help. Teaching kids to cook is a great way to get them interested in trying new foods.

Prep time: *About 5 minutes*

Cooking time: *15 minutes*

Yield: *5 servings*

2 tablespoons canola oil

1 pound baby carrots

2 teaspoons minced ginger (available already minced in jars)

³/₄ cup orange juice

Salt and pepper to taste

1 Heat oil in large skillet over medium heat. Add carrots, ginger, and orange juice, and bring to boil.

2 Reduce heat and simmer until carrots are tender, about 15 minutes. Add salt and pepper to taste.

Per serving: *Calories 108 (From Fat 49); Fat 6g (Saturated 1g); Cholesterol 0mg; Sodium 165mg; Carbohydrate 14g (Dietary Fiber 2g); Protein 1g.*

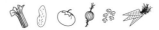

◔ Green Beans with Sun-Dried Tomatoes

Sun-dried tomatoes packed in olive oil contain lycopene, which is good for your heart (so is the olive oil). Green beans are low in calories and rich in vitamins and minerals. This side dish is easy to make, especially if you buy frozen green beans.

Prep time: *About 5 to 10 minutes*

Cooking time: *15 to 20 minutes*

Yield: *5 servings*

1 pound green beans, fresh or frozen

2 tablespoons olive oil

¹/₂ cup oil-packed sun-dried tomatoes, drained and minced

¹/₂ teaspoon oregano

2 tablespoons lemon juice

Salt and pepper to taste

1 Fill a pot with water and bring to a boil. Prepare green beans by boiling or steaming them until tender-crisp, about 5 to 10 minutes. Drain and set aside.

2 Add olive oil and tomatoes to a large skillet over medium heat and stir until tomatoes are heated through, about 1 to 2 minutes. Stir in green beans and oregano, and cook for 1 to 2 minutes.

3 Transfer to a serving dish and sprinkle with lemon juice. Add salt and pepper to taste.

Per serving: *Calories 95 (From Fat 53); Fat 6g (Saturated 1g); Cholesterol 0mg; Sodium 232mg; Carbohydrate 11g (Dietary Fiber 4g); Protein 3g.*

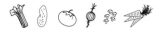

Creamy Feta Spinach

Dark green spinach is rich with calcium, vitamin K, folate, and antioxidants. This side dish also gives your family calcium and protein with the parmesan and feta cheese.

Prep time: *About 10 minutes*

Cooking time: *7 minutes*

Yield: *4 servings*

³/₄-ounce package of fresh dill, chopped

¹/₂ onion, minced

1 garlic clove, minced

1 tablespoon olive oil

7¹/₂-ounce can chopped spinach, drained; or 10-ounce box chopped frozen spinach, cooked according to package instructions and drained

¹/₄ cup grated parmesan cheese

¹/₄ cup crumbled feta cheese

Freshly grated parmesan cheese (optional)

1 In a large saucepan over medium heat, sauté the dill, onion, and garlic in olive oil for 5 minutes.

2 Mix in the spinach, and then fold in both cheeses.

3 Serve topped with more parmesan cheese, if desired.

Per serving: *Calories 74 (From Fat 34); Fat 4g (Saturated 2g); Cholesterol 12mg; Sodium 251mg; Carbohydrate 6g (Dietary Fiber 3g); Protein 6g.*

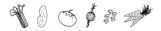

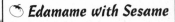 Edamame with Sesame

Edamame are young soybeans that are rich in fiber, vitamins, and omega-3 fats. Garlic is well-known for its health properties (see Chapter 9). Green onions, also known as scallions, are rich in vitamin K and lutein (a relative of vitamin A that works as a powerful antioxidant).

Prep time: *About 5 minutes*

Cooking time: *18 minutes*

Yield: *4 servings*

10 ounces fresh shelled edamame, or 16-ounce bag of frozen shelled edamame	⅛ teaspoon ground black pepper (or to taste)
	1 green onion, chopped
½ teaspoon salt	1 tablespoon olive oil
1 garlic clove, minced	1 tablespoon toasted sesame seeds

1 Fill a pot with water and bring to a boil. Boil edamame with salt for 10 minutes until tender. Remove from heat, drain, and set aside.

2 In a large saucepan over medium heat, sauté the garlic, pepper, and green onion in olive oil for 3 minutes.

3 Add the sesame seeds and edamame to the garlic and onion mixture. Sauté for 5 minutes, stirring occasionally.

Per serving: *Calories 198 (From Fat 81); Fat 9g (Saturated 1g); Cholesterol 0mg; Sodium 191mg; Carbohydrate 15g (Dietary Fiber 6g); Protein 13g.*

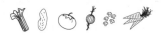

☞ Almond and Balsamic-Glazed Green Beans

Green beans are low in calories and a good source of vitamin C. The healthful fats found in olive oil and almonds turn this dish into a superfoods dish. Shallots are similar to onions, but with a milder flavor.

Prep time: *About 10 minutes*

Cooking time: *7 to 8 minutes*

Yield: *4 servings*

2 tablespoons olive oil

1 pound fresh, frozen, or canned green beans

1 shallot, chopped

2 tablespoons balsamic vinegar

Salt and ground black pepper to taste

¼ cup toasted almonds, chopped

1 In a large saucepan, heat olive oil over high heat until it starts to bubble. Add the beans and sauté until they begin to darken, stirring occasionally to prevent burning, about 4 minutes. Note that fresh green beans will take longer to sauté.

2 Add the shallot to the beans, and stir to combine. Transfer the bean mixture to a separate bowl.

3 Put the saucepan back on the heat, and add the balsamic vinegar to the pan. Scrape any bits of food from the bottom of the pan as the vinegar simmers, and then add the beans and shallot back to the pan and heat through.

4 Season with salt and pepper to taste. Sprinkle with almonds before serving.

Per serving: Calories 160 (From Fat 105); Fat 12g (Saturated 1g); Cholesterol Xmg; Sodium 154mg; Carbohydrate 13g (Dietary Fiber 5g); Protein 4g.

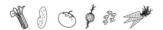

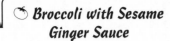 Broccoli with Sesame Ginger Sauce

The sweet and tangy sauce in this recipe is similar to the sauces found at Chinese restaurants, so kids and picky eaters will love it. This is a great way to get a superfood vegetable into your kids. Broccoli is rich in vitamins, minerals, and antioxidants that may help to prevent cancer and keep your heart healthy (see Chapter 5).

Prep time: *About 5 minutes*

Cooking time: *5 minutes*

Yield: *6 servings*

3 green onions, chopped	*¼ teaspoon red pepper flakes*
¼ cup soy sauce	*2 tablespoons sesame oil*
2 tablespoons sesame seeds	*1 pound broccoli florets, cut into bite-sized pieces*
2 tablespoons grated fresh ginger	
1 clove garlic, minced	*8-ounce can water chestnuts, rinsed and drained*

1 In a small bowl, stir together the green onions, soy sauce, sesame seeds, ginger, garlic, and red pepper flakes.

2 Heat the sesame oil in a wok or large frying pan over medium-high heat. Add the broccoli and stir-fry until tender, about 3 minutes, stirring continuously.

3 Add the water chestnuts and soy sauce mixture to the broccoli, and stir until heated through, about 2 minutes.

Tip: *Use low-sodium soy sauce to make this dish even healthier.*

Per serving: *Calories 102 (From Fat 56); Fat 6g (Saturated 1g); Cholesterol 0mg; Sodium 640mg; Carbohydrate 9g (Dietary Fiber 4g); Protein 5g.*

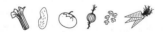

Chapter 19

Rounding Out the Menu: Super Snacks, Appetizers, and Desserts

In This Chapter

▶ Snacking on sensational superfoods

▶ Serving superfoods starters

▶ Dressing up your desserts

*Y*ou may think it isn't possible to eat snacks, appetizers, and desserts that are both delicious and healthy for you. Actually, though, these items offer a great way to incorporate superfoods into your day.

In this chapter, we provide some tips on choosing and preparing easy snacks, appetizers, and desserts, as well as the best ways to get the most superfoods in each portion. We also offer a few of our favorite healthy *and* yummy recipes to try out.

Satisfying Cravings with Superfoods

Many people who want to lose weight believe that snacking is their biggest problem. They think that snacking automatically means eating too much. The truth is that snacking can be good for you. Eating snacks throughout the day can help regulate your body's insulin response and control cravings.

It's not snacking that causes you to gain weight; it's the foods that you choose to snack on. Snacking can actually be a great way to watch your weight when you choose the right foods.

Many of the superfoods make the simplest, healthiest snacks in their natural, whole state. What could be easier than grabbing an apple from your fruit bowl, munching on a handful of mixed nuts, or dipping broccoli pieces into your favorite veggie dip?

When you combine two or more superfoods, you can use their different flavors and textures to satisfy most of your cravings, without ruining your healthy superfoods diet. The following are a few delicious examples:

- **Apples and almond butter:** Slice up a sweet-tangy apple, like a Gala, and serve with a little almond butter. The apple gives you crunchy and sweet, while the almond butter gives you savory, smooth, and just a little salt. Of course, if you don't have almond butter, you can use peanut butter and still get good nutrition.

- **Mixed berries with whipped topping and nuts:** Another great combination is a mix of fresh blueberries, strawberries, and raspberries with a dollop of low-calorie whipped topping and a sprinkling of walnuts or pecans. This is just as delicious as a fattening ice cream sundae and so much better for you.

- **Veggies and dip:** Raw vegetables can not only tame your craving for savory foods, but because superfood vegetables are loaded with fiber, they also keep you feeling full. Dip some carrot slices into your favorite salad dressing. Or, instead of regular chip dip, dip some baked chips into tomato salsa or guacamole.

Super Snack, Appetizer, and Dessert Recipes

Superfoods make great snacks just as they are, but we know there are times when you want something more. Maybe you need a great appetizer to take to a party, or maybe you just want something new to snack on. In that case, you've come to the right place. Here are some recipes for delicious snacks, appetizers, and desserts that feature superfoods, so you can serve healthy snacks to your family and make delicious desserts that won't bust your diet.

Snacking on superfoods

Snacks are great for tiding you over until your next meal. Here are some recipes that are easy to make when you need a little something to eat and it's not quite lunch or dinnertime.

☙ Strawberry Mocha Smoothie

Fruit smoothies have become wildly popular, but many of the ones you buy at coffee shops are made from mixes and don't even contain any real fruit. Make this deliciously healthy berry mocha smoothie at home.

Prep time: *About 10 minutes*

Yield: *2 servings*

¹/₂ cup cold coffee (brewed strong)	2 teaspoons sugar or sucralose
¹/₄ cup milk	1 banana, frozen and cut into 1-inch pieces
3 tablespoons unsweetened cocoa powder (not Dutch processed)	4 large strawberries
¹/₄ teaspoon cinnamon	¹/₂ cup ice cubes

1 Pour coffee and milk into electric blender. Add cocoa powder, cinnamon, and sucralose. Blend on high speed for 10 seconds.

2 Add the banana, strawberries, and ice cubes and blend on high speed until smooth.

Per serving: Calories 181 (From Fat 29); Fat 3g (Saturated 2g); Cholesterol 4mg; Sodium 20mg; Carbohydrate 42g (Dietary Fiber 7g); Protein 5g.

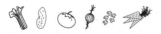

☙ Chia Fruit Smoothie

This chia smoothie makes a great snack for any time of the day. The chia seed can absorb ten times its weight, so it has a strong filling effect and a sustained release of energy. Of the plant-based superfoods, chia also has one of the highest concentrations of omega-3 and omega-6 fatty acids. This smoothie just gets more super with the banana and berries, which are rich in antioxidants, vitamins, and minerals.

Prep time: *About 20 minutes*

Yield: *2 servings*

1 to 2 tablespoons chia seeds	*1 banana, cut into 1-inch pieces*
12 ounces water	*½ cup berries, any types*

1 Grind chia seeds in a coffee grinder until finely ground. If you don't have a coffee grinder, you can use a hand grinder or put the seeds in a sealable plastic bag and break them up with a rolling pin. If none of these options appeals to you, you can use whole chia seeds.

2 In a blender, combine the seeds and water. Blend 4 to 10 seconds on low speed.

3 Add the banana pieces and berries to the blender. Blend on medium to high speed until smooth.

Tip: *Use frozen fruit for a thicker smoothie.*

Per serving: *Calories 86 (From Fat 12); Fat 1g (Saturated 1g); Cholesterol 0mg; Sodium 2mg; Carbohydrate 19g (Dietary Fiber 4g); Protein 2g.*

☙ Superfood Protein Shake

This protein shake contains more than 25 grams of protein and three superfoods, making it a great snack at any time of the day. With the added chia, it will surely fill you up!

Prep time: *5 minutes*

Yield: *1 serving*

8 almonds, chopped	*8 to 10 ounces regular, light, or low-carb vanilla soy milk*
1 scoop of your favorite berry- or vanilla-flavored protein shake mix (look for mixes with fewer than 5g carbs and near 25g protein per serving)	*1 tablespoon whole or ground chia seed*
	¼ cup frozen or fresh blueberries

Add the chopped almonds to blender and pulse a few times. Add the rest of the ingredients to the blender, and blend on low until smooth.

Per serving: Calories 266 (From Fat 87); Fat 10g (Saturated 2g); Cholesterol 0mg; Sodium 394mg; Carbohydrate 13g (Dietary Fiber 7g); Protein 34g.

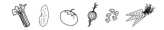

⌕ *Hummus and Pita*

Hummus is a spread made from garbanzo beans and sesame seed paste called *tahini*. Hummus is traditionally served with slices of pita bread. It makes a delicious appetizer that's high in protein, fiber, and minerals.

Prep time: *About 10 minutes*

Yield: *8 servings*

6 cloves garlic

15-ounce can garbanzo beans, rinsed and drained

3 tablespoons lemon juice

2 tablespoons olive oil

1¹/₂ tablespoons tahini

¹/₂ teaspoon salt

8 whole-wheat pitas, cut into 6 wedges

Process the garlic cloves in a food processer for 2 to 3 seconds. Add the remaining ingredients and process for 5 minutes, until smooth. Serve as a dip for pita wedges.

Tip: *You can buy tahini in the international foods aisles of many grocery stores, or you can make your own by combining 5 cups toasted sesame seeds with 1¹/₂ cups olive oil and blending for 2 minutes in a blender or food processor. Tahini stores well in the refrigerator for up to 3 months.*

Per serving: Calories 210 (From Fat 59); Fat 7g (Saturated 1g); Cholesterol 0mg; Sodium 509mg; Carbohydrate 33g (Dietary Fiber 5g); Protein 7g.

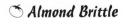 *Almond Brittle*

This snack is made with plenty of almonds, which are an excellent source of vitamin E, magnesium, tryptophan (an amino acid), and fats that help keep your heart healthy. This recipe is sugar-free (that makes it diabetes-friendly) and easy to prepare — a great idea for the holiday season. You can always double the recipe for bigger parties.

Prep time: *10 to 15 minutes*

Cooking time: *25 minutes*

Yield: *4 servings*

Nonstick cooking spray	*1 tablespoon cinnamon*
1 egg white	*¼ cup sugar-free pancake syrup*
¼ teaspoon salt	*2 cups roasted almonds*

1 Preheat oven to 350 degrees Fahrenheit. Line a baking sheet with foil, and spray the foil with nonstick cooking spray.

2 In a medium-sized metal bowl, beat the egg white until foamy and slightly thickened. You'll get the quickest results with a hand mixer as opposed to whisking the white by hand.

3 Add the salt, cinnamon, and syrup to the egg white, and mix well.

4 Stir in the almonds, and then spread the mixture on the baking sheet.

5 Bake for 25 minutes until dry. Break into pieces, and store in an airtight container.

Per serving: *Calories 435 (From Fat 329); Fat 37g (Saturated 3g); Cholesterol 0mg; Sodium 210mg; Carbohydrate 18g (Dietary Fiber 9g); Protein 16g.*

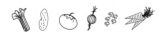

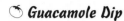 *Guacamole Dip*

Avocados are rich in monounsaturated fats that are good for your heart. Make this delicious dish extra-healthy by choosing omega-3 enriched mayonnaise.

Prep time: *10 to 15 minutes*

Refrigeration time: *30 minutes*

Yield: *4 servings*

2 avocados, peeled and pitted	*1 teaspoon grated onion*
1 teaspoon salt	*½ teaspoon chili powder*
1 tablespoon lemon or lime juice	*½ cup light mayonnaise*

1 In a large bowl, mash avocado with a fork.

2 Stir in salt, lemon or lime juice, onion, and chili powder, and then mix in the mayonnaise. Cover and refrigerate for 30 minutes before serving.

Per serving: Calories 260 (From Fat 202); Fat 22g (Saturated 4g); Cholesterol 11mg; Sodium 824mg; Carbohydrate 11g (Dietary Fiber 8g); Protein 3g.

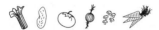

Starting off with superfood appetizers

An *appetizer* is a small amount of food or drink that is served before a meal to stimulate appetite. Sometimes when you order appetizers, they're so large and filling that instead of stimulating your appetite they satisfy your appetite altogether. Keep portion control in mind when you make these appetizers.

◌ Spinach & Artichoke Pizza

Pizza has never been healthier! This version contains garlic, flax, and spinach, so it has lots of vitamins, minerals, and healthy fats. You also can enjoy the rich flavor of the garlic, basil, and peppers.

Prep time: *20 minutes*

Cooking time: *5 to 8 minutes*

Yield: *4 to 6 servings*

1 tablespoon flax seed	*1 large portabella mushroom, thinly sliced*
2 cloves garlic, diced or pressed	*10 ounces fresh spinach leaves*
3 tablespoons olive oil, divided	*1 teaspoon fresh basil leaves*
4 low-carb or whole-wheat wraps or tortillas	*14-ounce can artichoke hearts, drained and chopped*
1 medium red bell pepper, seeded and cut into ¼-inch strips	*1 ½ cups shredded part-skim mozzarella cheese*

1 Preheat oven to 400 degrees Fahrenheit.

2 Grind the flax seed in a coffee grinder or small food processor. Combine it with the garlic and 1 tablespoon olive oil in a small bowl, and mix well.

3 Spread 1 teaspoon of the garlic mixture over each of the wraps.

4 In a medium skillet over medium heat, sauté the red pepper strips and mushrooms in the remaining olive oil for 5 minutes, until soft. Add the spinach leaves and sauté for another 2 minutes to absorb the olive oil and flavor.

5 Layer the pepper and spinach mixture with the basil leaves and artichokes over the garlic mixture on each wrap, and top with cheese.

6 Bake for 5 to 8 minutes until golden brown and the cheese is melted. Cut into small wedges before serving.

Per serving: Calories 379 (From Fat 187); Fat 21g (Saturated 6g); Cholesterol 23mg; Sodium 577mg; Carbohydrate 26g (Dietary Fiber 11g); Protein 23g.

Salmon Lettuce Wraps

This dish is a great way to eat salmon, which is rich in omega-3 fats and protein. This recipe could easily be added to the main dish section, but when sliced into finger food it makes a great starter. It also contains tomatoes, garlic, and other fine herbs. If you serve it as an appetizer, you can eat leftovers for a snack the next day.

Prep time: *20 minutes*

Cooking time: *20 minutes*

Yield: *4 servings*

2 tablespoons fresh ginger, roughly chopped

¼ cup fresh cilantro

1 jalapeño pepper, seeded and roughly chopped

1 small onion, roughly chopped

2 cloves garlic, roughly chopped

2 tablespoons olive oil, divided

3 tablespoons fresh-squeezed lime juice

1 large tomato, roughly chopped

2 fresh salmon fillets (about 6 ounces each)

1 head iceberg or Bibb lettuce, or large spinach leaves

Lime wedges, for serving

1 Preheat broiler to high.

2 Combine the ginger, cilantro, jalapeño pepper, onion, garlic, 1 tablespoon olive oil, and lime juice in a food processor, and process until chopped and mixed. Add the tomato and process again. Transfer to a bowl, cover, and refrigerate.

3 Lightly coat the salmon fillets with the rest of the olive oil, salt, and pepper. Place fillets on a foil-lined baking sheet and broil for 20 minutes, or until salmon is firm and pink.

4 Separate lettuce leaves from the head. Fill with small pieces of the flaked broiled salmon and the ginger mixture from Step 2. Top with fresh lime juice when serving.

Tip: *The salsa may seem watery if you let it sit too long before using it in the wraps (or if you have leftovers), but a quick stir will get it back to the right consistency.*

Per serving: *Calories 140 (From Fat 53); Fat 6g (Saturated 1g); Cholesterol 32mg; Sodium 50mg; Carbohydrate 9g (Dietary Fiber 2g); Protein 14g.*

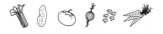

○ *Baked Spinach and Artichoke Dip*

This is another great spinach dish. With the addition of garlic and artichokes, it becomes an appetizer of choice to get you and your guests warmed up for the main meal. You can serve it with low-carb wraps for dipping (bake them for a few minutes until crispy), or substitute other superfoods as dippers, such as broccoli spears and celery.

Prep time: *20 minutes*

Cooking time: *20 minutes*

Yield: *4 servings*

Nonstick cooking spray	*½ cup mayonnaise*
1 pound frozen chopped spinach, thawed and drained	*½ cup sour cream*
	2 cups part-skim shredded mozzarella cheese
2 tablespoons olive oil	*2 cups crumbled feta cheese*
1 clove garlic, minced	*2 tablespoons ground pepper*
15-ounce can artichoke hearts, drained and chopped	*1 tablespoon red pepper flakes*

1 Preheat oven to 350 degrees. Spray a 1-quart casserole or baking dish with nonstick cooking spray and set aside.

2 In a large skillet over medium-high heat, sauté the spinach, olive oil, and garlic for 5 minutes.

3 Add to the skillet the remaining ingredients except for red pepper flakes, and mix well. Transfer the mixture to the casserole or baking dish, and bake for 20 to 25 minutes.

4 Sprinkle with red pepper flakes before serving.

Per serving: *Calories 699 (From Fat 510); Fat 57g (Saturated 21g); Cholesterol 100mg; Sodium 1,503mg; Carbohydrate 20g (Dietary Fiber 6g); Protein 31g.*

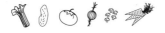

Salmon Cakes

You can serve this great starter with confidence. Even people who aren't big fish eaters usually enjoy canned salmon. It's a great source of omega-3 fatty acids and protein. Oatmeal adds fiber, and parsley is a terrific source of vitamin C.

Prep time: *About 20 minutes*

Cooking time: *8 minutes*

Yield: *5 servings*

¹/₃ cup nonfat milk	*2 tablespoons chopped green onions*
2 egg whites	*1 tablespoon chopped fresh dill*
15-ounce can salmon, drained	*1 tablespoon chopped fresh parsley*
1 cup whole-wheat bread crumbs	*¹/₄ teaspoon paprika*
³/₄ cup quick-cooking oats (not instant or old-fashioned oats)	*¹/₄ teaspoon salt*
	1 tablespoon olive oil

1 In a small bowl, beat together the milk and egg whites.

2 In a large bowl, combine the salmon, bread crumbs, oats, onions, dill, parsley, paprika, and salt, and mix well. Stir in the egg and milk mixture, and let it all stand for 5 minutes.

3 Shape the salmon mixture into 5 equally sized cakes, each about 1-inch thick.

4 Place a large skillet over medium heat, and add the olive oil. Sauté the salmon cakes until golden, about 4 minutes on each side.

Tip: *If the mixture is too crumbly when you start to form the cakes, add 1 or 2 more tablespoons milk to help it bind together.*

Tip: *Serve the salmon cakes with an easy, almost-homemade lemon dill sauce by combining ¹/₄ cup light dill veggie dip (such as T. Marzetti's) with 2 tablespoons lemon juice, ¹/₄ teaspoon Tabasco sauce, and 2 to 3 tablespoons nonfat milk.*

Per serving: Calories 173 (From Fat 88); Fat 10g (Saturated 2g); Cholesterol 54mg; Sodium 542mg; Carbohydrate 4g (Dietary Fiber 1g); Protein 19g.

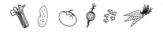

Delving into not-too-decadent desserts

It's what you've been waiting for — desserts. Yes, you can actually incorporate superfoods into desserts. If you think any dessert with superfoods must be super tasteless, think again. The important thing to remember is that anytime you can get some of the superfoods into your eating structure, you should do it. Read on for some super desserts that you can serve with a smile.

🍎 Strawberry-Banana Pudding

This quick dessert is low in calories and carbohydrates, yet rich in antioxidants, vitamins, and minerals thanks to the almonds and strawberries. And it's so easy to make!

Prep time: *10 minutes*

Yield: *1 serving*

3¹/₂-ounce container banana-flavored pudding (Snack Pack size)

4 strawberries, finely diced

1 tablespoon whipped topping

1 tablespoon finely crushed almonds

Stir together the pudding, strawberries, and whipped topping. Top with almonds.

Tip: *Feel free to use vanilla pudding also. If you are watching your weight, try "no sugar added" pudding.*

Per serving: Calories 199 (From Fat 78); Fat 9g (Saturated 3g); Cholesterol 0mg; Sodium 150mg; Carbohydrate 29g (Dietary Fiber 3g); Protein 3g.

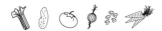

🍎 Almond Puffs

This is another great almond delight that's a delicious way to enjoy a superfood. Plus, it's diabetes-friendly! Although this recipe may not be as easy to make as the almond brittle, it's worth the wait. It uses healthy egg whites, and almonds contain fats and nutrients that are very good for you. Plus, your kids will love them!

Prep time: *20 minutes*

Cooking time: *20 to 30 minutes*

Yield: *4 to 6 servings*

Nonstick cooking spray

4 egg whites

¹/₈ teaspoon salt

1¹/₂ cups sucralose sugar substitute

1 tablespoon vanilla extract

¹/₂ teaspoon almond extract

¹/₂ cup toasted almonds, ground in food processor

1 Preheat oven to 250 degrees Fahrenheit. Spray 2 baking sheets with nonstick cooking spray.

2 Beat the egg whites with an electric mixer for a few minutes until they're creamy white and smooth. Add salt. Continue beating while slowly adding sugar substitute and extracts. Beat until the egg whites form stiff peaks (dip the tip of a spoon in them, invert it, and the resulting point of beaten egg white should stand up on its own).

3 Fold in chopped almonds.

4 Use a teaspoon to quickly drop batter onto cookie sheets, lifting the spoon at the end to create peaks.

5 Bake for 20 to 30 minutes until lightly brown and firm to the touch. Transfer to a wire rack to cool. Store in an airtight container.

Per serving: Calories 129 (From Fat 54); Fat 6g (Saturated 1g); Cholesterol 0mg; Sodium 128mg; Carbohydrate 12g (Dietary Fiber 1g); Protein 6g.

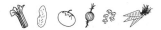

🍎 Low-Carb Parfait

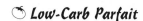

This is a quick and tasty snack for low-carb dieters and, of course, diabetics. It contains chia and bananas and is so good it will satisfy even the toughest critic's sweet tooth.

Prep time: *10 minutes*

Yield: *1 serving*

3 ½-ounce container pudding in your favorite flavor, low sugar if possible

1 tablespoon whole chia seeds (you can grind them if you prefer)

3 ½-ounce container low-carb yogurt in your favorite flavor

1 banana, cut into bite-sized pieces

1 tablespoon sugar-free whipped topping

1 In a small bowl, mix together the pudding and chia.

2 Layer yogurt and pudding in a dessert glass and top with banana and whipped topping.

Per serving: Calories 354 (From Fat 48); Fat 5g (Saturated 3g); Cholesterol 10mg; Sodium 828mg; Carbohydrate 61g (Dietary Fiber 6g); Protein 15g.

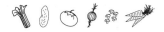

☕ Baked Apples

This old favorite is packed with some great superfoods. Furthermore, apples come in three colors to choose from, all of which are different in taste or texture. With almonds, cranberries, and even a touch of cinnamon, this recipe is great on everyone's table — but remember portion control!

Some types of apples don't cook as well as others, so pay attention to the apples that we suggest for this recipe. If you'd like to try another type of apple, ask your grocer for a recommendation, or just keep in mind that you may not get the same results.

Prep time: *20 minutes*

Cooking time: *60 minutes*

Yield: *4 servings*

2 tablespoons chopped almonds

2 tablespoons dried cranberries

2 tablespoons brown sugar or brown sugar sucralose

½ teaspoon ground cinnamon

⅛ teaspoon nutmeg

4 large apples, such as Gala, Rome, Golden Delicious, or Granny Smith

¾ cup apple juice

2 tablespoons canola oil

Light whipped topping, for serving

1 Preheat oven to 350 degrees Fahrenheit.

2 Combine almonds, cranberries, brown sugar, cinnamon, and nutmeg in bowl. Mix until all ingredients are coated with sugar.

3 Core the apples, and then slice off about ½ inch of each core and plug the bottom of each apple. Place apples upright in nonstick or glass baking dish.

4 Spoon ¼ of the sugar mixture into each apple.

5 Pour the apple juice into the dish, and drizzle canola oil over each apple. Cover the apples with aluminum foil and bake for 1 hour, or until apples are tender. Serve apples as they are, or add a small amount of light whipped topping.

Per serving: Calories 267 (From Fat 86); Fat 10g (Saturated 1g); Cholesterol 1mg; Sodium 4mg; Carbohydrate 49g (Dietary Fiber 7g); Protein 1g.

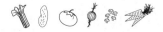

Part V
The Part of Tens

The 5th Wave   By Rich Tennant

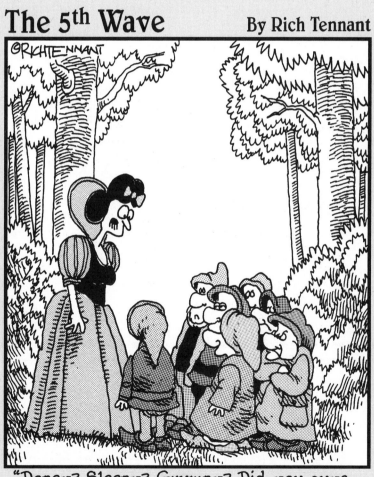

"Dopey? Sleepy? Grumpy? Did you guys forget to take your supplements again?"

In this part . . .

In this part we provide some information "snacks," so to speak, about superfoods. We list ten super-duper superfoods, our top choices for super supplements, and great tips for getting superfoods into your diet every day. Finally, we note ten almost-superfoods — runners-up to our list of superfoods that are worthy of honorable mention.

Chapter 20

Ten Super-Duper Superfoods

In This Chapter

▶ Exploring the health benefits of the best superfoods

▶ Discovering ways to incorporate the top superfoods in your diet

▶ Finding out where to buy the best superfoods

*T*he list of superfoods is long, and you may be wondering which foods pack the biggest nutritional punch. Or maybe you're just getting started with superfoods, and you want to choose a few that can make the biggest impact on your health.

Here, we list the best of the best: our top ten superfoods. We chose these ten foods based on nutritional content, versatility, availability, and ease of storage.

Blueberries

The rich dark color in blueberries provides lots of antioxidants that protect the cells in your body from damage by free radicals. This damage can come from a variety of factors, including too much sun exposure, pollution, foods with unhealthy fats, and even as a by-product of normal metabolism. In fact, blueberries have more antioxidants than any other commercially grown fruit (see Chapter 4).

Being good for you is one thing, but in order for a food to become a regular part of your diet, it has to taste good, too. Blueberries rise to the challenge. They don't require much preparation; just rinse them and enjoy. You can eat them plain or sprinkle a half cup of blueberries on your morning cereal. Blueberries add flavor and extra nutrition to warm, whole-wheat muffins, too.

Blueberries are available year-round, but the best time to buy them is during the summer months, when you can find them at local farmers' markets and sometimes at pick-your-own blueberry farms. Blueberries keep for a few days in the refrigerator, and they freeze very well.

Salmon

Many of the superfoods contain healthy fats, especially fish (see Chapter 7). Salmon stands head and shoulders (or should that be fins?) above the others because salmon has the most omega-3 fats of all the superfoods in the fish category. Salmon is also a source of several vitamins and minerals and has plenty of protein.

Grill or broil your salmon steaks to serve as a main dish. Salmon chunks work well in salmon cakes (see Chapter 19) or in salmon sandwiches (just take care not to overdo the high-fat mayonnaise).

Fresh salmon may be available in the seafood or meat department of your local grocery store, or you can buy frozen salmon steaks from the freezer section. You can buy cans of salmon chunks, too.

Some canned salmon contains skin and bones. If you don't mind, you can eat the salmon bones because they're a good source of calcium. Or you can check the label for cans of salmon meat only.

Spinach

The deep green pigments in spinach contain several antioxidants, including lutein, which helps keep your vision clear (see Chapter 5). You also get your daily dose of vitamins A and K and most of the manganese (an important trace mineral) and folate (water-soluble B vitamin) you need. Eating spinach even provides calcium and iron. And the calories in spinach are so few that they hardly count.

You can use raw spinach leaves in place of iceberg lettuce in your salads or on sandwiches. Spinach makes a delicious side dish (see Chapter 18 for a recipe), or you can use it to boost the nutritional value of spaghetti, pizza, and even macaroni and cheese.

Fresh spinach leaves are available at your grocery store in the produce section, and you can buy canned or frozen spinach, too. In the summer, you can find spinach at local farmers' markets, or you can grow it yourself in your own superfoods garden (see Chapter 14).

Tomatoes

The luscious red color of red tomatoes (especially in the form of heat-processed tomato sauces) contains an antioxidant called lycopene that helps keep your heart healthy (see Chapter 5). Eating one tomato gives you half the vitamin C you need for the day. Tomatoes are also a good source of fiber, which helps keep your digestive system healthy.

Slice a big tomato and serve it with mozzarella cheese, basil leaves, and a drizzle of olive oil for a salad, or add chunks of tomatoes to a traditional garden salad. Tomatoes are the base for many sauces, soups and stews, and condiments.

Your grocery store is likely to carry some interesting varieties of tomatoes. Large, round tomatoes can be sliced or cut into chunks and are very versatile, while plum tomatoes are smaller with less juice. There are several types of cherry or grape tomatoes — cute as can be, and perfect for perching on a salad. Whole, sliced, or stewed tomatoes (in the canned vegetables aisle of your grocery store) are useful for recipes.

You can grow many different varieties of tomatoes in your garden or in a large pot on your deck (see Chapter 14 for more on growing superfoods).

Olive Oil

Olive oil is rich in monounsaturated fats, which take care of your heart by decreasing your LDL cholesterol (the bad kind) and raising your HDL cholesterol (the good kind). Virgin olive oil also contains *polyphenols* (natural substances that have health benefits), making it even better for your heart (see Chapter 9).

Use olive oil to make salad dressings (just combine a little balsamic vinegar with the olive oil) or to add flavor to vegetables. You can use olive oil infused with herbs or peppers to add interesting flavors to many dishes — but don't attempt to make your own flavored oils, as botulism is a concern. Olive oil is good for cooking, too, because it has a high smoking point.

Olive oils differ in flavor (and even in color) depending on the varieties of olives used and even where they're grown. Virgin and extra virgin olive oils contain less acid than regular olive oil and have a much better flavor (and more of those polyphenols).

Almonds

Almonds contain vitamin E, minerals, and monounsaturated fats (like the kind found in olive oil) that fight bad cholesterol. Eating almonds may help to keep your heart healthy and protect you from diabetes (see Chapter 6).

Grab a handful of almonds to eat as a snack, or sprinkle sliced or slivered almonds on a salad. Almonds add a nice crunch to a bowl of berries and make a tasty topper for green vegetables.

Your grocery store should have both raw and roasted almonds. They may be whole, sliced, slivered, or chopped, which makes them very versatile. Some specialty stores also carry almond butter, a delicious alternative to peanut butter. Store your almonds in airtight containers or bags to keep them fresh.

If you only have whole almonds and you need smaller pieces, you can use your coffee grinder to chop them up.

Oats

Oats are our favorite whole grain. Eating oatmeal helps control cholesterol levels because it contains *beta-glucan,* a type of soluble dietary fiber that binds to and removes cholesterol from your body. Oats may also help to keep your blood vessels healthy (see Chapter 8).

Start your morning with a bowl of hot oatmeal or a whole-grain oat cereal, such as Cheerios. Choose low-fat and low-sugar oatmeal muffins and cookies. Substitute oats for breadcrumbs or part of the wheat flour in some of your recipes.

You can find a variety of oats in the cereal section of grocery stores — steel-cut, old-fashioned (rolled), quick-cooking, and instant. Steel-cut oatmeal takes the longest to cook. Old-fashioned oatmeal takes less time because the oats are rolled thin compared to the steel-cut variety. Quick-cooking oats are even thinner than old-fashioned oatmeal. Instant oatmeal has been cooked and dehydrated and is ready almost as soon as you add hot water.

When you buy instant oatmeal, be sure to read the label on the box. Some brands contain quite a lot of sugar and extra calories you may not want.

Garlic

Garlic may be best-known for keeping vampires away — at least in some old B movies — but in reality, garlic helps to ward off heart disease and cancer (see Chapter 9). Garlic lowers cholesterol and helps to lower your blood pressure if it's too high. Eating garlic regularly may also help you fight infections.

Make garlic bread by first drizzling olive oil on whole-wheat bread, then spreading some roasted garlic on the bread. Top off with a little parmesan cheese, and toast in the oven until golden brown.

Fresh garlic is available in the produce department. You can also buy pre-peeled and -chopped garlic in jars — talk about convenient. Garlic is easy to grow and can make a nice addition to your superfoods garden. Just be sure to let the garlic dry (or cure) for about two weeks after you harvest it.

Fresh garlic is easy to peel if you first put the cloves into the microwave for about 5 to 10 seconds. The papery skin slides right off.

Strawberries

The rich red color in strawberries provides antioxidants, and one serving gives you all the vitamin C you need for the whole day. Strawberries also contain *folate* — an important B vitamin — and potassium to keep your heart healthy. The phenols in strawberries may help to protect you from cancer, cardiovascular disease, and rheumatoid arthritis (see Chapter 4).

Strawberries are very sweet, so they don't need extra sugar. Add strawberries to cold or hot cereal or make them part of a salad (see Chapter 18). Combine fresh strawberries with blueberries and raspberries and top with light whipped topping for a sweet and healthy dessert, or dip some large strawberries into dark chocolate for a decadent treat.

Fresh strawberries are available year-round in the produce section of the grocery store, but they may be best during the spring and summer months, when, like blueberries, they're available at pick-your-own strawberry farms or local farmers' markets. You can also find strawberries in the freezer section (look out for added sugar), and you can grow strawberries in your own backyard garden.

Chia Seeds

These little seeds come from Mexico and are members of the mint family. Chia seeds are very high in omega-3 fatty acids (even higher than flax seeds) and rich in antioxidants (see Chapter 10). Chia seeds form a gel when exposed to liquids in your stomach. Experts believe eating chia seeds slows down carbohydrate absorption to keep you feeling full longer. This gel formation can also soothe heartburn and keep your stomach calm.

Chia seeds have a nutty flavor that goes well with many other foods. Sprinkle chia seeds on salads, vegetables, and cereals, and add them to recipes for baked goods, like muffins.

You may not find chia seeds in your local grocery yet, but look for them to be hitting major chains in the near future. In the meantime, you can find them online or in specialty health food stores. We know this requires a little extra effort, but chia seeds are so beneficial to your health, they're worth it.

Chapter 21

Ten Sensational Dietary Supplements

In this Chapter

▶ Looking at the top ten superfood supplements

▶ Seeing why these supplements are so special

▶ Finding out how much to take and where to buy them

*O*ne of the recurring themes in this book is the importance of getting your nutrition by eating whole superfoods whenever possible. But given today's busy lifestyles and people's various food preferences, getting great nutrition all the time can be difficult. Thus, adding a superfood supplement or two may be a great help.

With the availability of so many different supplements, how do you know which ones to choose? We give you our favorites here, but in general, look for supplements that offer a variety of vitamins, minerals, and extra antioxidants without a lot of added sugars and calories. You can choose pills, powders, or liquids — whichever works best for you and your family.

Because supplements vary in daily dosage recommendations, you may find one fits your needs better than another. You may not need as much as the label suggests, just remember that any research done with these supplements was based on specific amounts. More important, don't take more than what the labels recommend unless directed by a medical professional. See Chapter 3 for more information on taking dietary supplements.

Supplements don't replace real food; they simply fill in some of the nutritional gaps in your diet. Your first priority is to boost your diet with a variety of superfoods. Supplements take second place, because they often lack chemicals that are found in the raw foods and are important for absorption and digestion.

Vibe

Vibe is the signature product of the Eniva Corporation and is an excellent overall dietary supplement. The great thing about Vibe is that it's a bunch of superfood supplements all in one. Eniva takes pride in the quality of both the ingredients and the processing of its products.

Vibe meets the recommended daily amounts of many nutrients and, after much research, the Eniva team was able to formulate the product by a special process that enhances the absorption and *bioavailability* — the amount of nutrition value left after the supplement is metabolized by the body. Vibe was formulated to have a small particle size so it's easy for your body to absorb and use.

Vibe is one of the more complete supplements on the market. It contains the extracts of several superfoods, including green tea, blueberries, goji berry, tomatoes, and apples. One ounce of Vibe has:

✔ The antioxidant equivalent of 96 blueberries

✔ The vitamin A equivalent of 13 tomatoes

✔ The green tea extract equivalent of 5 cups of tea

✔ The selenium equivalent of 30 heads of broccoli.

VIBE gives you the power of many superfoods in a 1-ounce dose, and you can take one or two doses each day. Go to www.eniva.com for more information.

This liquid has a quick delivery system, and some people may experience flushing due to the fast absorption of the niacin. This reaction goes away quickly, but if you're sensitive to niacin, you should talk to you doctor about some things you can do to help reduce the symptoms of the niacin flush.

Prime One

The formulation of this supplement is based on research done by scientists from the Soviet Union. The research was focused on *adaptogens* (biologically active substances found in plants that help the body deal with various stressors). Adaptogens often contain high concentrations of antioxidants, too, which is part of the reason that they've been the center of so many clinical studies.

The potential benefits of Prime One make this supplement worth mentioning in our top ten. This liquid supplement is a blend of several plant extracts that were combined after doing tests on hundreds of plants. The studies revealed improvements in athletic performance, mental alertness, and improved general well-being. With a focus on reducing the effects of stressors on the body, this supplement helps the body heal and keeps it from expressing the normal negative effects of stress.

The recommended dose of Prime One is 1 to 2 tablespoons, depending on your age. (We recommend that you start with half the dosing for the first week.) Each 2-tablespoon serving has about 10 calories and about 2 grams of carbohydrates. It can be taken alone, or mixed with milk or juice. Prime One can be given to children beginning at age one. Check out the Web site www. iamams.com for more information on Prime One.

Dr. Shulze's SuperFood Plus

Dr. Schulze's has a whole line of reputable nutritional supplements that have been used by happy consumers for years. For the purposes of this book, our focus is on Dr. Shulze's SuperFood Plus Formula, which is an excellent fit for our top ten. Like Vibe, this product is a multi-superfood supplement with plenty of health benefits.

This formula contains a few of the exotic superfoods and is a great choice for those interested in supplementing with algae, seaweed, and wheat grass. Dr. Shulze uses three types of algae, including spirulina (see Chapter 10 for more info). Algae is one of the most concentrated sources of protein and has 40 times the amount of protein in another superfood, soybeans.

SuperFood Plus also contains wheat grass, which is a great source of many vitamins, minerals, and amino acids. Other healthful ingredients the supplement includes are blue-green algae, chlorella broken-cell algae, barley, alfalfa, Purple Dulse seaweed, Acerola cherry, rose hips, palm fruit, lemon and orange peels, beet root, and spinach leaf.

The recommended dose of Dr. Shulze's SuperFood Plus is 1 to 2 tablespoons per day. You can mix the powder with milk or juice, or even use it in a smoothie. You can also get this in tablet form, but the recommended dosage is up to 13 tablets per day, so many people find the powder easier to use. Go to www.dr-shulze.com for more information.

HD Food: Oranges

Do you want a substitute for your morning coffee? HD Food: Oranges from HealthDesigns is a powdered drink mix full of important nutrients that support energy, making it a great starter for people who need that pick-me-up in the morning. The amino acids, adaptogens, *catechins* (plant chemicals that have antioxidant properties), protein, and fiber are provided in a small (10-gram) serving size with less than 50 calories.

The drink contains green coffee bean and green tea extracts that provide energy-boosting polyphenols (caffeic and chlorogenic acids), while Panax ginseng helps control the release of stress hormones. HD Food: Oranges also contains good nutrition from a blend of fruits and vegetables that are provided in each serving:

- ✔ **Fruits:** Oranges, peaches, nectarines, tangerines, cantaloupe, pineapple, clementines, papaya, apricot, mango, kumquat, and persimmons
- ✔ **Vegetables:** Yams, pumpkin, carrots, butternut squash, and rutabaga

One serving provides 2 grams of soluble fiber and 6 grams of carbohydrates. Go to www.healthdesigns.com for more information on getting HD Food: Oranges into your daily routine.

Sambazon Power Scoop

Sambazon Power Scoop is a popular supplement because its star ingredient is a great superfood: açaí berries. Originating in Brazil, each açaí berry is about the size of a blueberry, but even more powerful. Açaí berries contain twice the antioxidant activity of blueberries and substantially more antioxidant power than red wine.

Sambazon has both liquid and powder supplements that contain the açaí berry. The açaí berry offers plenty of health benefits due to the *anthocyanins* — plant pigments found in the skins of fruits and vegetables that have high antioxidant activity. They add some important fatty acids, vitamins, and minerals to make this a great option for daily nutrition.

The recommended dose of Sambazon Power Scoop is 1 to 2 scoops a day added to your favorite juice, milk, or smoothie. You can also get the capsule form and take 2 to 4 capsules daily. Go to www.Sambazon.com for more information on this superfood supplement.

FRS Healthy Energy

FRS stands for Free Radical Scavengers, and the natural antioxidant *quercetin* (a bioflavonoid found in the skins of some fruits and vegetables) leads this supplement in the battle against free radical damage. Several studies, including one published in the *Journal of Sports Nutrition and Exercise Metabolism* in 2006, support the use of FRS for brain function, immune system support, and boosting athletic performance.

FRS Healthy Energy was developed by Harvard graduates to fight fatigue and to supplement general nutrition. They discovered that high levels of quercetin in the form of a supplement offered more than just an energy boost; they actually improved recovery time of elite athletes after heavy workouts. FRS Healthy Energy also includes green tea extract, B vitamins, vitamin C, and caffeine.

FRS is available in a few different supplemental forms to meet your needs. It comes in a ready-to-drink can, soft chews, powder, and liquid concentrate. The drinks are low-calorie and come in a few different flavors. Go to www.frs.com for more information on how to purchase this supplement.

FRS contains caffeine (about what you would find in half a cup of coffee) so if you're sensitive to caffeine, have any medical conditions, or take prescription medications, you should check with your doctor to see whether this supplement is safe for you.

Green Tea Extract

Green tea extract is often added to supplements such as HD Food: Oranges and FRS Healthy Energy (both discussed earlier in this chapter), but it also makes a great supplement by itself. This superfood supplement is prized for its high amounts of *polyphenols*, the plant-derived antioxidants that are the hallmark of green tea's health benefits.

The main polyphenols in green tea are called catechins. Studies have shown that consuming green tea may reduce your risk for several cancers and heart disease. Green tea has also been used for weight loss and diabetes control.

Although some people like to drink more than 6 cups of this superfood every day, you don't have to. Several great green tea supplements come in powders, capsules, pills, and liquid drops and can replace some of the tea you'd normally drink. You can compare the efficacy by the amounts of catechins in each serving. You may find a high dose of green tea in the multi-nutritional mixes, but if you're looking solely for green tea, there are several brands to choose from. Check out your local health food or grocery stores to find some green tea products.

Green tea supplements contain caffeine in varying amounts. If you're sensitive to caffeine, have any medical conditions, or use prescription medications, make sure you discuss the use of these supplements with your doctor.

Amazing Grass

Wheat grass is a superfood that has been used for thousands of years for health and nutrition. Taking a dose of Amazing Grass can make up for those days when you don't get enough servings of fruits or vegetables. Ounce per ounce, wheat grass has a higher content of nutrition than vegetables.

Amazing Grass is good for digestive health, immune boosting, and energy, and it's gluten-free. It contains high concentrations of phytonutrients, the driving force behind wheat grass's health benefits. It's a great source of vitamins and minerals and a complete source of amino acids. Amazing Grass is a low-calorie, low-carb liquid supplement that contains two grams of fiber per serving.

Amazing Grass comes in pills or a powder form to be mixed into a drink. The tablets are made from wheat grass powder and an organic binder. The serving size is 8 tablets per day or an 8-gram serving (a little over ¼ ounce) of the powder, and you can take 1 to 3 servings per day. Go to www.amazinggrass.com for more information on Amazing Grass. (See Chapter 10 for more information on wheat grass.)

Many people who are sensitive to wheat can actually use Amazing Grass. Wheat grass does not contain any wheat grain (which is where gluten is stored), so it has no gluten. If you have any questions about your ability to use wheat grass supplements, check with your doctor.

Trim Fuel Bar

The Trim Fuel Bar is a great source of omega-3 fatty acids. The main superfoods in this supplemental bar are chia seeds and soy. It also has extra vitamin B12, fiber, and protein.

Chia is the leading plant source of omega-3 fatty acids. Your body metabolizes the seeds slowly, so they can be used for sustained energy and for weight loss. The seeds can absorb 10 times their weight in water, so chia is very filling. Chia also stabilizes blood sugars so your body doesn't need to make more insulin. The bar tastes great; it's a great snack option for children and an easy way to give them their daily amount of omega 3s.

The bar is a great option for those who are watching their weight. The 34-gram (a little over 1 ounce) bar has only 130 calories, with 8 grams of protein, 5 grams of fiber, and less than 5 grams of impact carbohydrates. We recommend one or two bars every day as a meal replacement for weight loss, or as a healthy snack alternative. Go to www.trimlifestyle.com for more information on the Trim Fuel Bar (and see Chapter 10 for more information on chia and its benefits).

Lovaza

This is the only supplement on our superfood list that you can get only by prescription. We thought it was worth mentioning due to the medical benefit of Lovaza's main ingredient, omega-3 fatty acids. Although a prescription supplement, it's made from all natural fish oils.

Omega-3 fatty acids reduce _triglycerides_ (a type of cholesterol found in the blood stream that can lead to thickening of artery walls), so taking Lovaza can improve your cardiovascular health. It has also been associated with weight loss and may help to improve brain function. Studies have been done related to the roles of omega-3 fatty acids in diseases such as autism and Alzheimer's. See Chapter 7 for more information on fish and omega-3 fatty acids.

Each capsule of Lovaza contains 465 milligrams eicosapentaenoic acid (EPA) and 375 milligrams docosahexaenoic acid (DHA), the two forms of omega-3 fatty acids found in fish. Lovaza contains higher concentrations of EPA and DHA than most dietary supplements, so the recommended dose of Lovaza is 4 capsules per day. You can talk to your doctor to see whether you would benefit from getting a prescription for Lovaza.

Chapter 22

Ten (Plus) Ways to Make Sure You Get Your Daily Superfoods

● ●

In This Chapter

▶ Finding ways to eat more fruits and vegetables

▶ Snacking with superfoods

▶ Making a super healthy salad

● ●

*T*rying to incorporate superfoods into your diet may seem overwhelming, but there are easy ways to do it. Here we present our top ten (plus one) tips for making sure you get your daily superfoods.

You don't need to follow every single step we list here. Just choose the ones that work best for you and your family.

Making Over Your Recipes

Substituting or adding superfoods as ingredients in your recipes is an easy way to add superfoods to your diet. Start with a healthy recipe — one that doesn't use a lot of sugar or high-fat ingredients (or cooking methods, like deep frying). Look for ingredients you can replace with superfoods. For example, use olive oil in place of regular vegetable oil, or substitute tuna chunks for chopped chicken in your favorite sandwich. Tofu can be used in place of meat in a stir-fry. Alternatively, you can add a superfood to your recipe without subtracting anything in its place. For example, add cooked and drained spinach to mashed potatoes or add broccoli bits to spaghetti sauce. Add a handful of blueberries to your favorite oatmeal, or use them to top off a delicious salad.

Sometimes, you can adjust your recipes to enhance superfoods. When you make a beef stew, cut back on the amount of meat and add extra carrots and other vegetables to make up the difference. This makes your stew healthier by adding extra nutrients and more fiber, and it cuts calories, too.

Putting Superfoods in Easy Reach

Thank goodness for refrigeration — many of our superfoods would spoil quickly without it. But don't put all your superfoods in the bottom of the produce drawer. Keep a few of them out in the open where you can see them (and hide the cookie jar instead).

Fruits like bananas, apples, and oranges keep well at room temperature for several days, so load up a pretty fruit bowl and place it on the kitchen counter or your dining room table. This way, you and your family will be tempted by superfoods rather than not-so-healthy snacks like cookies and candy. You can also store mixed nuts such as almonds, pecans, and walnuts in a pretty glass jar on the counter instead of leaving them in a crumpled bag in the back of the cabinet. A fresh crisp apple with a handful of walnuts makes for a terrific midafternoon snack.

Going Vegetarian

You don't need to give up meat to get healthy. However, many vegetarian dishes are loaded with superfoods, so enjoying a vegetarian meal once or twice each week can help you increase your superfood intake. Vegetarian meals also tend to be very high in nutrients and fiber while being low in calories, so you can fill up with good-sized portions.

When you're looking for vegetarian meals to substitute for the usual meaty fare, look for dishes that include plenty of protein. A combination of protein and fiber keeps you feeling full long after the meal is done. Good sources of protein include

- Dry beans, such as black beans and navy beans
- Soy products, such as tofu
- Nuts, such as almonds and walnuts

You can go vegetarian at lunch by choosing a veggie sandwich with a side of carrot sticks, hummus, and vegetable dip rather than a greasy cheeseburger with fries. This delivers a lot more nutrition and fewer calories than a typical fast-food lunch.

Choosing Five to Nine Fruits and Vegetables

It's no secret that fruits and vegetables are good for you, and many of the superfoods fall in this category. Aim for a certain number of servings (we suggest seven or more — but at least five) every day. Here's a sample menu to give you ideas about how to get those servings of fruits and vegetables:

- ✔ **Breakfast:** Top your bowl of cereal with ½ cup of berries or a sliced banana, or have a vegetable omelet.

- ✔ **Lunch:** Add tomato, lettuce, onions, and sprouts to a sandwich and serve with a side salad or a cup of vegetable soup.

- ✔ **Dinner:** Divide your dinner plate into four equal sections. A serving of meat, chicken, or fish should take up one section. Another section is for a starchy vegetable like potatoes or corn, and the remaining two sections are for green or colorful vegetables or salad greens.

- ✔ **Snacks:** Select a fresh piece of fruit; raw carrots, broccoli, and cauliflower with veggie dip; or yogurt with ½ cup of berries.

- ✔ **Beverages count, too:** Four ounces of 100 percent fruit or vegetable juice count as a serving, so one large (12-ounce) glass of juice could equal three servings. (See the upcoming section, "Drinking Superfood Beverages.")

Keeping Healthy Snacks on Hand

Snacking is fine. In fact, it's a great way to boost your energy and tide you over until your next meal. And it offers a great opportunity to add superfoods to your diet.

Next time you go to the grocery store, look for snack items that will increase your intake of superfoods. Ready-to-eat, superfood snacks include frozen juice bars (without added sugar), dried berries, bananas and apples, nuts, and sun-dried tomatoes.

You can upgrade your regular snacks, too. If you normally dunk your tortilla chips into nacho cheese sauce while watching TV, switch to baked chips that are lower in unhealthy fats, and use them to scoop up superfood-rich guacamole or spicy salsa. Replace that nightly ice cream sundae with low-fat yogurt topped with lots of blueberries and strawberries.

Drinking Superfood Beverages

Many superfood juices are available in your grocery store, such as pomegranate, orange, apple, blueberry, and tomato juice. Read the labels and choose 100 percent fruit or vegetable juices that don't have added sugar or high-fructose corn syrup. Why? Sugar and corn syrup add calories but no nutrition, while 100 percent juices offer lots of vitamins, minerals, and phytochemicals.

Think about how your beverages can add to your daily superfood intake. Replace that bottle of soda with 100 percent fruit juice. If you miss the fizz, mix the juice with some sparkling mineral water. If you normally drink coffee or black tea, try brewing some green tea instead. Or make some refreshing iced green tea during the warm days of summer.

You can take your superfood juices one step further by buying a juicing machine so that you can make your own fruit and vegetable juices at home. Choose a machine that keeps the fiber and pulp in the juice for maximum nutrition.

Eating a Rainbow

Pay attention to the colors of the foods you eat. The pigments that give the fruits and vegetables their beautiful colors also give you healthful antioxidants. Different colors of fruits and vegetables may have slightly different health benefits, so eat a variety of colors.

Superfood vegetables are green, red, and orange; superfood fruits are red, blue, orange, and yellow. Fill out your food rainbow with superfood nuts and seeds (brown) and fish (pink or white).

Maybe your favorites are the greens and browns, but make sure you get some yellows and oranges in your daily intake of superfoods, too. You need all the colors of the superfoods rainbow to maximize nutrition and health.

By selecting a few different colors of superfoods every day, you can be sure you're getting an excellent assortment of phytochemicals and the number of servings of fruits and vegetables you need.

Planning for Superfoods on the Go

If you travel frequently, you know how easy it is to slip into the fast-food rut of low-cost, not-so-nutritious fare. But you don't need to sacrifice your health when you find yourself eating convenient travel meals.

Add superfoods at fast-food restaurants by choosing side salads instead of French fries, and order an orange juice instead of a soda. When you go to a sit-down restaurant, start with a salad or vegetable soup, choose baked fish when it's available, and don't forget to eat your vegetables.

As an alternative to restaurant meals, get a small cooler and stop at the grocery store to buy healthy snacks that can go on the road with you. No need to grab a candy bar or a bag of potato chips if you have a cooler filled with fresh berries, crunchy vegetables, and sweet juicy apples.

When you travel by air, you probably don't want to lug an extra cooler with you, so choose convenient dehydrated superfoods that won't take up much space in your carry-on bag. Blend your own trail-mix by choosing dried berries and fruits, almonds, walnuts, and some whole grain cereal. You can even toss in a few dark chocolate pieces to tame your sweet tooth.

Taking Advantage of Seasonal Superfoods

While much of the produce you buy in the grocery store is available year-round, there's something to be said for eating produce while it's in season. For one thing, fruits and vegetables are often less expensive when they're in season. (This is great news for preventing colds and flu, because orange and citrus season starts just before cold and flu season.)

Another reason for taking advantage of seasonal foods is the opportunity to support local farming. Plus, fresh, locally grown produce is bursting with flavor because it's harvested closer to peak ripeness.

When fresh seasonal superfoods are available, you can buy them in larger quantities and freeze or can them to enjoy throughout the year. See Chapter 15 for tips.

Dipping with Vegetables Rather than Chips

Instead of opening a bag of chips, serve sliced raw carrots, crunchy green beans, and broccoli florets with a variety of dips. If your family is getting tired of the same old veggie dip, bring out their favorite chip dips and cheese sauce.

The secret to making this work is to have the vegetables ready to go so they're ready when your family is hungry. You can prepare the veggies ahead of time and keep them in a container in the fridge, or, if you're pressed for time, you can buy them already cut and washed at the grocery store. (Remember, though, that you'll pay more for this convenience.)

Eating a Salad

Some people love salads, and others just see them as something to pick at before the real meal starts. But whether you enjoy a salad as a meal or are only grudgingly willing to eat one before a meal, a salad is a great way to add lots of superfoods to your diet.

Go beyond the typical small garden salad (iceberg lettuce, a slice or two of cucumber, little tomatoes, and lots of croutons, drowned in high-fat dressing) by choosing a superfood salad instead. You can do this whether you're in your own kitchen or serving yourself at a restaurant salad bar.

Start with spinach or dark greens along with your regular lettuce. Add lots of cherry tomatoes, carrots, broccoli, mushrooms, and olives, or other available vegetables. For extra flavor (and flavonoids), sprinkle some blueberries or dried cranberries on top. Skip the croutons and add some flax seeds or sunflower seeds. Finally, avoid that high-fat salad dressing. Keep it light with a little balsamic vinaigrette and olive oil or walnut oil.

Chapter 23

Ten (Plus) Almost-Superfoods that Can Help Round Out Your Diet

In This Chapter

▶ Rounding out your superfoods diet with other healthful foods

▶ Finding substitutes for high-fat red meats

▶ Enjoying even more healthful vegetables

Several foods fall short of the truly "super" standard, but they're still good for you. These are what we call almost-superfoods. We chose these foods using the same criteria we used for our superfoods — nutrient content, types of fats, and the availability of phytonutrients. Using the best preparation and cooking methods is the best way to keep these foods almost-super (see Chapter 15).

In this chapter, we've come up with ten almost-superfoods that are delicious, usually easy to find in grocery stores, and add variety to your diet while keeping you healthy.

Whole Grains

Most of the bread, buns, cereals, and pasta you see lining the shelves in your local grocery store are made from refined white wheat flour. When flour is refined, the fiber- and nutrient-rich bran and covering are removed, leaving flour that yields a softer texture for baked goods and a milder flavor for pasta. Most flour is enriched with iron and B vitamins, which is good, but you're still missing a good bit of fiber.

Whole-grain products retain the fiber and natural nutrients found in grains, such as wheat, barley, and spelt (similar to wheat but with a sweeter, nuttier flavor). Eating 100 percent whole-grain cereal, baked goods, and pasta adds fiber to your diet and helps slow down the digestion and absorption of the starches in the grain. Most people consume grains on a daily basis; we recommend incorporating at least three servings of whole grains every day.

Look for "100 percent whole wheat" or "100 percent whole grain" on the ingredients list to be sure the product you're buying is really made from the whole grain.

Increase your intake of whole grains by substituting whole-wheat flour for part of the refined flour in your favorite recipes. Chapters 16 through 19 include several recipes with whole-wheat flour and no refined white flour.

Poultry

Chicken and turkey are lower in saturated fats than beef and are often used in place of red meat in low-fat diets to reduce the cholesterol-raising and inflammatory effects of eating saturated fat. Much of the fat in poultry is contained in the skin, so you can keep your chicken or turkey low-fat by removing the skin.

One cup of cooked chicken breast meat without the skin has only 1 gram of saturated fat and slightly more than 200 calories (dark meat from the legs and thighs has a little more fat and calories). Turkey has even less saturated fat than chicken.

Buy a whole chicken or turkey and roast the bird in the oven, and then remove the skin before serving (roasting with the skin on makes the meat more flavorful). You'll have enough for dinner and lots of leftovers that you can use for other meals. Add cooked, chopped turkey or chicken to a regular garden salad to turn it into a full meal. Or make healthful sandwiches on 100 percent whole-grain bread, with a slice of cheese, tomatoes, and lettuce.

You can also find organic, free-range poultry, which means the birds were raised in healthier conditions and were not exposed to hormones or antibiotics. Organic and free-range poultry is more expensive, but it's becoming more popular every year.

Bison

The meat from American Bison (and game meat such as venison and elk) is much lower in fat than other red meat, and can serve as a delicious substitute for beef. Bison tastes very similar to beef, but is actually a bit richer.

Bison can be used in most dishes that call for beef; however, since bison is lower in fat, you'll have better results if you use lower temperatures for cooking, especially for ground bison. Bison steaks can be prepared just like beef. They're best if not cooked past medium doneness (about 145 degrees Fahrenheit measured with a meat thermometer), meaning the steak is still pink in the middle.

Depending on where you live, bison may be available in your local grocery store, or you may have to travel to a larger store or purchase it online. You can also use venison (deer meat) or elk to replace beef in your diet. They have similar nutritional profiles, but a slightly gamier (but still delicious!) flavor.

Yogurt

Eating yogurt is a great way to get calcium into your diet, plus yogurt contains friendly bacteria that happily populate your digestive system. The bacteria help to keep your digestive system healthy by keeping the bad bacteria and yeast at bay, while the good bacteria make short-chain fatty acids that help to maintain and repair the walls of your digestive tract.

Some brands of yogurt contain added live bacterial cultures called *probiotics* that increase the amount and type of friendly bacteria in the yogurt. Eating these brands of yogurt may improve regularity, and may even reduce the symptoms of other digestive disorders.

Yogurt is available in a wide variety of flavors. You need to read the label to be sure you're not ruining the nutritional value of your yogurt by adding too many calories. One cup of non-fat yogurt has less than 90 calories, but sugar and high-fructose corn syrup can ratchet the count up to over 200 calories.

To save calories, choose brands that are sweetened with Splenda, or buy plain yogurt and add just a touch of sweetness with a little honey and plenty of freshly sliced fruit.

Snap Beans

The nutritional content of green and yellow snap beans makes them a great addition to any superfoods diet. The mild flavor and versatility means that fussy eaters can enjoy these vegetables. Snap beans are low in calories and are a good source of vitamin C, potassium, and folate. Green snap beans are also rich in vitamin A, lutein, and beta-carotene, which trigger antioxidant activity to help prevent damage to the cells in your body.

Green and yellow snap beans are easy to find in the grocery store. Fresh or frozen are best; however, they're available in cans, too — just watch out for added sodium. Snap beans are frequently cooked and served as a side dish (top them with some almonds and olive oil — two of our superfoods). Green beans are also a favorite ingredient in many casseroles (just beware of added fat and calories).

Raw snap beans taste great and have a wonderful crunch. Try serving them with your favorite vegetable dip or as a healthful ingredient in your salads.

Cabbage

Cabbage is a good source of vitamin C, vitamin K, and *sulphorophane,* a phytochemical that may help to fight cancer. According to the journal *Cancer Letter* in 2008, diets rich in cruciferous vegetables, including cabbage, reduce the risk of colon and prostate cancer.

You can find fresh cabbage (and possibly red cabbage) in the produce section of every grocery store; look in the deli for premade slaws and salads. Store-bought cole slaw is usually fattened up with creamy dressings, but you can make a healthier slaw at home by using a wine or vinegar-based dressing instead.

Add cabbage pieces to soups and stews, or sauté some cabbage in a little olive oil with onions. You can eat a lot of cabbage without harming your diet: One cup of raw shredded cabbage has only 18 calories.

Winter Squash

You can find fresh squash in the produce section of your grocery store. Winter squash comes in several varieties, including butternut, acorn, and turban squash, plus pumpkins. The bright orange flesh contains lots of vitamin A and *carotenoids* (phytochemicals related to vitamin A) such as beta-carotene and lutein, which help to keep your vision normal.

Winter squash is also a good source of calcium, potassium, and vitamin C, while remaining low in calories. One cup of cooked, cubed squash has fewer than 100 calories.

To cook a squash, slice it in half, scoop out the seeds and pulp, and place both halves, cut side down, in a baking dish. Then add one inch of water. Bake at 350 degrees Fahrenheit until the flesh is soft when you pierce the rind with a sharp knife. Serve the orange flesh with a little olive oil or walnut oil, salt, and pepper.

Save the seeds and toast them for a healthy snack. Pumpkin seeds are rich in omega-3 fatty acids (see Chapter 6 for information on how to toast pumpkin seeds).

Cauliflower

Like the other cruciferous vegetables (kale, broccoli, and cabbage), cauliflower contains sulphorophanes that help reduce your risk of some cancers. Cauliflower is rich in vitamin C and potassium, contains substantial amounts of folate (a B vitamin), and is very low in calories.

In addition to finding cauliflower in the produce section of the grocery store, you can find it in the frozen foods section. It's available as a single vegetable or in a variety of blends with other vegetables like broccoli. Just watch out for high-calorie sauces and sodium.

Add raw cauliflower florets to salads or use them to scoop up a tasty vegetable dip. Or serve steamed cauliflower as a side dish. Simply remove the outer green leaves, break the florets into bite-sized pieces, and steam for about eight minutes.

Canola Oil

Canola oil is good for you because it's rich in both monounsaturated fats (like olive oil) and omega-3 fatty acids (like flax oil). The healthful fats in canola oil are good for your cardiovascular system and help reduce inflammation. Canola oil is also low in omega-6 fatty acids. These kinds of fatty acids are good for you in small amounts, but they may increase inflammation in your body when consumed in large amounts.

Canola oil is good for cooking because it has a very light flavor compared to the stronger taste of olive oil, and canola oil stands up to heat much better than flax oil, which breaks down quickly when exposed to the high temperatures of cooking.

You can avoid saturated fats when you use canola oil in place of butter because canola is very low in saturated fat. There are also several products made with canola oil, such as mayonnaise and margarine (look for foods marked "trans-fat free").

Grapes

Grapes contain polyphenols such as resveratrol, anthocyanins, and other flavonoids that help reduce inflammation. According to an article published in 2001 in the journal *Circulation,* subjects who drank grape juice every day for two weeks had better blood flow. Red wine remains the superfood because the fermentation improves the absorption of the polyphenols (see Chapter 9). However, grapes are close behind, and grape juice is a good choice for those who don't drink alcohol.

Grapes contain B vitamins, vitamin C, and potassium. One cup of grapes has only 62 calories, so eating a cup of grapes may help tame your sweet tooth without adding a lot of calories.

Choose grapes with dark purple colors because they have the highest concentrations of phytochemicals. You should store your grapes in the refrigerator; you also can freeze grapes, which turns them into a cool summertime treat. Enjoy grapes as a snack or drink grape juice as a beverage.

Raisins are dehydrated grapes. They're very sweet because the natural sugars are more concentrated. However, a study published in 2008 in the journal *Nutrition Research* found that raisins don't have the same negative impact on your blood sugar as other sweets, which may be important for people who have diabetes.

Raisins don't have the same nutritional content as grapes because some nutrients are lost during dehydration. Raisins do, however, retain some of the phytochemicals like oleanolic acid, which may fight tooth decay by reducing the bacteria in your mouth.

Mangos

Mangos are sometimes considered to be an exotic fruit, but they're becoming more popular and therefore easier to find in grocery stores. Their golden yellow flesh tastes something like a cross between a peach and a pineapple.

Mangos are rich in vitamin A and vitamin C, plus a phytochemical called *lupeol* that, according to a 2008 article in the journal *Nutrition and Cancer,* combats prostate cancer cells in the lab. Mangos also contain another phytochemical called *mangiferin* that may help to prevent cancer and immune system diseases, according to research published in the journal *Biochemical Pharmacology* in 2003.

Mangos can be eaten alone or used in salads, fruit smoothies, and salsas. Ignore the color of the mango when you're picking one out. Instead, gently squeeze the fruit; it should be slightly soft when it's ripe. Firm mangos can ripen at home at room temperature. Once they're ripe, they can be stored in the refrigerator for up to five days.

Index

BUSINESS, CAREERS & PERSONAL FINANCE

Accounting For Dummies, 4th Edition*
978-0-470-24600-9

Bookkeeping Workbook For Dummies†
978-0-470-16983-4

Commodities For Dummies
978-0-470-04928-0

Doing Business in China For Dummies
978-0-470-04929-7

E-Mail Marketing For Dummies
978-0-470-19087-6

Job Interviews For Dummies, 3rd Edition*†
978-0-470-17748-8

Personal Finance Workbook For Dummies*†
978-0-470-09933-9

Real Estate License Exams For Dummies
978-0-7645-7623-2

Six Sigma For Dummies
978-0-7645-6798-8

Small Business Kit For Dummies, 2nd Edition*†
978-0-7645-5984-6

Telephone Sales For Dummies
978-0-470-16836-3

BUSINESS PRODUCTIVITY & MICROSOFT OFFICE

Access 2007 For Dummies
978-0-470-03649-5

Excel 2007 For Dummies
978-0-470-03737-9

Office 2007 For Dummies
978-0-470-00923-9

Outlook 2007 For Dummies
978-0-470-03830-7

PowerPoint 2007 For Dummies
978-0-470-04059-1

Project 2007 For Dummies
978-0-470-03651-8

QuickBooks 2008 For Dummies
978-0-470-18470-7

Quicken 2008 For Dummies
978-0-470-17473-9

Salesforce.com For Dummies, 2nd Edition
978-0-470-04893-1

Word 2007 For Dummies
978-0-470-03658-7

EDUCATION, HISTORY, REFERENCE & TEST PREPARATION

African American History For Dummies
978-0-7645-5469-8

Algebra For Dummies
978-0-7645-5325-7

Algebra Workbook For Dummies
978-0-7645-8467-1

Art History For Dummies
978-0-470-09910-0

ASVAB For Dummies, 2nd Edition
978-0-470-10671-6

British Military History For Dummies
978-0-470-03213-8

Calculus For Dummies
978-0-7645-2498-1

Canadian History For Dummies, 2nd Edition
978-0-470-83656-9

Geometry Workbook For Dummies
978-0-471-79940-5

The SAT I For Dummies, 6th Edition
978-0-7645-7193-0

Series 7 Exam For Dummies
978-0-470-09932-2

World History For Dummies
978-0-7645-5242-7

FOOD, GARDEN, HOBBIES & HOME

Bridge For Dummies, 2nd Edition
978-0-471-92426-5

Coin Collecting For Dummies, 2nd Edition
978-0-470-22275-1

Cooking Basics For Dummies, 3rd Edition
978-0-7645-7206-7

Drawing For Dummies
978-0-7645-5476-6

Etiquette For Dummies, 2nd Edition
978-0-470-10672-3

Gardening Basics For Dummies*†
978-0-470-03749-2

Knitting Patterns For Dummies
978-0-470-04556-5

Living Gluten-Free For Dummies†
978-0-471-77383-2

Painting Do-It-Yourself For Dummies
978-0-470-17533-0

HEALTH, SELF HELP, PARENTING & PETS

Anger Management For Dummies
978-0-470-03715-7

Anxiety & Depression Workbook For Dummies
978-0-7645-9793-0

Dieting For Dummies, 2nd Edition
978-0-7645-4149-0

Dog Training For Dummies, 2nd Edition
978-0-7645-8418-3

Horseback Riding For Dummies
978-0-470-09719-9

Infertility For Dummies†
978-0-470-11518-3

Meditation For Dummies with CD-ROM, 2nd Edition
978-0-471-77774-8

Post-Traumatic Stress Disorder For Dummies
978-0-470-04922-8

Puppies For Dummies, 2nd Edition
978-0-470-03717-1

Thyroid For Dummies, 2nd Edition†
978-0-471-78755-6

Type 1 Diabetes For Dummies*†
978-0-470-17811-9

***** Separate Canadian edition also available
† Separate U.K. edition also available

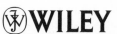

INTERNET & DIGITAL MEDIA

AdWords For Dummies
978-0-470-15252-2

Blogging For Dummies, 2nd Edition
978-0-470-23017-6

Digital Photography All-in-One Desk Reference For Dummies, 3rd Edition
978-0-470-03743-0

Digital Photography For Dummies, 5th Edition
978-0-7645-9802-9

Digital SLR Cameras & Photography For Dummies, 2nd Edition
978-0-470-14927-0

eBay Business All-in-One Desk Reference For Dummies
978-0-7645-8438-1

eBay For Dummies, 5th Edition*
978-0-470-04529-9

eBay Listings That Sell For Dummies
978-0-471-78912-3

Facebook For Dummies
978-0-470-26273-3

The Internet For Dummies, 11th Edition
978-0-470-12174-0

Investing Online For Dummies, 5th Edition
978-0-7645-8456-5

iPod & iTunes For Dummies, 5th Edition
978-0-470-17474-6

MySpace For Dummies
978-0-470-09529-4

Podcasting For Dummies
978-0-471-74898-4

Search Engine Optimization For Dummies, 2nd Edition
978-0-471-97998-2

Second Life For Dummies
978-0-470-18025-9

Starting an eBay Business For Dummies, 3rd Edition†
978-0-470-14924-9

GRAPHICS, DESIGN & WEB DEVELOPMENT

Adobe Creative Suite 3 Design Premium All-in-One Desk Reference For Dummies
978-0-470-11724-8

Adobe Web Suite CS3 All-in-One Desk Reference For Dummies
978-0-470-12099-6

AutoCAD 2008 For Dummies
978-0-470-11650-0

Building a Web Site For Dummies, 3rd Edition
978-0-470-14928-7

Creating Web Pages All-in-One Desk Reference For Dummies, 3rd Edition
978-0-470-09629-1

Creating Web Pages For Dummies, 8th Edition
978-0-470-08030-6

Dreamweaver CS3 For Dummies
978-0-470-11490-2

Flash CS3 For Dummies
978-0-470-12100-9

Google SketchUp For Dummies
978-0-470-13744-4

InDesign CS3 For Dummies
978-0-470-11865-8

Photoshop CS3 All-in-One Desk Reference For Dummies
978-0-470-11195-6

Photoshop CS3 For Dummies
978-0-470-11193-2

Photoshop Elements 5 For Dummies
978-0-470-09810-3

SolidWorks For Dummies
978-0-7645-9555-4

Visio 2007 For Dummies
978-0-470-08983-5

Web Design For Dummies, 2nd Edition
978-0-471-78117-2

Web Sites Do-It-Yourself For Dummies
978-0-470-16903-2

Web Stores Do-It-Yourself For Dummies
978-0-470-17443-2

LANGUAGES, RELIGION & SPIRITUALITY

Arabic For Dummies
978-0-471-77270-5

Chinese For Dummies, Audio Set
978-0-470-12766-7

French For Dummies
978-0-7645-5193-2

German For Dummies
978-0-7645-5195-6

Hebrew For Dummies
978-0-7645-5489-6

Ingles Para Dummies
978-0-7645-5427-8

Italian For Dummies, Audio Set
978-0-470-09586-7

Italian Verbs For Dummies
978-0-471-77389-4

Japanese For Dummies
978-0-7645-5429-2

Latin For Dummies
978-0-7645-5431-5

Portuguese For Dummies
978-0-471-78738-9

Russian For Dummies
978-0-471-78001-4

Spanish Phrases For Dummies
978-0-7645-7204-3

Spanish For Dummies
978-0-7645-5194-9

Spanish For Dummies, Audio Set
978-0-470-09585-0

The Bible For Dummies
978-0-7645-5296-0

Catholicism For Dummies
978-0-7645-5391-2

The Historical Jesus For Dummies
978-0-470-16785-4

Islam For Dummies
978-0-7645-5503-9

Spirituality For Dummies, 2nd Edition
978-0-470-19142-2

NETWORKING AND PROGRAMMING

ASP.NET 3.5 For Dummies
978-0-470-19592-5

C# 2008 For Dummies
978-0-470-19109-5

Hacking For Dummies, 2nd Edition
978-0-470-05235-8

Home Networking For Dummies, 4th Edition
978-0-470-11806-1

Java For Dummies, 4th Edition
978-0-470-08716-9

Microsoft® SQL Server™ 2008 All-in-One Desk Reference For Dummies
978-0-470-17954-3

Networking All-in-One Desk Reference For Dummies, 2nd Edition
978-0-7645-9939-2

Networking For Dummies, 8th Edition
978-0-470-05620-2

SharePoint 2007 For Dummies
978-0-470-09941-4

Wireless Home Networking For Dummies, 2nd Edition
978-0-471-74940-0